# CYLINDER DAT

D1433435

| | B | C | D | E | F | **AF | G | J |
|---|---|---|---|---|---|---|---|---|
| mm<br>in | 330 x 76<br>13 x 3 | 430 x 89<br>17 x 3 | 535 x 102<br>21 x 4 | 865 x 102<br>34 x 4 | 930 x 140<br>37 x 5 | 670 x 175<br>26 x 7 | 1320 x 178<br>52 x 7 | 1520 x 229<br>60 x 9 |
| kg<br>lb | 1.6<br>3½ | 2<br>4½ | 3.4<br>7½ | 5.4<br>12 | 14.5<br>32 | 9.9<br>22 | 34.5<br>76 | 68.9<br>152 |
| *Contents — (litres)<br>Valve — | | 170<br>Pin-Index | 340<br>Pin-Index | 680<br>Pin-Index | 1360<br>Bullnose | 1360<br>Bullnose | 3400<br>Bullnose | 6800<br>Pin-Index<br>(side spindle) |
| *Contents — (litres)<br>Valve — | | 450<br>Pin-Index | 900<br>Pin-Index | 1800<br>Pin-Index | 3600<br>Handwheel | | 9000<br>Handwheel | |
| *Contents — (litres)<br>Valve — | | | 500<br>Pin-Index | | 2000<br>Pin-Index | | 5000<br>Pin-Index | |
| *Contents — (litres)<br>Valve — | | | | 640<br>Pin-Index | 1280<br>Bullnose | | 3200<br>Bullnose | 6400<br>Pin-Index<br>(side spindle) |
| *Contents — (litres)<br>Valve — | | | | | 1360<br>Bullnose | | 3400<br>Bullnose | |
| *Contents — (litres)<br>Valve — | | | | 600<br>Pin-Index | 1200<br>Bullnose | | | |
| *Contents — (litres)<br>Valve — | | 450<br>Pin-Index | | 1800<br>Pin-index | 3600†<br>Handwheel | | | |
| *Contents — (litres)<br>Valve — | | | 300<br>Pin-Index | | 1200<br>Bullnose | | | |
| *Contents — (litres)<br>Valve — | 180<br>Pin-Index | | | | | | | |

e nominal          ** Domiciliary use only          † Also supplied with dip tube for liquid outlet,
                                                       identified by white lines down the body of the cylinder

ital' are available from BOC medical gas branches

MGM/4152/BB/9.90/1.5M

# Ward's Anaesthetic Equipment

# Ward's Anaesthetic Equipment

## 3rd edition

**Andrew Davey** FCAnaes
Consultant Anaesthetist
Royal Sussex County Hospital
Brighton, UK

**John T. B. Moyle** MB, BS, MIElecIE, MInstMC, IEng, FCAnaes
Consultant Anaesthetist
Milton Keynes General Hospital

Consultant in Palliative Care
Willen Hospice,
Milton Keynes, UK

Honorary Senior Research Fellow in Bioengineering
Nuffield Department of Anaesthetics, University of Oxford
Oxford, UK

**Crispian S. Ward** MB, BS, FFARCS
Consultant Anaesthetist (retired)
The Royal Infirmary
Huddersfield, UK

**W. B. Saunders Company Ltd**
London · Philadelphia · Toronto
Sydney · Tokyo

W. B. Saunders    24–28 Oval Road
Company Ltd       London NW1 7DX, UK

Baillière Tindall

The Curtis Center
Independence Square West
Philadelphia, PA 19106–3399, USA

55 Horner Avenue
Toronto, Ontario M8Z 4X6, Canada

Harcourt Brace Jovanovich Group
(Australia) Pty Ltd
30–52 Smidmore Street
Marrickville, NSW 2204, Australia

Harcourt Brace Jovanovich Japan Inc.
Ichibancho Central Building,
22–1 Ichibancho
Chiyoda-ku, Tokyo 102, Japan

First edition published 1975
Second edition published 1985
Third edition published 1992

A catalogue record for this book is available from the
British Library

ISBN 0–7020–1435–4

This book is printed on acid-free paper

Typeset by Columns Design & Production Services Ltd, Reading
Printed in Great Britain by The Bath Press, Avon

# Contents

# Preface

This book is written primarily for the trainee anaesthetist, particularly for those studying for the FCAnaes and similar examinations. However we have not forgotten the needs of others such as the anaesthetist responsible for designing and running anaesthetic departments, the anaesthetic nurse, the operating department technician, the Electronic and Biomedical and the hospital engineers, as well as the manufacturers' representatives and engineers.

While much of what we have included refers to the UK, Europe, the USA and Canada, we have remembered the needs of those working elsewhere with special consideration for those who have to contend with limited facilities in developing and remote areas.

Two new co-authors, Dr Andrew Davey and Dr John Moyle, have rewritten or revised most of the chapters, brought much new material to the book and greatly extended the scope of this edition.

Inevitably, a multi-author approach leads to some reiteration of material in various chapters, but this has been kept to a minimum. There are instances where such repetition is necessary; a reader may not have consulted an earlier chapter before referring to a later one and the duplicated information will be essential to the understanding of the topic under discussion.

Equipment is described as it is used for general anaesthesia and analgesia for surgical procedures, but not for intensive care. However, those engaged in the latter will find much information which will assist them.

Essentially, this book considers the principles by which anaesthetic equipment works, and how to use it safely, as opposed to giving a catalogue of the latest models of a few manufacturers. For this reason, some items of equipment which are obsolete in many parts of the world are described, because they demonstrate principles which may be embodied in modern and future developments.

The basic physical and mechanical principles have not changed a great deal since the last edition of this book, though the accepted meaning of some terms has, and these are shown in 'Terminology'. However, the use of electronic and logical devices has advanced greatly. Chapters 2 and 8, describing electronics and how they will be used in the anaesthetic machine of the future, will prove a welcome addition to those readers who, hitherto, have found this subject somewhat bewildering.

Monitoring has been divided into two parts. Chapter 15 concerns the machine and its output, and Chapter 16 describes the non-invasive monitoring of physiological functions of the patient. It has been reintroduced since this monitoring has become mandatory and equipment for this purpose has now become an important and integral part of modern anaesthetic machines.

Chapters 10 and 11 refer to intermittent flow machines and equipment for dental chair anaesthesia. Although these are not often seen in the teaching establishments, nor even in many regional hospitals, they are still widely in use in UK and elsewhere. They have become unfamiliar to many highly experienced anaesthetists.

Chapter 12 has been largely rewritten to give a new approach to the classification of ventilators. Previous classifications have often been difficult to understand. It is hoped that this new classification will prove easier to apply.

A further addition to this book is a chapter on intravenous infusion, since this is now frequently controlled electronically and supervised by the anaesthetist.

Regrettably, mishaps still occur and therefore Chapter 24, on accidents, has been expanded, with particular reference to the warning devices available and the causes of human error.

In more developed parts of the world 'do-it-yourself' service and repairs to the now very complicated equipment are wisely depricated. All engineering matters should be referred to trained engineers. Anaesthetists are increasingly at risk of litigation if there are mishaps. In no way should this book be considered as a passport for the uninitiated enthusiast to meddle with anaesthetic equipment.

Gone for ever are the days when every anaesthetist had a pipe-dream of building his own machine, and the principle of 'flying by the seat of one's pants' is no longer acceptable.

*Andrew Davey*
*John Moyle*
*Crispian Ward*

# Acknowledgements

We are indebted to many manufacturing companies who have provided us with essential data and illustrations. Of the latter, some have been reproduced in their original form, but others have been altered to ensure that they conform to a uniform style. Space would not permit us to acknowledge our gratitude for each illustration, but all the companies which have assisted us are listed in Appendix V. To all these manufacturers we extend our warmest thanks.

We are also grateful to the Department of Health (formerly the Department of Health and Social Security) and the British Standards Institution for providing several texts, tables and diagrams and permission to reproduce the 'Permit to Work' document.

Many of the original diagrams which we have retained from the previous editions and some new ones have been prepared by Mrs C. Barrett of the Department of Medical Illustration at the Huddersfield Royal Infirmary, and Mr Stephen Lunn and Mr Kevin Conroy have kindly undertaken the arduous task of correcting proofs.

The Association of Anaesthetists of Great Britain and Ireland has kindly consented to the reproduction of the Checklist in Appendix IV.

Finally we wish to thank Mr B. R. Sugg for his invaluable advice, help and encouragement.

# Terminology

The interpretation of the various terms employed in anaesthetic practice tend to vary from one anaesthetist to another. Some terms that were incorrectly derived have become so common in usage that they are likely to remain. To prevent confusion a few definitions are given below:

*Pulmonary ventilation* (breathing) may be spontaneous or passive and is also known as respiration. Passive ventilation may be achieved by rhythmically inflating the lungs by applying gases at fluctuating pressure to the patient's airway. This is usually abbreviated to *IPPV* (intermittent positive pressure ventilation).

*Breathing.* This is divided into three phases:
(a) *Inspiration* or inhalation;
(b) *Expiration* or exhalation;
(c) A period after the end of expiration and before the next inspiration, when no movement takes place, known as the *expiratory pause* or *end-expiratory pause*. During IPPV there may be a pause after inspiration, before expiration commences, known as *plateauing* (the airway pressure curve shows a plateau).

The following terms are also employed:
(d) *Tidal volume* — the volume of a single breath.
(e) *Stroke volume* — the volume delivered by a ventilator during the inspiratory phase of IPPV. Part of this volume may fail to enter the patient.
(f) *Minute volume* — the sum of the tidal volumes of all the breaths in one minute.
(g) *PEEP* (positive end-expiratory pressure) — which implies that a positive pressure is maintained in the breathing system during the expiratory pause.
(h) *NEEP* (negative end-expiratory pressure) — which implies that a negative pressure is maintained in the breathing system during the expiratory pause.

*Respiratory exchange* is the process in which oxygen in the alveolar air passes into the plasma and carbon dioxide is given up by the plasma to the alveolar air.

*Rebreathing* is the reinhalation of any gas that has previously entered the patient's respiratory tract. The rebreathed gases may have previously occupied only the patient's dead space, and therefore this does not constitute functional rebreathing, which is the rebreathing of gases that have already taken part in respiratory exchange. Note, however, that exhaled gas, which has had the carbon dioxide removed (by an absorber) and fresh oxygen added, is not regarded as rebreathed gas if it is subsequently reinhaled.

*Positive pressure* indicates a pressure above the ambient, and *negative pressure* one below it.

*Upstream* is the direction from which gases are flowing. *Downstream* is the direction to which gases are flowing.

The *back bar* is that part of a continuous flow anaesthetic machine which dispenses gases and vapours. It includes flowmeters, vaporizers and an outlet.

The *Breathing system* is that part of the anaesthetic apparatus which is normally attached to the common gas outlet of an anaesthetic machine, and into which gases are passed at, or not far from, atmospheric pressure and through which the patient breathes or is ventilated.

Whereas oxygen is a true *gas* (see p. 1), nitrous oxide, carbon dioxide and cyclopropane are strictly speaking *vapours*. They are, however, frequently termed gases, see below.

*Mixed gas flow* is the mixture of gases (and vapours) that have been metered through the flowmeters.

*Fresh gas flow (FGF)* consists of the mixed gas flow and vapours of the volatile agents from the vaporizers, which are supplied from the back bar to the breathing system.

*Back pressure* is the pressure that has to be overcome by the mixed gas flow as a result of it having to do work, for example by driving a minute volume divider ventilator or passing through a constriction.

The term does not imply that the gases flow in a reverse direction to normal.

*Apparatus dead space* is that portion of a breathing system in which exhaled gases remain, and are destined to be inspired at the next breath. The rate and direction of the fresh gas flow into the breathing system may well remove some of the gas within this area, and that which remains is termed the *functional apparatus dead space*.

*Anatomical dead space* is that part of the patient's respiratory tract (Oro- and naso-pharynx, trachea and large bronchi, etc.) into which fresh gases enter, but where they do not take part in respiratory exchange. They may be warmed and humidified, but no carbon dioxide is added nor oxygen removed, so they may be usefully reinhaled.

*Rotameter* is a commonly used name for a flowmeter with a rotating bobbin. In fact, 'Rotameter' is the trade name for one particular manufacturer.

*Expiratory valve* is a valve through which all expired gases pass, or should pass, either to the external atmosphere or to part of the breathing system.

*APL valve*. The adjustable pressure limiting valve allows the escape of excess gases from the breathing system.

*Overpressure valve* is a valve which will open under fault conditions to allow the escape of gases if the pressure in it exceeds a preset limit.

*Underpressure (air-entrainment) valve* is a valve which will open under fault conditions to allow the ingress of atmospheric air to a breathing or scavenging system if the pressure within it falls below a preset limit.

A *Dumping valve* allows the escape to atmosphere of excess gases in a breathing system, to prevent them causing overpressure therein. It may also be called a *Spill valve*. (Note this change of definition.)

*Scavenging* is the collection and removal of waste anaesthetic gases from the operating theatre or recovery room. This is usually achieved by attaching hoses and other components to the breathing system.

*Regulated pressure* is the pressure within the reduced pressure circuitry of the anaesthetic machine.

*Compliance* is a measure of the ease with which gas may be introduced into a system. It is measured in unit volume per unit increase in pressure. With regard to the lung, physicians usually refer to the lung alone, whereas anaesthetists usually refer not only to the lung, but also the chest wall and any other factors which may impede the inflation of the lungs. The unit used is litres per cm $H_2O$ pressure.

*MAC*. This is a measure of the potency of a volatile anaesthetic agent. It is the *Minimal Alveolar Concentration* of an agent which, at equilibrium, will prevent 50% of experimental animals from reacting to a standard surgical stimulus. It may thus be used to compare the potency of various agents.

*Parameter*. In Anaesthesia it is, strictly speaking, a factor common to a number of equations or situations, and may be used as an arbitrary constant that defines or assists in defining the relationship between other variables, and quantifies them. However, it has recently been used to refer to repeated measurements of physiological functions.

*Module*. Correctly used, this is a standard unit of length or area common to a number of situations: as for example, in architecture the 9" × 3" brick which the builder takes as the standard unit of measurement. It then became a term for conglomerate equipment where all the units were of the same size, so that they could be interchanged within the main structure. Now it is used, quite erroneously, for anything that can be plugged in or attached, regardless of its dimensions.

*Transducer*. This is a device which converts one signal, or form of energy, into another, usually so that it may be processed and eventually used to control a function or to give an indication of a value. It is usually associated with electronic equipment.

# Abbreviations

| | | | |
|---|---|---|---|
| ADC | Analogue to Digital Converter | ISO | International Standards Organization |
| ANSI | American National Standards Institute | K | Degrees Kelvin (always stated without °) |
| APL | Adjustable pressure limiting (valve) | Kg/cm$^2$ | Kilograms per square centimetre |
| atm | Atmosphere (unit of pressure) | KPa | Kilopascal (European standard measurement for pressure) |
| BOC | British Oxygen Company | | |
| BP | British Pharmacopoeia | LMA | Laryngeal Mask Airway |
| BS | British Standard | l/min | Litres per minute |
| BSP | British Standard Pipe (screw thread) | MDM | Monitored Dial Mixer (Quantiflex flowmeter) |
| cmH$_2$O | Centimetres of water (unit of pressure) | | |
| °C | Degrees Celsius | MGI | Medical Gas Installations Ltd |
| COSHH | Control of Substances Hazardous to Health | ml/min | Millilitres per minute |
| | | M&IE | Medical and Industrial Equipment Ltd |
| CSSD | Central Sterile Supply Department | mmHg | Millimetres of mercury (unit of pressure) |
| DAC | Digital to Analogue Converter | MMV | Mandatory minute volume |
| DoH | Department of Health (Replaces DHSS, Department of Health and Social Security) | MV | Minute volume |
| | | NAD | North American Dräger |
| | | NEEP | Negative end-expiratory pressure |
| DISS | Diameter Indexed Safety System (USA) | NIOSH | National Institute for Occupational Safety and Health (USA) |
| EBME | Electronic and Biomedical Engineering (Department) | | |
| | | NIST | Non-interchangeable screw threaded (connection) |
| EPROM | Eraseable programmable read only memory | | |
| | | OD | Outside diameter |
| EXH | Exhaust | ODA | Operating Department Assistant (UK) |
| EXP | Expiratory (valve) | OMV | Oxford Miniature vaporizer |
| FGF | Fresh gas flow | Pa | Pascal (unit of pressure) |
| HEI | Health Equipment Information (issued by the DoH) | PEEP | Positive end-expiratory pressure |
| | | PI | Pin index |
| HFPPV | High frequency positive pressure ventilation | PMGV | Piped medical gas and vacuum (system) |
| | | ppm | Parts per million |
| HME | Heat and moisture exchanger | PPM | Planned preventative maintenance |
| HSC | Health and Safety Commission (UK) | psi | Pounds per square inch (US standard measurement for pressure) |
| HTM | Hospital Technical Memorandum (issued by HM Stationery Office) | | |
| | | PTFE | Polytetrafluorethylene (= Teflon; = Fluon) |
| i.c. | Integrated circuit | RAM | Random Access Memory |
| ICU/ | Intensive care unit/ | R.h. | Relative humidity |
| ITU | Intensive therapy unit | ROM | Read Only Memory |
| ID | Internal diameter | SI(units) | Système International d'Unites (International System of Units) |
| IEC | International Electrotechnical Commission | | |
| IMV | Intermittent Mandatory Ventilation | SIMV | Synchronized Intermittent Mandatory Ventilation |
| INSP | Inspiratory (valve) | | |
| IPPR | Intermittent positive pressure respiration (IPPV is the preferred term) | SVP | Saturated vapour pressure |
| | | TILC | Temperature indicated, level compensated (vaporizer) |
| IPPV | Intermittent positive pressure ventilation | | |

| | | | |
|---|---|---|---|
| Torr | (Torricelli) mmHg pressure (also used for subatmospheric pressures) | VIBS | Vaporizer in breathing system |
| | | VIC | Vaporizer in circle |
| TSSU | Theatre Sterile Supply Unit | VIE | Vacuum insulated evaporator |
| TV | Tidal volume | VOC | Vaporizer out of circle |
| USP | United States Pharmacopoeia | | |

# 1 Physical Principles

## Introduction

The art of anaesthesia is essentially practical. For this reason the anaesthetist must have an understanding of the physical aspects of the apparatus he uses, not only so that he can use it efficiently but also so that he may understand its limitations and use it safely. Many unnecessary accidents and near-misses have occurred as the result of the misuse of equipment because the anaesthetist did not understand the basic principles of its operation.

The first two chapters of this book are therefore devoted to the basic physics of gases, liquids, vapours and solids, and to the principles of modern control systems, which are increasingly a part of the latest anaesthetic machines. The principles of the electromagnetic spectrum are also discussed at the end of the chapter.

One of the problems besetting the medical profession today is the clinician's inability to discuss his requirements with the engineer in terms that they both understand. This problem occurs not only with the development of new equipment, but in discussing faults and difficulties with older equipment.

## States of Matter

In order to understand the functioning of an anaesthetic machine it is necessary to appreciate the difference between the three states of matter — solid, liquid and gas.

A *solid* is compact and relatively dense. It maintains its shape unless subjected to comparatively large forces and is not easily compressed. Its molecules, although in a state of constant agitation, do not change their position relative to one another; hence a solid tends to maintain its shape. Different solids, in contact with each other, do not normally mix.

A *fluid* is a substance that cannot sustain shearing forces or mechanical stress — it easily changes shape when a force is applied to it. Liquids, vapours and gases are all therefore fluids.

A *liquid* is also compact. Its molecules are constantly moving relative to each other and, owing to their being densely packed, there are frequent collisions between them. Because its molecules move freely, a liquid takes the shape of the container in which it is confined and moves from one part of it to another under the influence of gravity. Its shape may be distorted by small forces. Different liquids, in contact with each other, may or may not mix.

*Vapours* and *gases* are best characterized as having no inherent boundary or volume, they expand to fill evenly the space within which they are confined. Different vapours or gases in contact with each other normally mix. The terms *vapour* and *gas* are synonymous but vapour is usually used for the gaseous state at a temperature and pressure close to those at which it would condense into a liquid. The scientific distinction between a vapour and a gas is as follows. For any substance there is a maximum temperature at which it can be compressed so as to convert it from a gas to a liquid. Above that temperature, known as the *critical temperature*, no amount of pressure will liquefy it. At temperatures lower than the critical temperature the substance may exist as a vapour or as a liquid or, indeed, as a mixture of both depending on its pressure and volume. The relationship between pressure, volume and temperature is usually displayed as a family of *isotherms*. Figure 1.1 shows an isotherm family for nitrous oxide. Each isotherm shows the relationship between pressure and volume at a given temperature. Nitrous oxide may exist as a liquid or a vapour below the critical temperature of +36.5°C; above the critical temperature it may exist only as a gas. It follows that if a gas is stored below its critical temperature and hence in its liquid/vapour state, assessment of the contents of its container cannot be made from the pressure therein. If a gas is stored

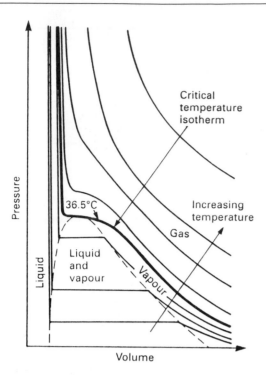

**Figure 1.1** Isotherms for nitrous oxide.

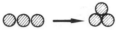

**Figure 1.2** The cohesion between three molecules arranged in a straight row causes them to take up a more compact form.

called *surface tension*. With an even larger quantity of mercury, the sphere would be so large that it would be distorted by the force of gravity (*G*) and the force of the surface upon which it rests (Fig. 1.3). Note that the edges of the blob are still circular. This may be observed when a small quantity of mercury is spilled and blobs of various sizes are formed. The small ones are nearly spherical whereas the larger ones are flattened.

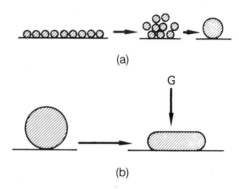

**Figure 1.3** (a) The cohesion between a number of molecules causes them to group together in the most compact form, a sphere. (b) The sphere is distorted by the effect of gravity.

above its critical temperature, for example, oxygen which has a critical temperature of −118°C and therefore is in its gaseous state, the quantity of gas will be proportional to the pressure inside its container. The *critical pressure* is that which is required to liquefy a gas at its critical temperature. The critical temperatures and pressures of various gases are shown in Table 3.1 in Chapter 3.

# Behaviour of Molecules of Solids and Liquids

The molecules of a solid or a liquid attract each other. They may also be attracted by the molecules of another substance. The mutual attraction between the molecules of a substance is termed *cohesion*, and their attraction to those of another substance is called *adhesion*. Let us suppose that there are three molecules of mercury in a straight row. Each molecule will attract its neighbour, but the first will also attract the third, so that they will at once move to take up a more compact form (Fig. 1.2).

If we now consider a much larger number of molecules of mercury, each one attracting the others, they will tend to take up the shape of a sphere. The force that preserves the periphery of the sphere is

The molecules of other substances may exert less mutual attraction and so the force of adhesion to another substance may be stronger than the force of cohesion. Thus, if there are a number of water molecules, for example, on a glass surface, the outer molecules have a greater force of attraction for the glass than for the inner ones, so they 'wet' the surface (Fig. 1.4). However, water will not wet a greasy surface, upon which it takes up a globular form.

If a vertical dry glass tube of about 1-cm diameter is dipped into a vessel of water, the upper surface within the tube forms a *meniscus* with an upturned edge because the water wets the surface of the tube (Fig. 1.5a). Water is drawn a little way up the tube by molecular attraction, against the force of gravity. However if the water is replaced by mercury, which does not wet the glass, the shape of the meniscus is reversed and the edges are depressed (Fig. 1.5b) since the edge of the meniscus is pulled inwards by cohesion and it resembles the blob of mercury described above (Fig. 1.3).

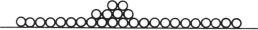

**Figure 1.4** The molecules of a substance for which the force of adhesion is greater than the force of cohesion spread out as they wet the surface on which they rest.

Returning to the case of the tube filled with water, if it has a very narrow bore it is known as a *capillary* tube and the water may be drawn up a considerable amount by the wetting effect on the inside of the tube. The force of attraction of the wall of the tube on the column determines the height to which the column of water will be raised. This phenomenon is known as capillary action or *capillarity*. It may also occur, for example, when two closely fitting smooth surfaces of any shape are separated by a thin film of water. Considerable force may be needed to prise them apart.

Use is made of capillarity when a wick is used in a vaporizer. Since it dips into the liquid agent, the liquid rises up the wick and so presents a larger surface area from which vaporization may occur.

# Heat and Temperature

## Temperature

Temperature means relative hotness or coldness of a substance and is actually a measure of the average kinetic energy possessed by its molecules. Temperature is indicated in degrees on a defined scale. At sea level, at normal atmospheric pressure, pure water freezes at 0°C (degrees Celsius, formerly known as Centigrade) and boils at 100°C. Other scales of temperature in common use are Kelvin (Absolute) and Fahrenheit

*Kelvin (Absolute) scale.* The SI unit of temperature is the Kelvin (K) and is based on the absolute temperature scale where zero K is the temperature at which molecular motion ceases. It is equivalent to −273°C on the Celsius scale which is also allowed as an SI scale of temperature. It will be seen from Charles' law (see Properties of Gases) that the volume of an ideal gas (whose molecules have zero volume) is proportional to its temperature. Zero Kelvin is known as absolute zero, as though if a gas could be cooled to 0 K it would disappear. Of course this does not happen as the gas liquefies before this low a temperature is reached. Table 1.1 compares Absolute, Celsius and Fahrenheit scales.

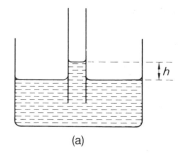

(a)

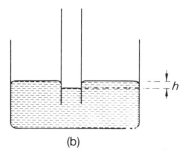

(b)

**Figure 1.5** (a) If a narrow tube is dipped into a vessel of water, the wetting effect causes the water to rise up the tube and the edge of the meniscus is turned up. The height $h$ of the water column depends, apart from other factors, on the diameter of the tube. (b) If the same tube is dipped into a vessel of mercury, the level of mercury in the tube is depressed and the edge of the meniscus is turned down, because it does not wet the glass.

## Heat

In order to raise the temperature of a substance, energy, in the form of heat, must be added to it. The SI unit of heat is the *joule* but the most commonly used unit is the *calorie*. One calorie raises the temperature of 1 g of water by 1°C from 14.5 to 15.5°C. The calorie is a very small amount of heat and therefore heat energy is usually expressed in kilocalories (kcal), which is often written as Calories.

$$1 \text{ Cal} = 1 \text{ kcal} = 1000 \text{ calories} = 4200 \text{ joules}$$

Heat may be transferred from one object or substance or from one part of an object or substance to another by conduction, convection or radiation.

In *conduction*, heat simply travels along a substance from molecule to molecule. Metals, such as copper, are good conductors of heat, whereas, for example, glass and expanded polystyrene are poor conductors. Very poor conductors of heat are termed thermal insulators (Table 1.2).

**Table 1.1**   Comparison of the Absolute, Celsius and Fahrenheit temperature scales

| Reference point | Temperature | | |
|---|---|---|---|
| | Absolute | Celsius | Fahrenheit |
| 'Absolute zero' | 0 K | −273°C | −459°F |
| Freezing point of water | 273 K | 0°C | 32°F |
| Boiling point of water (at sea level) | 373 K | 100°C | 212°F |

*Conversion formulae:*
K = °C + 273
°C = ⅝(°F − 32)
°F = ⅑°C + 32

**Table 1.2**   Relative thermal conductivity at 0°C

| Good conductors | | Poor conductors | |
|---|---|---|---|
| Silver | 428 | *Liquid state* | |
| Copper | 403 | Nitrous oxide | 1.5 |
| Gold | 319 | Carbon dioxide | 1.45 |
| Aluminium | 236 | Glass | 1.0 |
| Nickel | 94 | Water | 0.561 |
| Iron | 84 | Asbestos | 0.11 |
| Bronze | 53 | Paper | 0.06 |
| Lead | 36 | Wool | 0.05 |
| Stainless steel | 25 | Polystyrene | 0.035 |
| | | *Gaseous state* | |
| | | Oxygen | 0.0245 |
| | | Nitrous oxide | 0.015 |

## Convection

If part of a fluid, be it a liquid or a gas, is heated, it expands and becomes less dense than the fluid around it. Being free to move, it rises, and as it travels upwards, its place is taken by the cooler, denser fluid from around it, which in turn is heated and rises. There is, therefore, a constant rising stream above the source of heat and the heat is carried by *convection*.

## Radiation

The amount of heat radiated from a surface depends not only on its temperature but on its nature. A matt black surface radiates far more than a smooth, shiny one. Radiated heat 'rays' can be focused and directed, as is seen in the electric radiant heater with a reflector. Radiation is defined as energy that is transferred directly from a source, and propagated as wave energy in straight lines from a source.

## Specific heat

The quantity of heat required to raise the tempera-ture of a given mass of a substance by a certain amount varies from one substance to another. This is termed *specific heat capacity*, which is defined as the amount of heat required to raise the temperature of 1 kg of the specified substance by 1 K.

## Latent heat

Considerably more heat is required to vaporize a liquid than to raise its temperature from room temperature to its boiling point. The heat required to vaporize a liquid is called the *latent heat of vaporization*. For water, this is 539 cal/g at 100°C and normal atmospheric pressure. The heat required to melt a solid is known as the *latent heat of fusion*. For ice this is 80 cal/g at 0°C and normal atmospheric pressure.

## Vaporization

Molecules of a liquid are in constant motion, but they also have a mutual attraction for each other.

If the liquid has a surface exposed to air or other gases, or to a vacuum, some molecules will escape from the surface when their energy exceeds that of their mutual attraction for other molecules at the surface. This is the process of *evaporation*. Its rate is increased if the temperature of the liquid is raised, since the molecules move faster and possess more energy. If the atmosphere is enclosed, some of the molecules that have escaped while moving freely in the gaseous state will impinge on the surface of the liquid and re-enter it. The vapour formed by the molecules exerts a pressure which is known as *vapour pressure*. Within a confined space there may occur an equilibrium in which the number of molecules re-entering the liquid equals the number leaving it. At this stage the vapour pressure is at a maximum for the temperature and is called *saturated vapour pressure* (SVP). Figure 1.6 shows the vapour

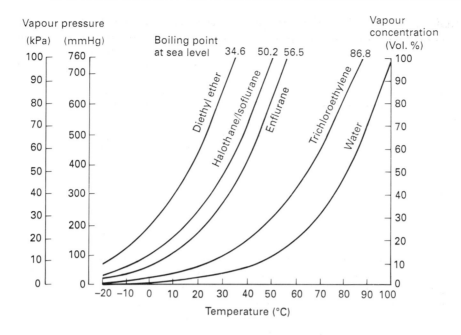

**Figure 1.6** Vapour pressure curves for anaesthetic agents and water vapour.

pressure curves of volatile anaesthetic agents and water vapour and shows how they vary with temperature.

If the liquid is heated, a point is reached at which the SVP becomes equal to ambient atmospheric pressure. Vaporization now occurs not only at the surface of the liquid but also in the bubbles that develop within its substance. The liquid is *boiling* and this temperature is its *boiling point*. From this it is evident that the boiling point of a liquid depends on the ambient pressure. At high altitudes there is a significant depression of the boiling point. This may render the use of agents such as ethyl-chloride, divinyl ether and diethyl ether difficult. Figure 1.7 shows the variation of boiling point with atmospheric pressure.

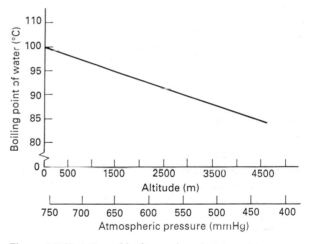

**Figure 1.7** Variation of boiling point of water with atmospheric pressure or altitude.

## Expansion of solids

As any substance is heated it expands and different metals expand to a different extent. There is a considerable difference between the *coefficients of expansion* of various metals, as shown in Table 1.3.

If strips of two dissimilar metals are bonded together side by side and heated, one expands more than the other, causing a deflection of the bimetallic strip that they form (Fig. 1.8). This principle is used in thermostats, some dial thermometers and the temperature-compensating mechanisms of many vaporizers.

**Table 1.3** Coefficients of linear expansion of metallic solids in units of $10^{-6}/°C$

| | |
|---|---|
| Aluminium | 23 |
| Copper | 16.7 |
| Iron | 12 |
| Lead | 29 |
| Nickel | 12.8 |
| Platinum | 8.9 |
| Silver | 19 |
| Tungsten | 5 |
| Zinc | 30 |

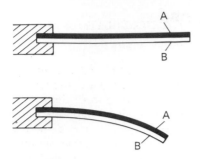

**Figure 1.8** A bimetallic strip. Two strips of dissimilar metals (A and B) are bonded together. Initially A and B are the same length, but when heated A expands more than B, causing the deflection shown.

## Expansion of gases

The molecules of a gas are far more widely separated than those of a solid. This results in two phenomena that do not occur in the case of solids or liquids.

- A gas expands to fill evenly the space within which it is confined.

- Gases expand to a greater extent when heated than do solids or liquids.

# Properties of Gases

As is the case with all substances, the smallest particle of a gas that can exist separately is a molecule. Gas molecules are in constant motion, moving about in all directions and occasionally bombarding the walls of the space in which they are confined. It is this bombardment of the walls that exerts the pressure due to the gas.

A vessel may be occupied by more than one gas, in which case the total pressure within it is the sum of the pressures exerted independently by each of the gases. Each gas is said to exert a *partial pressure*. If a gas is heated, the movement of its molecules becomes more energetic and this leads to a rise in pressure. If the volume in which it is confined is constant, its pressure varies directly with temperature. These facts are expressed in Dalton's, Boyle's and Charles' laws as follows.

*Dalton's law relating to vapours.*

- The pressure exerted by a vapour or a gas in a closed space, at a given temperature, depends only on that temperature, and is independent of the pressure of other vapours or gases (provided they have no chemical action upon it).

- When several vapours or gases, having no chemical action upon each other, are present in the same space, the pressure exerted by the mixture is the sum of the pressures that would be exerted by each of its constituents if it was separately confined in the same space.

*Boyle's law.* Boyle's law states that, at a constant temperature, the volume of a mass of gas is inversely proportional to the pressure.

*Charles' law.* Charles' law states that the coefficient of expansion of any gas at a constant pressure is 1/273.

From the last two laws we may derive the equation

$$\frac{P_1 V_1}{T_1} = \frac{P_2 V_2}{T_2}$$

where $P_1$, $V_1$ and $T_1$ are the pressure, volume and temperature of one case and $P_2$, $V_2$ and $T_2$ are the corresponding quantities of a second case. $T$ must be expressed on the absolute scale (i.e. in Kelvin). The above formula may be used to calculate the results of a change of pressure, temperature or volume of a gas.

## The Poynting effect

The Poynting effect is also known as the *overpressure effect*.

The critical temperature and critical pressure of one gas may be affected by its admixture with another. If a cylinder is partially filled with liquid nitrous oxide, inverted, and then further filled from a high-pressure source of oxygen, an unexpected phenomenon occurs. This may be viewed through the glass observation window of a high-pressure rig. The bubbles of oxygen diminish in size as the gas is partially dissolved in the liquid nitrous oxide through which it passes. Simultaneously, the volume of the liquid nitrous oxide diminishes as it evaporates and mixes with the oxygen. Eventually the cylinder, filled to a pressure of nearly 137 000 kPa (2000 psi), contains mixed oxygen and nitrous oxide both in the gaseous state. A 50 : 50 mixture of these two gases is marketed under the name 'Entonox'. Further details of the use of this mixture and the correct handling of the cylinders are given (see page 44). Precautions concerning cooling of cylinders of the mixture are necessary as the critical temperature of the nitrous oxide changes from 36.5°C to a *pseudocritical* temperature of −6°C.

## Viscosity

The *viscosity* of a fluid is a measure of its resistance to flow. If we consider a fluid passing along a tube, the fluid in the centre of the tube flows more rapidly than that at the periphery, which tends to adhere to the walls of the tube. We can imagine that there are layers of fluid slipping over each other. It is the friction between these layers that causes viscosity. Viscosity is measured in *poise* (1 poise = 0.1 pascal second), named after the French physiologist Poiseuille, but a more useful measure for both liquids and gases is the coefficient of viscosity as compared with that of water.

# Temperature Changes in Anaesthetic Apparatus

The performance of some items of anaesthetic equipment is affected by changes in temperature. A rise in temperature:

- increases the vaporization rate of volatile agents;
- causes a fall in density of fluids due to expansion;
- reduces viscosity of liquids;
- increases the viscosity of gases owing to the increased molecular activity.

As vaporization proceeds, there is a fall in the temperature of the liquid and of the vaporizer in which it is contained, owing to the latent heat required, so that unless there is some form of compensation, the vapour concentration falls.

Three different measures may be taken to counteract this effect.

- The temperature of the vaporizer may be indicated by a thermometer so that the anaesthetist can make appropriate adjustments to maintain the desired concentration.
- Automatic compensation for temperature changes may be made within the vaporizer by making use of the properties of the bimetallic strip.
- An external supply of heat may be made available to satisfy the needs of the latent heat of vaporization, as a rule either by physically attaching a large mass of metal such as copper or by immersing the vaporizing chamber in a large mass of water which may be warmed. Alternatively, heat may be gained by the attachment of fins, which increase the area of the external surface of the vaporizing chamber to the surrounding air and so assist in heat transfer by conduction and convection. Some vaporizers are electrically heated.

# Force and Pressure

It is important to understand the terms force and pressure. *Force* causes an object to move in a certain direction. The amount of force does not vary with the area over which it is exerted. The unit of force is the *newton*. One newton causes a mass of 1 kg to accelerate by 1 m per second per second (1 m/s$^2$). Other units are the kilogram-force kgf and the pound-force lbf, a thrust of 1 kg and 1 lb respectively.

*Fluid pressure* is exerted in all directions and is a measure of force *per unit area*, i.e.

$$\text{Pressure} = \frac{\text{Force}}{\text{Area}}$$

Hydrodynamic pressure (in a fluid) is exerted in all directions. Consider the hypodermic syringe. The user exerts a force on the plunger in one particular direction. The pressure of the fluid in the syringe is exerted in all directions, and if there were a leak in the barrel of the syringe, the liquid would squirt out sideways (Fig. 1.9). If a wide-bore syringe is used, the same force exerted by the thumb acts over a large area and so the pressure in the syringe is lower than it would be if the same force were exerted on the plunger of a narrower bore syringe.

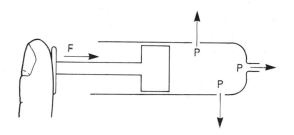

**Figure 1.9** When the user exerts a force *F* on the plunger of an intravenous syringe, it is applied in one direction only, but the resulting fluid pressure *P* is exerted in all directions.

## Pressure and partial pressure

The air in which we live exerts a pressure. At the surface of the earth, this *atmospheric* pressure is due to the influence of gravity on the mass of air supported, as may be demonstrated as follows.

A long transparent tube, closed at one end, is filled with mercury and then inverted so that its

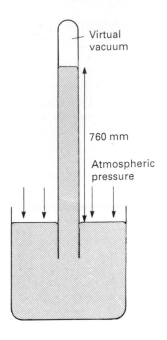

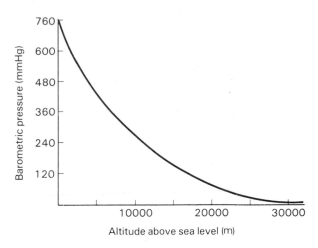

Figure 1.11 The relationship between barometric pressure and altitude above sea level.

Figure 1.10 A simple barometer. The long tube is closed at the top and, although it was filled with mercury before being inverted and placed in the mercury reservoir, the mercury level in the tube has fallen, leaving a virtual vacuum at the top of the tube. The height of the column of mercury indicates the atmospheric pressure.

open end rests in a reservoir of mercury, as shown in Fig. 1.10. The column of mercury falls until its meniscus is about 760 mm above the level in the reservoir. Above the meniscus is a vacuum (or near vacuum). The atmospheric pressure acting on the reservoir supports a column of mercury 760-mm high and is said to be 760 mmHg (or 760 Torr).

If the column had a cross-sectional area of 1 cm$^2$, it would weigh 1033 g, so the pressure can be said to be 1.033 kg/cm$^2$. The average atmospheric (barometric) pressure at sea level is therefore 1033 kg/cm$^2$ = 15 psi = 1.01 × 10$^5$ newtons/m$^2$ (pascals) = 1 bar = 1000 millibars.

*Partial pressure.* As already stated, the pressure (or partial pressure) of a gas is the result of energy expended by its molecules impinging on its confines, and if two or more gases are mixed the total pressure is the sum of all the partial pressures measured as if they were acting independently of each other.

If the pressure of a mixture of two gases is 760 mmHg, the partial pressures of each of the two gases added together equals 760 mmHg. If, for simplicity, we consider that air contains 20% oxygen and 80% nitrogen, then the partial pressures

of these two gases at sea level are:

> Oxygen:  20% of 760 = 152 mmHg
> Nitrogen: 80% of 760 = 608 mmHg

(disregarding other gases and water vapour) and the barometric pressure equals 760 mmHg (152 mmHg + 608 mmHg).

As the altitude above sea level increases, the barometric pressure decreases because for each unit of area a shorter column of air is being supported. The relationship between altitude and average barometric pressure is shown in Fig. 1.11.

When treating patients at high altitudes, a larger percentage of oxygen in the inspired gas mixture is required to maintain the same partial pressure, and it is the partial pressure rather than the percentage of oxygen that is important (refer to the oxygen-dissociation curve). The relationship between altitude and the partial pressure of the components of the atmosphere is shown in Fig. 1.12.

### Direct methods of measuring pressure

*Simple manometer.* Figure 1.13 shows the principle of a simple manometer, which is a U-tube partially filled with liquid, in this case water. A gas at pressure $P$ has been applied to end A of the tube and end B is open. The pressure $P$ causes the water to be pushed across to the opposite limb of the tube. At *a* the water level has been depressed by 5 cm from its former position and at *b* it has been raised by 5 cm. The pressure $P$ is therefore 10 cm of water. If the U-tube were filled with mercury, the pressure would be expressed in millimetres of mercury (Torr). Figure 1.14 shows the basic principle of the

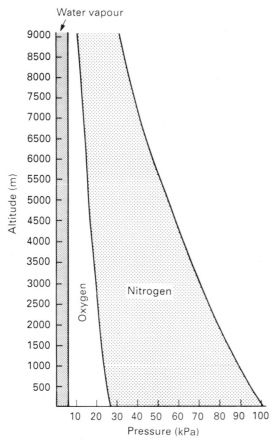

Water vapour

Oxygen

Nitrogen

Altitude (m)

Pressure (kPa)

**Figure 1.12** Variation with altitude of components of inspired air. Saturation with water vapour by upper airways is assumed.

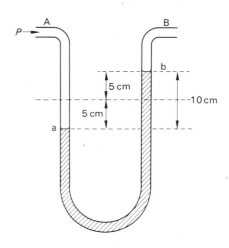

**Figure 1.13** A simple manometer. A pressure $P$ is applied at A. This causes a depression of the fluid level at $a$ and a corresponding rise of the fluid level at $b$. In this case the tube is filled with water and the pressure is 10 cm of water.

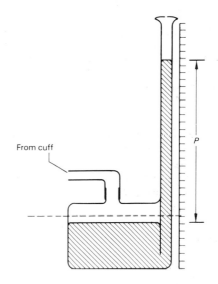

From cuff

**Figure 1.14** The principle of the mercurial sphygmomanometer.

mercurial sphygmomanometer, in which the two limbs are of different diameter. The pressure reading is still taken as the difference between the levels of the two columns of mercury, but the reservoir limb, being so very much wider than the other, exhibits a very much smaller change in level.

*Pressure gauges.* A simple type of diaphragm gauge is shown in Fig. 1.15. The gas enters at C and the diaphragm D is distended against the force of the spring S. The rod attaching the diaphragm to the spring has a rack R which turns a pinion on which is mounted the pointer. In practice the rack and pinion is replaced by a sophisticated train of gear wheels, and the spring is not needed if the elastic recoil of the diaphragm itself is sufficient. There may, however, be a hair spring to steady and improve the performance of the pointer. The larger and more compliant the diaphragm, the lower are the pressures that can be measured.

The Bourdon tube is a development of the diaphragm pressure gauge. It is normally used for much higher pressures, such as those in a full oxygen cylinder, and may be calibrated up to 137 000 kPa (2000 psi) or even higher. As will be seen in Fig 1.16, the chamber with the diaphragm has been replaced by a curved and flattened tube. When the pressure is applied to it, the tube expands and the curvature is partially straightened out, thus moving the rack and the pinion. Again the rack and pinion is usually replaced by a compound train of gear wheels and there is a hair spring. The inlet to the gauge is fitted with a constriction to prevent sudden surges of pressure damaging the mechanism.

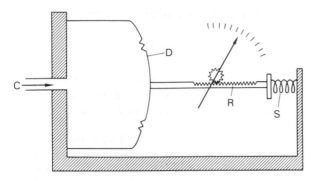

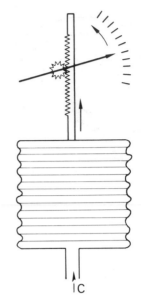

**Figure 1.15** A diaphragm pressure gauge. Pressure exerted at C causes deflection of the diaphragm D. This pushes the rack R against the pressure of the spring S, thereby turning the cogwheel so that the pressure is indicated on the scale by the pointer.

**Figure 1.17** A low-pressure aneroid gauge.

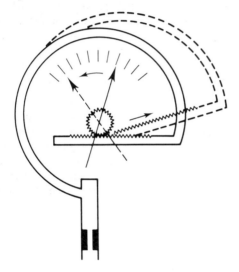

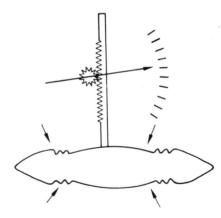

**Figure 1.16** The principle of the Bourdon tube pressure gauge. Note the constriction at the inlet.

**Figure 1.18** A typical arrangement for a barometer. Note that the capsule is closed and the atmospheric pressure acts on its exterior.

Another type of pressure gauge for both high and low pressures is the aneroid gauge. This is frequently used in barometers. Figure 1.17 shows a typical low-pressure aneroid gauge, and Fig. 1.18 is a typical arrangement for a barometer. Note that in the latter case the capsule is completely sealed; it expands and contracts as pressure changes are applied to its exterior. Changes in atmospheric pressure compress it or allow it to expand, thereby causing movements of the pointer. Gauges for very low pressure have diaphragms made of neoprene or rubber; these may perish. In some low-pressure and all high-pressure gauges the diaphragm, tubes or capsules are made of various types of metallic alloy.

*Pressure transducers.* Electronic devices may measure pressure, or changes in pressure, by means of a transducer, which converts the pressure into electrical units. Often, the transducer consists of a semiconductor, the shape of which is deformed by the application of pressure, thus altering its electrical conductivity.

### Calibration of pressure gauges

Pressure gauges for high pressures are usually calibrated in psi, kg/cm², atmospheres (1 atm = 15 psi = 1.03 kg/cm²), kPa or bar. They are normally calibrated in *gauge pressure*, i.e. the pressure above

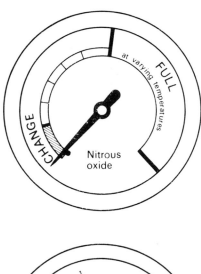

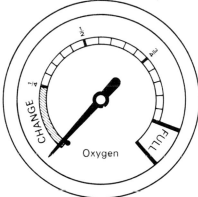

**Figure 1.19** Nitrous oxide and oxygen cylinder contents gauges.

## Pressure regulators (reducing valves)

Pressure regulators are used on anaesthetic and oxygen therapy apparatus for three main reasons.

- The pressure delivered from a cylinder is far too high to be used with safety in apparatus where a sudden surge of pressure might accidentally be delivered to the patient.
- If the pressure were not reduced, flow-control (fine-adjustment) valves, tubing and various other parts of the apparatus would have to be very much more robust, and a fine and accurate control of gas flow would be difficult to achieve. There would also be a danger of pressure building up and damaging other components of the apparatus.
- As the contents of a cylinder are exhausted, the pressure within the cylinder falls. If there were no regulator mechanism to maintain a constant reduced pressure, continual adjustment would have to be made of the flow-control valve in order to maintain a constant flow rate.

Not only is the pressure reduced, but it is also kept constant, and for this reason the correct term for this type of valve is a *pressure regulator*. The working principle of a pressure regulator is shown in Fig. 1.20. The chamber C is enclosed on one side by the diaphragm D. As gas enters the chamber through the valve V, the pressure in the chamber is

atmospheric pressure. In this case 'g' may be written after the pressure.

In some circumstances gauges are calibrated in *absolute* pressure ($P_{abs}$). In such a case a pressure gauge open to the air would indicate a pressure of 15 psi or 1 atm. Examples are the barometer and gauges used, in connection with hyperbaric oxygen therapy. Where it is not stated which of these units is used, as in this book, it is usually understood that *gauge* pressures are being described. It is important to make this distinction in apparatus such as hyperbaric oxygen equipment, where a gauge pressure of, say, 2 atm may be used, which equals an absolute pressure of 3 atm.

For lower pressures, gauges are often calibrated in millimetres of mercury (mmHg) or centimetres of water ($cmH_2O$). The term 'Torr' is now commonly used in place of millimetres of mercury (normal atmospheric pressure = 760 Torr).

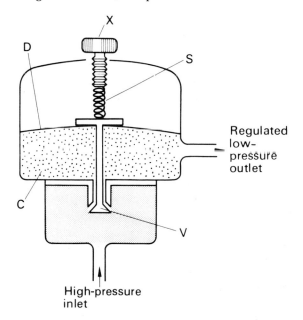

**Figure 1.20** A simple pressure regulator. D, diaphragm; S, spring; C, low-pressure chamber; V, valve seating; X, adjustment screw.

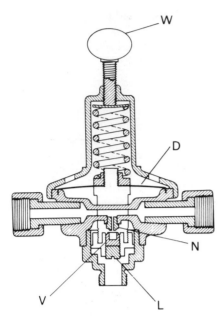

**Figure 1.21** A McKesson regulator. W, wing screw; N, nozzle; V, valve seat; L, lock screw; D, diaphragm.

increased and the diaphragm is distended against its own elastic recoil plus the tension in the spring S. Eventually the pressure rises so much and the diaphragm moves so far that valve V is closed. The pressure at which this occurs may be varied by adjusting the screw X so as to alter the tension in the spring S. If gas is allowed to escape from the outlet of the chamber, the pressure falls and valve V reopens. When the regulator is in use a steady pressure is maintained in the chamber by the partial opening of valve V.

There are several types of pressure regulator available, the choice being dependent on the maximum flow rate required, the regulated pressure to which it is to be set and the maximum input pressure that it is to handle. For low-pressure regulators, the diaphragms are frequently made of rubber or neoprene, whereas in those for higher pressures, such as the McKesson regulator shown in Fig. 1.21, the diaphragm is made of metal. Where there is to be a considerable pressure reduction and at the same time a high flow rate is required, it is common practice to use a two-stage regulator, as shown in Fig. 1.22. Adjustments to alter the regulated pressure should normally be made only by service engineers, except in the case of the McKesson regulator, which is provided with means for easy adjustment to equalize the pressures of nitrous oxide and oxygen. Adjustments should be made with the gas flowing.

On some anaesthetic machines 'universal' regu-

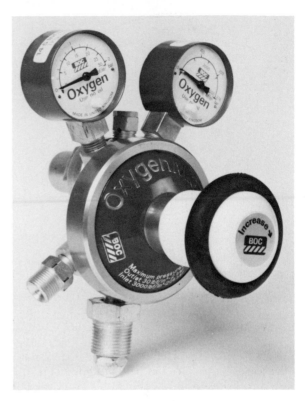

**Figure 1.22** A two-stage regulator.

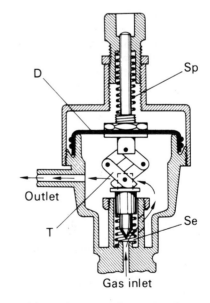

**Figure 1.23** The Adams regulator. D, diaphragm; Sp, spring; Se, seat; T, toggle levers.

lators are used. These operate equally well from an input of 420 kPa (60 psi) from the pipeline, as from a maximum of 140 000 kPa (200 psi) from cylinders. They are of the Adams type (see Fig. 1.23). The

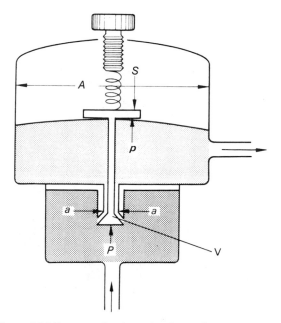

**Figure 1.24** Forces acting in a simple regulator.

British Standard stipulates a pressure of 420 kPa which is 61.3 psi. This has been rounded off in the text to 60 psi. The term 'universal' is also used in a different context (see page 14).

*The accuracy of regulators.* If we consider Fig. 1.24, the push-rod is pushed downward by two forces, the tension in the spring and the elastic recoil of the diaphragm. Let these be added together and represented by $S$. The force that opposes $S$ consists of two parts: the high pressure ($P$) of the gas pushing on the valve V over an area of $a$; and the low pressure ($p$) acting on the diaphragm over an area $A$, so:

$$S = Pa + pA$$

Thus if $S$ remains constant, as $P$ falls, $p$ rises so that as the cylinder empties, the regulated pressure increases. In fact, as $P$ falls, the valve V will have to open further to permit the same flow rate. The spring expands and therefore the tension in it is reduced, and in the same way the tension in the diaphragm is reduced. Therefore as $P$ falls, there is a small reduction in $S$, which partially reverses the effect shown here.

In the case of the Adams valve, however, the formula is different, since the push-rod is replaced by a 'lazy tongs' toggle arrangement, which reverses the direction of the thrust transmitted from the diaphragm.

In Fig. 1.25 it will be seen that the pressure $P$ exerted by the high-pressure gas on the valve V to

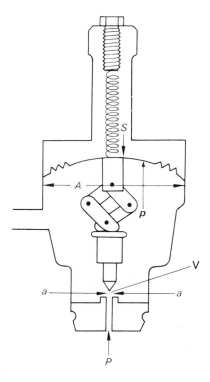

**Figure 1.25** Forces acting in an Adams regulator.

open it is assisted by the spring and the recoil of the diaphragm $S$. These forces jointly oppose the force exerted by the low-pressure gas on the diaphragm, so:

$$Pa + S = pA$$

Now as $P$ falls, so does $p$; therefore the regulated pressure falls slightly as the cylinder pressure drops. At the same time the valve V opens slightly and this, by allowing the spring to *expand*, reduces $S$, which slightly accentuates the fall in $p$. The fall of $p$ can be minimized by making $S$ great compared with $Pa$.

A more accurate regulated pressure may be more easily produced by using a two-stage regulator. The pressure is considerably reduced in the first stage. In the second stage there is little variation in the input pressure and therefore the final regulated pressure is relatively constant.

*Effect of flow rate on the performance of regulators.* The above description of a regulator shows what happens in static conditions or when there is a low flow rate. However, when there is a high flow rate the input to the valve may not be able to keep pace with the output, in which case the regulated pressure will fall. For this reason a sufficiently

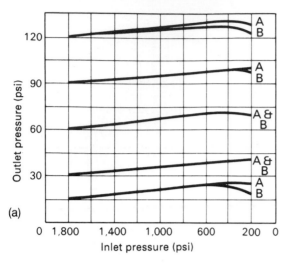

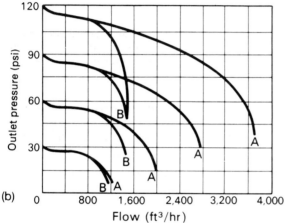

**Figure 1.26** Performance of an oxygen therapy regulator. (a) Note that as the cylinder (inlet) pressure falls, the regulated pressure rises. A, 50 ft³/h flow; B, 500 ft³/h flow. (b) The outlet pressure falls as the flow rate increases. A, 1800 psi inlet (when the cylinder is full); B, 200 psi inlet (when the cylinder is nearly empty).

heavy-duty regulator for the flow rate required must be used. For high gas flows, two-stage regulators are usually employed; these are sometimes referred to as 'endurance' regulators. Examples of the performance of an oxygen therapy regulator are shown in Fig. 1.26.

*Interchangeability of regulators.* Regulators for different gases may have individual design features and should be used only for the gas for which they are intended. One make of regulator is called 'universal' in that the same body is used for all gases, but different seatings and springs are fitted for each particular gas. This should not be confused with the regulators for universal use at input

pressures of 60 or 2000 psi (400 or 137 000 kPa), as described earlier.

*Common faults in regulators*

- Damage to the soft seating of valves may occur as a result of the presence of grit or dust, usually from a dirty cylinder. This may cause a steady build-up of pressure in the apparatus when the cylinder is left turned on but with no gas flowing.
- A hissing noise may indicate a leaking or burst diaphragm. The regulator will need replacing or repairing by the manufacturer or service engineer.
- Adams valves (Fig. 1.23) sometimes develop a fault that causes continual 'jumping' of the flowmeter bobbin — indicating an intermittent change of pressure and flow rate. This is usually due to the 'lazy tongs' sticking as a result of wear, but it may also be caused by small particles of grit or metal in the lazy tongs or the valve seating.

On older patterns of the Adams valve there were fins on the nitrous oxide regulator to conduct heat from the surrounding air to prevent excessive cooling of the valve. It was not uncommon for the nitrous oxide to contain a significant quantity of water vapour as an impurity, and this condensed upon the valve seating and then froze, jamming the valve. The extra heat conducted by the fins was sufficient to prevent this freezing. Another method of preventing freezing was to install a small heater adjacent to the regulator. This was more commonly used in dental anaesthetic apparatus where high gas flows were usual. Water vapour is no longer a problem, but the fins remain as a relic.

*Flow restrictors.* Where anaesthetic machines are supplied from the pipeline at a pressure of 420 kPa (60 psi), it had become a common practice to omit regulators. Sudden pressure surges at the patient end of the anaesthetic machine were prevented by flow restrictors. These consist of constrictions in the regulated pressure pipework upstream of the flowmeters (Fig. 1.27). The disadvantage of using flow resitrictors without regulators is that changes in pipeline pressure are reflected in changes of flow rate, which makes readjustment of the flow control valves necessary. Also, there is a danger that if there is an obstruction at the outlet from the anaesthetic machine, pressure could build up in the vaporizers and cause damage. This is normally prevented by the inclusion of a 'blow-off' safety valve (as shown in Fig. 7.23). Flow restrictors do not normally

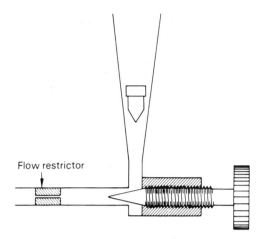

**Figure 1.27** A flow restrictor. The narrow orifice causes a considerable pressure drop when there is a high flow rate, thus protecting the patient from sudden surges at the supply pressure of 420 kPa (60 psi).

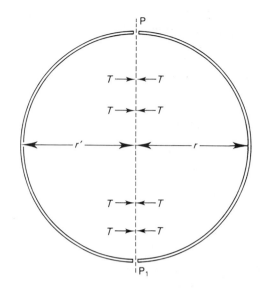

**Figure 1.28** A soap bubble bisected by an imaginary plane PP$_1$; $r$ = internal radius; $r'$ = external radius; $T$ = surface tension holding the two halves together around the cut circumference.

require any maintenance. A different form of flow restrictor may be fitted in the downstream end of the vaporizers to maintain them under some pressure and so reduce the effect of back pressure when controlled ventilation of minute volume divider ventilators are used.

*Relief valves on regulators.* Safety blow-off valves are often fitted on the downstream side of regulators to allow the escape of gas if by accident the regulators fail and allow a high-output pressure. With a regulator designed to give a pressure of 60 psi, the relief valve may be set at 100 psi. These valves may be spring loaded, in which case they close when the pressure falls again, or they may operate by rupture, in which case they remain open until repaired.

### The pressure within a bubble or a balloon

A bubble or droplet is maintained intact by the effect of *surface tension* ($T$) acting on its surface as if it were enclosing it in a capsule. Since the sphere is the shape that has the smallest surface area per unit volume, a bubble or droplet will tend to take this form. In the case of a bubble, the wall may have two surfaces, an inner and an outer one, as for example when it is floating free in air.

If we consider a soap bubble bisected by an imaginary plane PP$_1$ (Fig. 1.28), the force preventing the separation of the two halves is the surface tension ($T$), which acts over the whole of the circumference, i.e. over a length of $2\pi r$ for the inner surface and $2\pi r'$ for the outer. It is usually measured in dynes/cm although this is not an SI unit (N/m$^2$).

In practice $r$ and $r'$ are so nearly equal that they may be taken as identical, so the total force preventing the separation of the two halves of the bubble, $2\pi r T$ plus $2\pi r'T$, may be written as $4\pi r T$.

Pressure may be expressed as force/area, i.e.

$$P = \frac{F}{A}$$

$A$, the area of the cut face of the bubble, is $\pi r^2$, so

$$P = \frac{4\pi r T}{\pi r^2} = \frac{4T}{r}$$

In other words, the pressure in a bubble is inversely proportional to its radius. This was first demonstrated by Laplace and is of particular importance in pulmonary physiology and open chest anaesthesia.

Note that when the anaesthetist inflates the patient's lungs by squeezing the breathing or reservoir bag, if the bag is nearly empty, a greater pressure is exerted on the patient by the same manual effort than when the bag is relatively full.

There is a difference between a gas bubble within a liquid and a balloon constructed of a material such as rubber. In the former, the wall is fluid and the surface tension remains the same however much the bubble is increased in size. In the case of the balloon (i.e. a reservoir bag), as it is distended there is a preliminary stage when the wall assumes a progressively more spherical shape but is not under appreciable tension. Then there comes a time when the material of the wall becomes stretched against its own elastic recoil. Hooke's law of elasticity which states that the length of extension (or compression) of a spring is proportional to the force applied to it (within the elastic limit of the material) now begins to apply, and the pressure within the balloon becomes related to the elastic recoil of its walls and therefore to its diameter. This occurs when ventilators such as the East–Freeman Automatic Vent are used, but on the Mapleson A system the expiratory valve usually opens first. Eventually either the elastic limit of the rubber is reached or there is rupture. In this respect the nature of the material from which the bag is constructed is important, since some types of rubber are easily stretched, and in the case of accidental closure of the expiratory valve the reservoir bag becomes distended to an alarming degree, yet the pressure within it does not rise sufficiently (in the short term) to injure the patient. On the other hand, there have been disposable reservoir bags, constructed of other materials, that were by no means so distensible, and dangerously high pressures could develop very quickly within them. Some reservoir bags — such as that in the Flomasta ventilator — are surrounded by a net or similar device to limit distension, since in these cases it is the intention to develop sufficient pressure to inflate the patient's lungs.

# The Flow of Fluids Through Tubes and Orifices

By definition a tube has a length considerably greater than its diameter, whereas an orifice has a diameter greater than its length.

Three factors affecting the rate of flow of a fluid through a tube or orifice are its density, its viscosity and the pressure difference across the tube or orifice. The resistance to flow also depends on the diameter and length of the tube, or the diameter of the orifice.

Both the viscosity and density of a fluid are affected by changes in temperature. In the case of an orifice it is the density that has the most effect, and in the case of a tube, the viscosity.

### The flow of fluids through a tube

The relationships between the factors relating to a fluid (which may be a liquid or gas) flowing with laminar flow (see below) through a tube are:

Flow rate $\propto \dfrac{1}{L}$   where $L$ = length of tube

Flow rate $\propto P$   where $P$ = the pressure difference between the two ends of the tube

Flow rate $\propto \dfrac{1}{V}$   where $V$ = the viscosity of the fluid

Flow rate $\propto r^4$   where $r$ = the radius of the tube (Poiseuille's Law).

Thus

$$\text{Flow rate} \propto \frac{P \times r^4}{L \times V}$$

*Laminar and turbulent flow.* The above formulae refer to fluids when the entire stream flows in a straight line. This is known as *laminar flow*. However, under certain circumstances, although the general flow is in a straight line, eddy currents occur. This is known as *turbulence*. These eddy currents cause resistance to flow. For any system there is a *critical velocity*, above which the flow becomes turbulent and below which it remains laminar.

Turbulence may also be caused by the flow being deflected by rough areas, passing through a tube of irregular diameter, or passing around sharp bends (Fig. 1.29). As examples, the design of the inlet to a flowmeter tube is important, since turbulence would render the reading inaccurate, and in breathing systems, especially those of the circle type, it increases the resistance and therefore increases the work done in spontaneous breathing. Where there is turbulence a greater pressure is required to maintain the same rate of flow.

The wider the tube, the lower the flow velocity for the same flow rate (volume per unit time) and therefore the less the likelihood of turbulence.

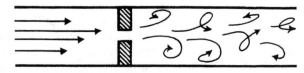

**Figure 1.29** Laminar flow becoming turbulent as its smooth pathway is obstructed by an obstacle.

## The flow of fluids through an orifice

When a fluid passes through an orifice there is usually turbulence. The flow rate is determined by the pressure difference across the orifice, the density of the fluid and the area of the orifice. Thus:

Flow rate $\propto \sqrt{P}$  where $P$ = the pressure difference across the orifice,

Flow rate $\propto \dfrac{1}{\sqrt{D}}$  where $D$ = the density of fluid

Flow rate $\propto r^2$  where $r$ = the radius of the orifice.

Thus

$$\text{Flow rate} \propto \frac{\sqrt{P}(r^2)}{\sqrt{D}}$$

## The effect of changing the bore of a tube

Where the bore of a tube is diminished, the flow velocity is increased, since the flow rate (volume per unit time) must remain the same. The change in diameter acts to some extent as an orifice, and because of this, and the fact that turbulence may occur, the density of the fluid becomes significant. The kinetic energy required to accelerate the fluid through the narrower part of the tube can be calculated and may be expressed as resistance or the pressure difference required to overcome it.

It will be seen, therefore, that for any system through which fluids flow there are three elements of resistance to overcome: (a) those due to the dimensions of the tube, (b) those of an orifice, and (c) those associated with initiating the flow and changing its velocity. A combination of all three is always present, but one or another tends to dominate under different circumstances.

The fact remains that the passages in anaesthetic equipment should be as wide, short, smooth, straight and uniform as possible.

## The Bernoulli effect and the venturi

Let us consider a tube that has a constriction along part of its course. When a gas passes through the tube it will accelerate when it encounters the constriction.

If pressure gauges are attached at various parts of the tube it is found that as the gas accelerates, the pressure falls (Fig. 1.30a). This is known as the Bernoulli effect. When the gas emerges from the constriction into the wider tube the linear velocity of flow decreases and the pressure increases again.

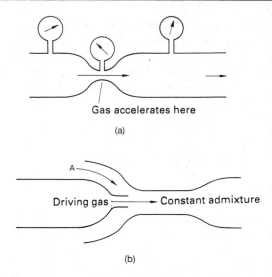

**Figure 1.30** (a) The Bernoulli effect. (b) The venturi.

The pressure may rise to a level almost as high as that before the constriction, the extent of this rise being dependent on the design of the tube and the constriction.

Advantage of this phenomenon was taken by Venturi, who found that if the shape of this constriction was suitably designed, and there was a side branch to the tube in a suitable position, fluid from the branch would be entrained by the main stream (Fig. 1.30b). In order to achieve this, not only must the constriction be of suitable shape, but also the distal limb of the tube needs to be of gradually increasing diameter.

The rate of flow of fluid per unit time is a function of the cross-sectional area of the tube and the flow velocity. Energy is expended in accelerating the flow of fluid to increase its velocity as it passes into the constriction. When it leaves the constriction it will tend to continue to flow at the same velocity, but since the cross-sectional area of the tube is gradually increasing, either it will be slowed down or further fluid may be entrained through the side branch mentioned above or the fluid close to the walls of the tube of expanding diameter will stagnate.

It is one of the features of a venturi that provided the velocity of the driving gas is adequate, and there is no change in the configuration of the orifice from which it emerges, or of the side branch, the volume of gas entrained will bear a constant proportion to the driving gas. It may, therefore, be used for the mixing of nitrous oxide and oxygen in an anaesthetic machine or in mixing valves such as some oxygen/air blenders.

Apart from their use in mixing of gases, venturis may also be used to provide a medical vacuum.

Very often the extra cost of using oxygen to drive the venturi is considerably less than the capital expense of installing a separate vacuum line.

Venturis have also been used for assisting the circulation of gases in a breathing system.

## The Joule–Kelvin Principle (Joule–Thompson Effect)

Work has to be done to compress a gas and the energy expended is converted into heat. In some circumstances, such as the compression–ignition (diesel) engine, the compression is sufficiently rapid to cause a considerable rise in temperature, resulting in ignition of the fuel vapour. In the same way, if a part of an anaesthetic apparatus contained oil, grease or some other flammable material and was subjected to a sudden rise of pressure in the presence of oxygen, as when a cylinder is turned on suddenly, an explosion could occur. For this reason all apparatus using high-pressure oxygen must be free of oil, grease or other flammable material. Pressure gauges are fitted with a constriction in the inlet to reduce the shock wave that occurs when a cylinder is turned on.

Conversely, when a gas expands, it does work and the temperature drops. Under normal circumstances in anaesthetic practice, the expansion of

a gas leaving the cylinder is not sufficiently rapid to cause a great fall in temperature. The fall in temperature is, for example, much less than that due to the latent heat of vaporization, which is the main cause of cooling of cylinders of nitrous oxide when in use.

## The Electromagnetic Spectrum

Radio waves, heat, light and X-rays are all part of a family of electromagnetic waves called the electromagnetic spectrum (Fig. 1.31). All members of the spectrum travel with the same velocity of $3 \times 10^8$ m/s in a vacuum. Although the various members of the spectrum have different properties and different methods of generation, absorption and detection, they all have in common the phenomena of *reflection*, *refraction*, *interference*, *diffraction* and *absorption*. The electromagnetic spectrum may be described by wavelength ($\lambda$), wavenumber ($1/\lambda$), frequency ($v$) or photon energy ($hv$). A basic grasp of the electromagnetic spectrum helps the anaesthetist to understand the principles behind the various forms of gas analysis, pulse-oximetry and other monitoring techniques as well as those of surgical diathermy, radiology and nuclear medicine with which he or she is likely to come in contact during the course of the working day.

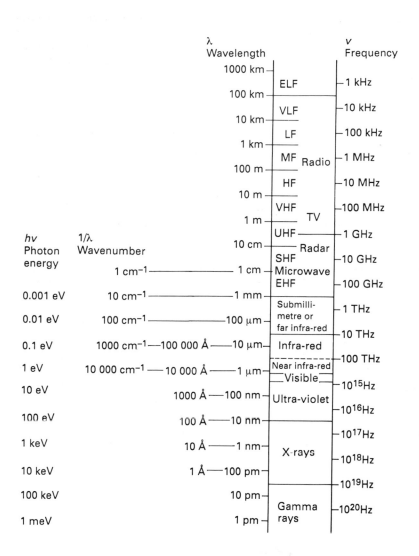

**Figure 1.31** The electromagnetic spectrum.

# 2 Pneumatics, Fluidics and Electronics

## Pneumatics and Fluidics

Pneumatics and fluidics are concerned with the behaviour of fluids as they flow through chosen pathways and orifices. As applied to anaesthesia, they are concerned with air and/or other gases in the manner by which they may be used to control or actuate equipment such as anaesthetic machines or lung ventilators. In other applications fluidic devices may be used to handle liquids rather than gases, but they function in the same manner.

Pneumatic and fluidic equipment may perform functions somewhat analogous to those of electrical and electronic devices, but as will be seen below the analogy often breaks down when details are considered.

### Pneumatics

The principal components in pneumatic equipment are spool valves, which perform switching functions and activators such as cylinders with pistons. Both of these contain moving parts in which wear and damage may occur, requiring service maintenance and replacement. The pressure of the driving gas is between 200 kPa (30 psi) and 1000 kPa (150 psi). In all the earlier equipment the compressed air that operated it contained a specially added oil mist to lubricate the components — but more modern developments have obviated the need for this lubrication in many instances and 'dry' devices, more appropriate to medical applications, have been developed. High-pressure equipment using oxygen rather than air should not be lubricated with flammable materials. If lubrication is required, a non-flammable grease such as Fomblin should be used. This substance is similar to a hydrocarbon, except that the hydrogen atoms have been replaced by those of fluorine.

In the industrial field, where large-diameter cylinder activators are employed, heavy-duty tasks may be performed. For instance, if a cylinder of 200 mm bore is operated at a pressure of 1000 kPa (150 psi), there is a thrust of over 30 kN. In anaesthetic equipment, much smaller cylinders are employed and the activating pressure is between 200 kPa (30 psi) and 400 kPa (60 psi).

The spool valve operates by means of a shuttle, usually in the shape of a cylinder of varying diameter, which moves from one end to the other in a passageway divided by seals into a number of chambers, the sides of which are pierced by inlet and outlet ports. By means of the recesses and seals, the gases passing through the valve are directed in

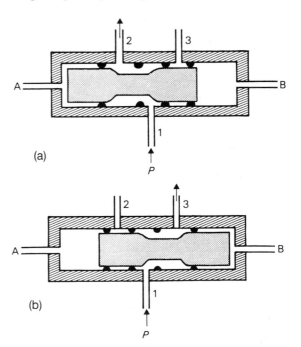

**Figure 2.1** A three-port spool valve. (a) When the spool is to the left-hand side the driving gas passes from port 1 to port 2. A pneumatic or mechanical force applied at A will cause the spool to travel to the right, as seen in (b), so that the driving gas now emerges from port 3. P, Driving gas supply.

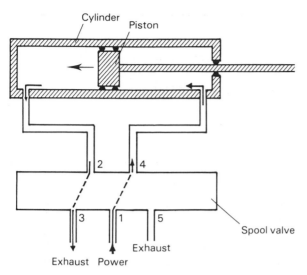

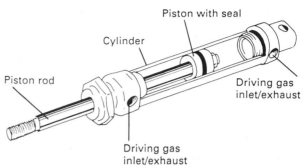

**Figure 2.3** A pneumatic cylinder. Note that there are ports at either end which, according to the direction of movement of the piston, act as the inlet or exhaust for the driving gas.

The driving gas passes from the spool valve to an activator, which is usually a double-acting cylinder (Fig. 2.3). The fact that the cylinder can be driven from either end permits it to be used in a reciprocating manner, with the strokes in each direction doing work.

Advances in technology have led to the development of pneumatic logic components. There are now logics with many functions, and these, with their fluidic and electrical equivalents are described later.

Fig. 2.4 shows the type of pneumatic logic circuit that might be used to control a lung ventilator.

The actual work of driving the bellows in the breathing system may be done by a reciprocating cylinder. The driving gas is applied alternately to its two ends via a spool valve, the action of which is controlled by two other valves, which are in turn activated, via levers, by the movement of the piston rod of the cylinder. The timers determine the interval between the end of one stroke and the start of the return stroke, i.e. the length of inspiratory and expiratory pauses, while the restrictors regulate the speed at which the piston travels, i.e. the inspiratory and expiratory flow rates. Note that the restrictors control the gas flow in the exhaust direction only, since they are connected in parallel with low-resistance diodes, which present little resistance to the flow of gas in the reverse direction.

## Fluidics

Pneumatic equipment has been used for many years, but the scope of fluid engineering was greatly enhanced by the exploitation, during the development of space rockets, of the discovery published in 1932 by Henri Coanda of the phenomenon of *wall attachment* (also see page 250). Coanda described the behaviour of a jet of fluid emerging from a nozzle.

**Figure 2.2** The pneumatic power is applied to port 1 of the spool valve. With the spool valve in one position the power passes through port 4 to the right-hand side of the cylinder, thus causing the piston to move to the left. At the same time the gas from the left-hand end of the cylinder escapes to the atmosphere via ports 2 and 3 of the spool valve. When the spool valve moves so as to alter the direction, the power passes to the left-hand side of the cylinder via ports 1 and 2 and the gases from the right-hand end of the cylinder are exhausted through ports 4 and 5.

one direction or the other. By virtue of there being multiple sections with inlets and outlets, these valves may control several operations simultaneously. Figure 2.1 shows a three-port spool valve, which is analogous to a two-way electric switch. In the 'on' position, gases pass from port 1 to port 2, while in the 'off' position they pass from port 1 to port 3. Here lies the essence of the difference between electrical and pneumatic functions. In the former, when the signal ceases, the effect becomes zero; whereas in the latter, when the signal ceases, it may still be stored in the position of the activator (as a 'trapped signal') until it is exhausted to atmosphere.

Spool valves with three, five or more ports are commonly employed, as will be seen in Fig. 2.2. The importance of the five-port valve will be seen when the activator cylinders are considered.

Spool valves may be operated by:

- a pilot air pressure (between 30 and 60 psi);
- a low-pressure air signal acting on a diaphragm;
- a toggle or push rod;
- an electric solenoid.

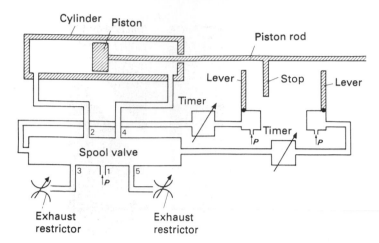

**Figure 2.4** A pneumatic logic ventilator cycling system. The output of the spool valve drives the piston in the cylinder. The piston rod may have a stop which operates triggers on the actuators for inspiration and expiration. The output of these actuators may pass through timers that can delay the onset of inspiration or expiration. The exhaust from each end of the cylinder may be controlled by flow restrictors which may be used to slow down the movement of the piston during either the inspiratory or expiratory phase. The piston rod might be used to operate a bellows that is part of the breathing system. *P*, driving gas supply.

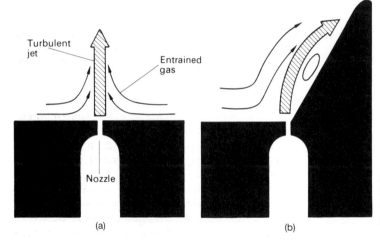

**Figure 2.5** (a) A turbulent jet entrains gas from around it. (b) If the supply of gas to be entrained is limited, a 'bubble' of reduced pressure is produced.

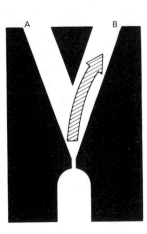

**Figure 2.6** If there is a choice of two walls, the entire jet will attach itself to one of them.

For present purposes a jet of gas is considered, but the same phenomenon occurs with liquids. Being turbulent, the jet entrains with it molecules of the surrounding gas (Fig. 2.5a). The presence of a wall on one side of the jet, thus limiting the availability of molecules of gas to be entrained, causes a 'bubble of reduced pressure' to develop. This results in the jet being diverted towards the wall and, under favourable conditions, becoming attached to it (Fig. 2.5b).

If there is a choice of walls to which it might become attached, the entire jet goes either one way or the other; it does not split (Fig. 2.6). These devices may, therefore, be described as digital logics, having two possible outlets only, 'on' and 'off'. (Splitting logics, operating on an analogue rather than digital basis, also exist and are described below.) Referring again to Fig. 2.6, when the jet is flowing through the right-hand limb B it may, by

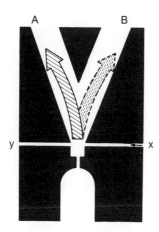

**Figure 2.7** A small control port has been drilled at each side. A signal at x will cause the jet to be deflected to the left-hand limb A.

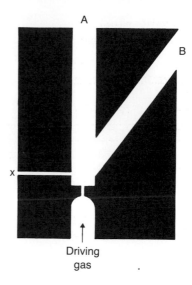

Driving gas

**Figure 2.9** A monostable in which the main jet will emerge at A, except when a control signal is applied at x, when it will transfer to B. When the signal at x ceases, the jet will return to A.

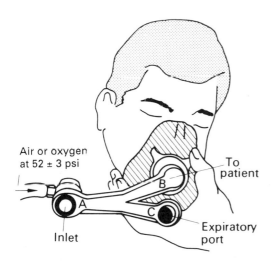

**Figure 2.8** A fluidic ventilator, consisting of one large fluidic element. The gas enters at A and, this being a monostable element, passes via B to the patient. However, when the airway pressure rises sufficiently, the jet from A changes over to C, allowing expiration to occur. When the pressure in B falls sufficiently, the jet returns to that side. Note that the input pressure must be within narrow limits.

the Venturi effect, entrain gas from the left-hand limb, A. Obstruction of the jet as it passes to one outlet may, by back pressure, cause it to transfer to the other. More important, however, is the fact that a small puff of gas injected at the site of the bubble will deflect the main jet to the opposite wall (Fig. 2.7).

The signal required to deflect the jet is very much smaller than the main jet itself, so this device may be regarded as not only a switch but also an amplifier. Switching frequency of up to 100 kHz

may be obtained. The dimensions of such a fluidic device may vary enormously from control units with very fine passages, measuring 2.5 cm in their largest dimension, to large pipes conducting liquids such as corrosive chemicals.

Anaesthetists were interested originally in designing single fluidic elements through which the actual patient gases pass. An example of this is shown in Fig. 2.8. This simple device, constructed of clear plastic, is driven by oxygen or other gas at a pressure of $52 \pm 3$ psi ($3.6 \pm 0.2$ bar). It is monostable, the preferred direction for the jet being towards the port attached to the facemask. When the lungs are inflated, the back pressure increases to a point where it causes the jet to switch to the other limb. Both the driving gas and the expired air escape via the expiratory port. At the end of expiration the jet switches back to the original direction and the cycle starts again. This type of system is not very satisfactory in anaesthetic practice owing to its lack of fine control and its dependence on driving gas at a precise pressure. It is more appropriate to employ fluidic logic systems to control ventilators, usually using gas that is not destined to be breathed by the patient.

By changing the design of the passages through which the jet passes, 'gates' or switching devices with various functions have been elaborated. For instance, in Fig. 2.9 the jet will normally pass to output A, but when a signal is applied at x it will be deflected to B and remain there only as long as the

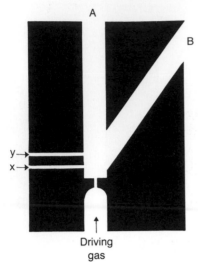

Figure 2.10 A monostable in which the main jet will switch from A to B only as long as a signal is applied at x or y or both. An OR gate.

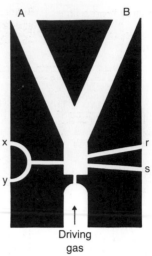

Figure 2.11 AND/OR flip-flop gate. Signals at x *and* y will cause the jet to pass to output B, whereas signals at r *or* s will cause it to return to A.

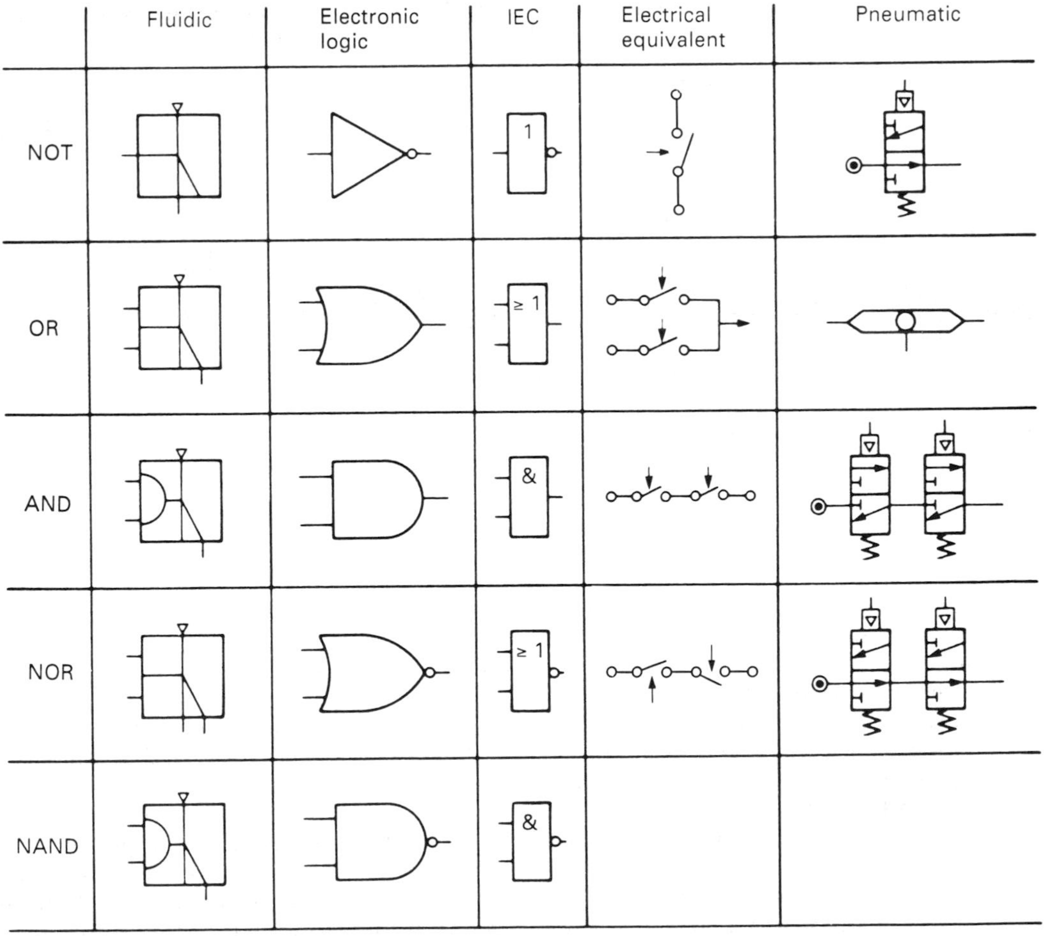

| | Fluidic | Electronic logic | IEC | Electrical equivalent | Pneumatic |
|---|---|---|---|---|---|
| NOT | | | | | |
| OR | | | | | |
| AND | | | | | |
| NOR | | | | | |
| NAND | | | | | |

Figure 2.12 Examples of logic symbols. IEC = International Electrotechnical Commission.

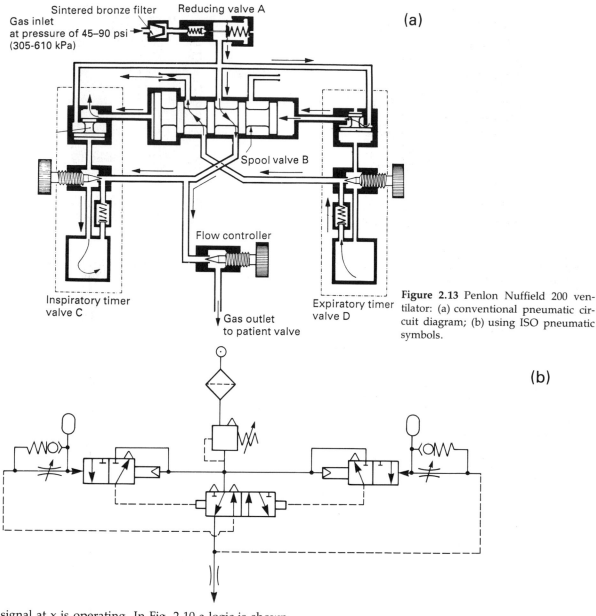

Gas inlet
at pressure of 45–90 psi
(305-610 kPa)

Sintered bronze filter    Reducing valve A

(a)

Spool valve B

Inspiratory timer
valve C

Flow controller

Gas outlet
to patient valve

Expiratory timer
valve D

**Figure 2.13** Penlon Nuffield 200 ventilator: (a) conventional pneumatic circuit diagram; (b) using ISO pneumatic symbols.

(b)

signal at x is operating. In Fig. 2.10 a logic is shown with two signal inputs, either of which will cause the jet to switch to output B.

In Fig. 2.11 the main gate is a flip-flop, but the signal ports on the two sides are different. A signal at x *or* y on its own will have no effect since it exhausts via y or x. The operation of x *and* y together will switch the output to B. On the other hand a signal at r *or* s, or at both, will result in an output at A.

The input signal may be derived from various devices, including a push button with a small balloon, a plunger, a proximity sensor or the output from another element.

## Logic

The term *logic* has been used fairly loosely so far. Logic elements in pneumatic, fluidic, and electronic form may be assembled to perform *logical functions*. Some of the conventional symbols of the various logics are shown in Fig. 2.12. The gas circuit in Fig. 2.13 is that of the Pneupac ventilator oscillator, which is the basis of the Penlon Nuffield 200 ventilator, shown in both conventional and pneumatic symbols.

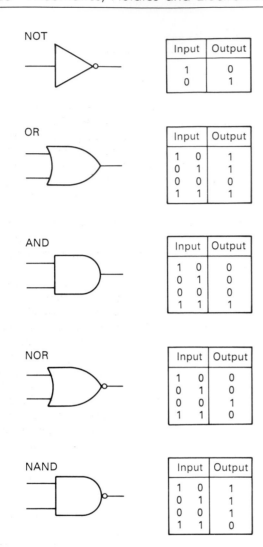

**Figure 2.14** Logic truth tables.

## Digital logic

*Combinational digital logic* circuits or elements are those in which the output state depends only on the present input states in some predetermined fashion and are designed to perform logical functions using only *two states*, based on the concepts of 'and', 'either–or', 'neither–nor' and 'inversion'. The so-called *gates* performing these logical functions are most commonly constructed as electronic integrated circuits but many of the simpler functions may also be performed by pneumatic equivalents. The AND gate is a circuit with two or more inputs and one output at which the output signal becomes high if and only if (sometimes written by engineers as 'iff') all the inputs are simultaneously high. The OR gate has two or more inputs and one output, which goes into the high state if any one or more of the inputs becomes high. An *inverter*, often referred to as a NOT-gate is a circuit with a single input and a single output the state of which is always the opposite to the input. NAND and NOR gates are equivalent to AND and OR gates respectively but with the addition of an inverter at the output. *Truth tables* for these circuit elements are shown in Fig. 2.14. Examples of the use of digital logic using combinational logic with these elements are safety interlocks, and change-over valves in ventilators, and similar situations where there are only two states. However, these simple logic elements also form the building blocks of simple and highly complex multistate digital computing sytems.

*Sequential logic* is a second class of digital electronics which is used where it is necessary to take into account not only the current inputs alone but also knowledge of past inputs as well. The building block of sequential logic is the *multivibrator* or *flip-flop*, a logic element with two outputs, one of which is always in the opposite state, high or low, of its partner. There are three basic types of multivibrator: astable, monostable and bistable. The *astable*, as its name implies, has no stable state and the outputs continuously oscillate in state at a predetermined frequency. A typical application of the astable could be the timer operating the valves in a simple ventilator, where one output controls the inspiratory valve and the other controls the expiratory valve. The *monostable multivibrator* usually has a single input. Its output has a single stable resting state which reverses for a pre-set period of time when the input is switched from one state to another but always returns to the original stable state. Thus, whatever the length of the input pulse, the output pulse is always of the same period. The *bistable* has two opposing outputs — two stable states — and may have one or two inputs. The outputs toggle between the two states, which are both stable. The bistable multivibrator is commonly used in fairly simple logic circuits but also forms the basic element of the electronic memory. Microprocessor integrated circuits are composed of many thousands of logic gates and sequential logic elements.

## Proportional (analogue) logic

Not all fluidic devices are digital, i.e. 'on/off'. The splitter (mentioned above) operates proportionally. Figure 2.15 at first resembles a flip-flop, but on closer inspection it will be seen that the power jet passes through a chamber so shaped as to prevent wall attachment. In the absence of any control signal

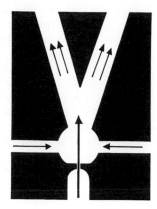

**Figure 2.15** The proportional splitter.

the jet is divided into two equal parts by the splitter. A control jet from one side deflects the power jet towards the opposite side to an extent proportional to its power. The flow from each output is therefore proportional to the power of the control signal applied to the opposite side.

## Turbulence amplifiers

Turbulence amplifiers are not currently in favour and are mentioned only for the sake of completeness. They operate on the principle of a low-pressure *laminar* jet (15–25 cmH$_2$O) passing across a chamber with side ports (Fig. 2.16a). In the absence of a side signal the jet passes into a chosen orifice and an output signal is registered. A side signal (Fig. 2.16b) interferes with the signal and interrupts the output. The advantage that these devices operate on so low a pressure is offset by the fact that on this account they are liable to interference by stray air currents and are therefore unreliable.

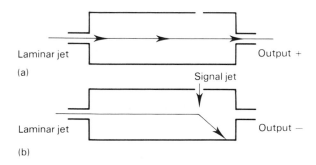

(a)

(b)

**Figure 2.16** The turbulence amplifier. (a) With no signal. (b) With a signal.

# Electronics

## Analogue versus digital

Modern electronic techniques have invaded almost every area of technology in medicine. The reason for this is that logic and computing power of great complexity is now feasible, economically and with high reliability. Electronic techniques may be subdivided into two broad groupings, namely *analogue* and *digital*, both of which are employed in most equipment.

*Analogue* circuits are those that handle *continuously variable* quantities (i.e. without discrete steps) such as pressure, flow, temperature, voltage or current. *Digital* circuits may handle the same variables but do so in discrete steps, of which there may be only two states (yes/no, high/low, go/no-go), or in many steps that may be very small — so small that the impression is given of a smooth transition. Most variables are expressed in *decimal* form, that is with a *base* of 10, i.e. using the digits 1, 2, 3, 4, 5, 6, 7, 8, 9, 10. This would require digital electronics to have ten stable states in each of its circuit elements, which would be extremely difficult to implement. As digital electronics is based upon *two* stable states, it requires the conversion of the variable into a *binary* or base-2 number code, see Fig. 2.17.

| | Binary | | | | | | | |
|---|---|---|---|---|---|---|---|---|
| | MSB | | | | | | | LSB |
| Decimal | $2^7$ | $2^6$ | $2^5$ | $2^4$ | $2^3$ | $2^2$ | $2^1$ | $2^0$ |
| 0 | 0 | 0 | 0 | 0 | 0 | 0 | 0 | 0 |
| 1 | 0 | 0 | 0 | 0 | 0 | 0 | 0 | 1 |
| 2 | 0 | 0 | 0 | 0 | 0 | 0 | 1 | 0 |
| 3 | 0 | 0 | 0 | 0 | 0 | 0 | 1 | 1 |
| 4 | 0 | 0 | 0 | 0 | 0 | 1 | 0 | 0 |
| 5 | 0 | 0 | 0 | 0 | 0 | 1 | 0 | 1 |
| 6 | 0 | 0 | 0 | 0 | 0 | 1 | 1 | 0 |
| 7 | 0 | 0 | 0 | 0 | 0 | 1 | 1 | 1 |
| 8 | 0 | 0 | 0 | 0 | 1 | 0 | 0 | 0 |
| 9 | 0 | 0 | 0 | 0 | 1 | 0 | 0 | 1 |
| 10 | 0 | 0 | 0 | 0 | 1 | 0 | 1 | 0 |
| 200 | 1 | 1 | 0 | 0 | 1 | 0 | 0 | 0 |
| 255 | 1 | 1 | 1 | 1 | 1 | 1 | 1 | 1 |

MSB = Most Significant Bit
LSB = Least Significant Bit

**Figure 2.17** Binary representation of decimal numbering.

An analogue signal is converted into a digital format using a circuit-block called an *analogue-to-digital converter* (ADC). An ADC integrated circuit has a single input connection for the analogue signal and multiple pins for the digital output. ADC integrated circuits may have 8, 12, 16 or even more output pins, each representing an output *bit*; the higher number of bits allows higher precision of conversion, i.e. each step represents a smaller change in the analogue signal: 256 steps with 8 bits. 4096 with 12 bits and 32 768 with 16 output bits.

A *digital-to-analogue converter* (DAC) has the reverse function of converting a signal in a digital format into an analogue form.

Almost all modern electronic instrumentation and control systems use a combination of analogue and digital circuitry. An input pressure flow or temperature (*a measurand*) is converted to a voltage or current whose magnitude is an analogue function of the measurand by a *transducer*. However, in all but the most simple cases, computation or manipulation of this signal is more conveniently carried out by digital techniques, usually by use of a *microprocessor*. The analogue signal from the transducer is converted to a digital format by an ADC. The output of the microprocessor, which is also in a digital format, may directly control solenoids, solenoid valves, motors, etc., or may be re-converted back to an analogue format by a DAC. The reasons for this seemingly complex conversion from analogue to digital and back again are as follows.

- Complex mathematical and logical functions between input and output are easier to implement with digital circuitry.
- The calibration and 'zero' of digital circuits do not drift as analogue circuits tend to.
- The calibration of digital circuitry is easier and more accurate.
- Major or minor changes in any mathematical functions can be enacted simply by software changes.
- Digital circuitry is cheaper and easier to design and manufacture.
- Digital circuitry tends to be more reliable than its analogue counterpart.

## Microprocessor systems

*Embedded microprocessors* are microprocessors which, although the integrated circuits comprising them are identical to those of a small computing system, are an integral part of the equipment into which they have been built, and the user will not necessarily appreciate their presence in the equipment. Such microprocessors are all composed of

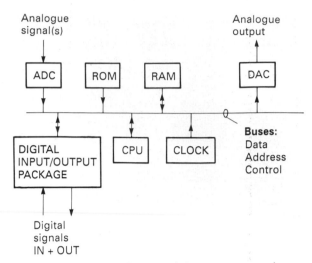

**Figure 2.18** Schematic diagram of the components of any microprocessor based system.

similar components (Fig. 2.18).

The central component of any microprocessor system is the *central processing unit* (CPU), which is a single integrated circuit (IC) with 40 or even 64 connection pins. The CPU is the heart of the system where all the mathematical and logic functions are carried out. However, the CPU is useless without its support ICs. *Input* and *output* (I/O) *packages* control the already digitized signals for the CPU. Input packages allow a number of different signals to be applied in turn to the CPU. Output packages similarly allow the output of the CPU to be applied between, say, solenoid valves, motors and display systems. This switching may be so rapid that the user is unaware that the CPU is carrying out many functions sequentially. The CPU cannot carry out any functions at all without a *program* or *software* which is held in *non-volatile memory*. Non-volatile memory is permanent memory unaffected by the equipment being switched off, in which the program is stored in binary digital form, usually in a *read only memory* (ROM), so called because it cannot be altered by the functioning of the microprocessor system. Embedded microprocessors also need *volatile memory* which can be altered by the CPU. It is said to be volatile because this form of memory, *random access memory* (RAM), is cleared by the disconnection of the power supply. It is used as a 'scratch-pad' by the CPU for making its calculations, 'remembering' trends, and assembling information for any display device. As microprocessor systems use the binary numbering system, it is necessary to use multiple connections between each of the ICs, usually 8, 16 or 32. These interconnections are

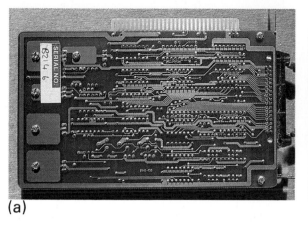
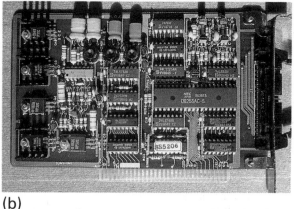

(a)

(b)

**Figure 2.19** Printed circuit board. (a) Track side. (b) Component side. Note that tracks are also on the component side of the board.

usually referred to as *buses* — a contraction from the term bus-bar used in the electrical industry. There are three buses in a microprocessor based system: a *data bus* which carries the actual data being manipulated; an *address bus* which carries the *addresses* of the 'pigeon holes' containing data stored in the memories; and a *control bus* which, as the name implies, carries all the control and timing signals. Synchronism is maintained by a crystal controlled *clock* or oscillator, which is usually at a fixed frequency of usually greater than 5 MHz. Because of the complexity of the interconnections involved in modern electronics, these interconnections are always made by use of *printed circuitry* (Fig. 2.19). Once the printed circuit has been designed it has the advantage of ease of economic manufacture without wiring errors and with high reliability.

# Appendix: Graphical Symbols for Pneumatic Components

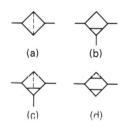

(a)      (b)

(c)      (d)

**Directional control valves**

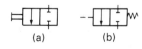

(a)      (b)

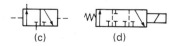

(c)      (d)

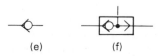

(e)      (f)

(a) Filter or strainer.
(b) Manually controlled water trap.

(c) Manually controlled filter with water trap.
(d) Air dryer.

(a) Manually controlled 2/2 directional control valve.
(b) Pilot pressure operated, spring return, normally closed, 2/2 directional control valve.

(c) Double pressure operated 3/2 directional control valve.
(d) Solenoid operated, spring return 3/2 valve, with intermediate condition.

(e) Non-return valve.
(f) Shuttle valve.

**Control methods**

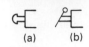

(a)      (b)

(a) Push button.
(b) Lever.

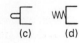

(c)      (d)

(c) Plunger.
(d) Spring.

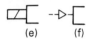

(e)      (f)

(e) Solenoid.
(f) Air pressure.

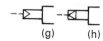

(g)      (h)

(g) Pilot air pressure.
(h) Release of pilot pressure.

**Pressure control**

(a)

(a) Pneumatic relief valve (safety valve).

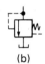

(b)

(b) Relief valve with remote pilot control.

(c)

(c) Sequence valve.

(d)

(d) Pressure regulator or reducing valve.

**Flow control**

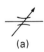     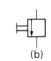

(a)      (b)

(a) Simplified symbol for throttle valve.
(b) Manually controlled throttle valve.

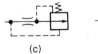

(c)      (d)

(c) Flow control valve with fixed output.
(d) Simplified symbol for (d).

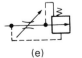     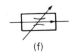

(e)      (f)

(e) Flow control valve with variable output.
(f) Simplified symbol for (f).

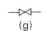

(g)

(g) Shut-off valve.

**Cylinders**

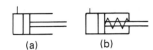

(a)  (b)

(a) Single acting cylinder.
(b) Single acting cylinder with spring return.

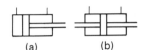

(a)  (b)

(a) Double acting cylinder with single piston rod.
(b) Double acting cylinder with double ended piston rod.

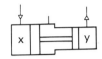

Pressure intensifier.

**Energy converter**

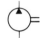

Fixed capacity compressor.

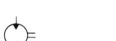

(a)  (b)

(a) Fixed capacity pneumatic motor.
(b) Fixed capacity pneumatic motor with two directions of flow.

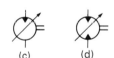

(c)  (d)

(c) Variable capacity pneumatic motor.
(d) Variable capacity pneumatic motor with two directions of flow.

# 3 The Supply of Anaesthetic Gases

## Introduction

The gases used in anaesthesia* may be supplied in cylinders small enough to be man-handled or in bulk in liquid form which is vaporized and transmitted to the anaesthetic machine via pipelines.

## Cylinders

Modern cylinders are manufactured from molybdenum steel and, because of the greater strength of this alloy, they have thinner walls than their larger carbon steel predecessors and are therefore lighter. Aluminium alloy cylinders are not, as yet, widely used in the medical field in the UK.

Oxygen, nitrogen, air, and helium are stored in cylinders as compressed gas (see the inside front cover). Nitrous oxide, carbon dioxide and cyclopropane, being strictly speaking vapours and not gases, liquefy at the pressures to which the cylinders are filled. Indeed, the greater part of the contents of cylinders of these 'gases' is in the liquid form when full. The cylinder is not completely filled with liquid since, if it were, a comparatively small rise in temperature would lead to a very large rise in pressure, which would result in rupture. It is filled to a *filling ratio* which is the weight of the substance with which it is actually filled divided by the weight of water that it could hold. In the UK, which has a temperate climate, nitrous oxide and carbon dioxide cylinders are filled to a ratio of 0.75; in tropical climates this is reduced to 0.67. For cyclopropane the figures are 0.51 and 0.48 respectively. Since they contain liquid, it is important that cylinders of nitrous oxide, carbon dioxide and cyclopropane are mounted in the vertical position,

with the outlets uppermost, when in use. The temperature of the cylinder and its contents drops during vaporization, and where high flow rates of nitrous oxide are taken from a small cylinder, the fall of temperature, and consequently pressure, may be marked. Water vapour from the surrounding air condenses on the exterior of the cylinder as it cools and if the temperature falls still further this may freeze. In a 'dental gas session' the pressure in a 3600-litre cylinder may fall from 750 to 500 psi (~ 50 000 to 35 000 kPa) before the liquid nitrous oxide is exhausted.

In the case of oxygen and other gases that do not normally liquefy, the contents of the cylinder may be estimated with a pressure gauge, since the amount of gas is proportional to the pressure. Fluctuations of pressure due to changes of ambient temperature are not usually of a significant order in clinical practice. However, in the case of nitrous oxide, carbon dioxide and cyclopropane, it is not until all the liquid content has evaporated that the pressure within the cylinder falls appreciably, provided that there has not been significant cooling. Therefore, in this case the contents gauge falls rapidly only when the contents are nearly exhausted. Some contents gauges for these gases are therefore calibrated with a wide segment marked 'Full at varying temperatures'. The pressure of gases in full cylinders is shown in Table 3.1.

The contents of nitrous oxide, carbon dioxide and cyclopropane cylinders are more accurately determined, if required, by weighing the cylinders. As shown in Fig. 3.1a, the weight of the empty cylinder (Tare) is stamped on the side of the valve block. The weight of the gas in terms of its density in ounces per gallon or grams per litre is shown on the label on the neck of the cylinder, and by weighing the cylinder and subtracting its empty weight, the weight of the contents of the cylinder can be estimated at any time. The densities of various gases are shown in Table 3.1.

The cylinder for each gas is painted in a distinctive colour, as shown in the inside front

---

* Including nitrous oxide, carbon dioxide and cyclopropane which are, strictly speaking, *vapours*.

**Figure 3.1** The four faces of a pin index cylinder valve block. Note on (a) the weight of the empty cylinder, 'tare' in pounds and ounces (or kg); on (b) the symbol for nitrous oxide; on (c) the pressure of the hydraulic test; on (d) the outlet and pin index holes.

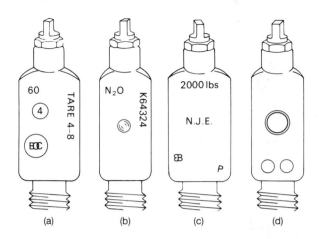

(a)          (b)          (c)          (d)

**Table 3.1** Physical properties of compressed vapours and gases

|  | Oxygen | Nitrous oxide | Entonox | Carbon dioxide | Cyclopropane |
|---|---|---|---|---|---|
| Symbol | $O_2$ | $N_2O$ | $O_2 + N_2O$ | $CO_2$ | $C_3H_6$ |
| Physical state in cylinder | Gas | Liquid | Gas | Liquid | Liquid |
| Pressure when full (15°C) |  |  |  |  |  |
| psi | 1980 | 639.5 | 1980 | 723 | 64 |
| kg/cm² | 139.2 | 44.9 | 139.2 | 50.8 | 4.5 |
| atm | 134.7 | 43.5 | 134.7 | 49.2 | 4.3 |
| $10^3 \times kPa$ | 136.5 | 4.4 | 136.5 | 5 | 436 (kPa) |
| Type of cylinder valve* | PI BN HW | PI HW | PI | PI | PI |
| Critical temperature (°C) | −118.4 | 36.5 | (Gases separate at −6°C) | 31 | 125 |
| Critical pressure (atm) | 50.14 | 71.7 | — | 72.85 | 54 |
| Boiling point (°C at 1 atm) | −183 | −89 | — | −78.5 | −33 |
| Flammability | Supports combustion | Supports combustion | Supports combustion | No | Yes |
| Approximate weight (for calculation of cylinder contents) |  |  |  |  |  |
| g/litre | — | 1.87 | — | 1.87 | 1.8 |
| oz/gallon | — | 3.3 | — | 3.3 | 3.5 |

* PI, pin index; BN, bull nose; HW, handwheel.

cover. They are also marked with the chemical symbol for the gas they contain. Throughout the equipment the colours shown in Table 3.2 are used to identify the gaseous pathways.

Medical gas cylinders are hydraulically tested every five years and this test is recorded by a mark which is stamped on the neck of the cylinder. Other marks on the neck and the valve block (Fig. 3.1) relate to the name of the owner, the serial number of the cylinder and the pressures to which the cylinder has been tested and may safely be filled.

### Pin-index system (International Standard)

This system has been devised in order to prevent the accidental fitting of a cylinder of the wrong gas to a yoke, thus making interchangeability of cylinders of different gases impossible. One or more pins

**Table 3.2** Colour codes for medical gases and vacuum

| Gas | Symbol | ISO & UK | USA | Germany |
|---|---|---|---|---|
| Oxygen | $O_2$ | White on black | Green | Blue |
| Nitrous oxide | $N_2O$ | Blue | Blue | Grey |
| Carbon dioxide | $CO_2$ | Grey | Grey | — |
| Cyclopropane | $C_3H_6$ | Orange | Orange | — |
| Air (medical) | AIR | White and Black on black | Yellow | Yellow |
| Entonox 50/50 $N_2O/O_2$ | $N_2O + O_2$ | Blue and White on blue | — | — |
| Vacuum | — | Yellow | — | — |

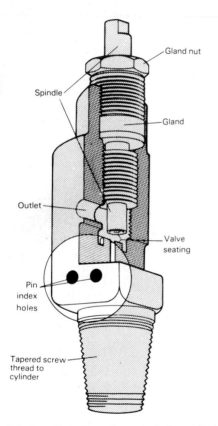

**Figure 3.2** A section through a pin index cylinder valve block, showing the position of the pin index holes.

project from the yoke, and these locate in holes bored in the valve block of the cylinder (Fig. 3.2). The configuration of the pins varies for each gas, as illustrated in Fig. 3.3. If the wrong cylinder is accidentally offered up to a yoke it is impossible to fit it. When piped medical gas systems were first employed, the supply hose to the anaesthetic machine often terminated in a block similar to the valve block of a cylinder and drilled for the appropriate pin index. Full details of the pin index system are given in British Standard 1319 of 1955.

The then Department of Health and Social Security advised in 1973 that pipeline hoses should be connected permanently to anaesthetic machines using a union such as a cap and liner (see page 95).

Medical gases are also supplied in cylinders other than those with pin index outlets, and those still available in the UK are shown in Fig. 3.4. Note that the 'handwheel' type cylinders (Fig. 3.4b) of nitrous oxide and oxygen, used commonly in dental practice, have different sizes of thread on the outlet and are therefore non-interchangeable. The British Oxygen Company (BOC) has now replaced handwheel cylinders for oxygen by 'bull-nosed' cylinders, but other companies such as Kingston Medical Gases have retained the handwheel type.

Full cylinders are usually supplied with plastic dust-covers over the outlet in order to prevent contamination by dirt or grit; these should be removed immediately before fitting the cylinder. When a cylinder is fitted, care should be taken to see that the sealing washer is present and in good order. If it is not so, it should be replaced by a new one, and this must be of non-combustible material. ('Bodok' seals supplied by BOC have a metal periphery, which keeps them in good order for a long period (Fig. 3.5).) The screw or clamp securing the cylinder in the yoke should not be tightened excessively, or damage to the washer or even the cylinder may occur. Immediately before fitting it is advisable to open the valve gently and to allow some gas to escape, in order to blow from the outlet any dirt or grit which might cause damage to the pressure regulator or could even lead to an explosion. The cylinder valve should be opened slowly so as to prevent a sudden surge of pressure (shock wave) on the contents gauge and regulator. It should be closed with no more force than is sufficient, or damage to the seating of the valve may result. If, after a cylinder has been turned on, there appears to be a leak, this may be tested for with water or a soapy solution. Occasionally there is a leak of gas around the spindle of the valve; this can be

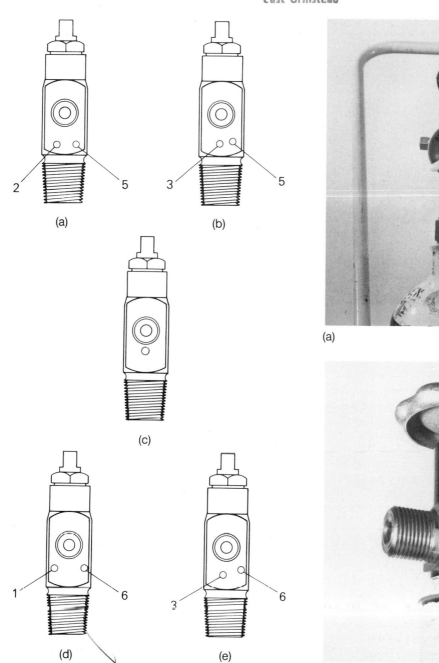

Figure 3.3 Pin index configuration. (a) Oxygen ($O_2$); (b) nitrous oxide ($N_2O$); (c) Entonox (50% $N_2O$ + 50% $O_2$); (d) carbon dioxide ($CO_2$); (e) cyclopropane ($C_3H_6$).

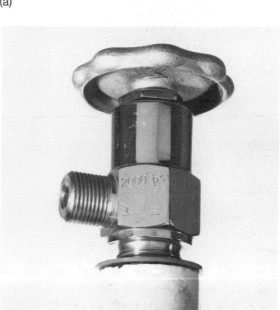

Figure 3.4 (a) A bull-nosed cylinder valve. (b) A hand-wheel cylinder valve. These are for larger cylinders.

prevented by gently screwing down the gland nut (see Fig. 3.2). If high-pressure oxygen is allowed to come into contact with combustible materials, especially oil or grease, fire or an explosion is liable to occur.

In the USA, cylinders are fitted with a Wood's metal fusible plug in the valve block which melts at low temperature. This is to prevent the risk of explosion if the cylinders are exposed to very high temperatures, such as in a fire. (In the UK the

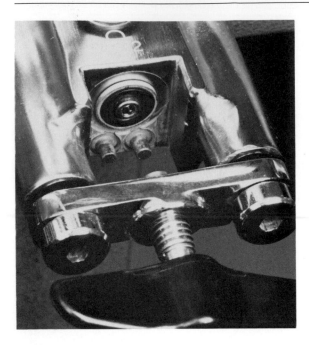

**Figure 3.5** A Bodok seal shown in position on a pin index yoke.

sealing material between the valve and the neck of the cylinder is often made of a fusible material that in the event of involvement in a fire would melt and allow the contents of the cylinder to escape around the threads of this joint.)

Cylinders should be stored in a clean place in order to prevent the admission of dirt and possible infection to the operating theatre. They should be kept in a rack in such a manner that they are used in rotation, to prevent any being stored for a long period, thereby reducing the possibility of their being empty when brought into use. Cylinders of Entonox (50% nitrous oxide plus 50% oxygen) should never be stored under conditions in which the temperature might fall below 0°C, since if the temperature falls below the pseudocritical (condensation) temperature for this mixture, the nitrous oxide and oxygen could laminate (separate). If this does happen, the instructions for remixing the contents, printed on the neck of the cylinder, should be followed. This involves gentle rewarming and repeated inversion of the cylinder.

Empty cylinders should be stored separately from full ones and marked accordingly. The valves of empty cylinders should be closed to avoid the ingress of water vapour, water or dirt. Faulty cylinders should be appropriately marked and returned to the supplier. Cylinders should not be stored under conditions where very high temperatures may occur.

# Oxygen Concentrators

The desirability of the local 'manufacture' of oxygen, obviating the need for the provision of cylinders or liquid oxygen has led to the development of methods of separating oxygen from air. Oxygen concentrators may be required for the following reasons:

- economy
  (a) very large bulk users
  (b) domestic users;
- convenience
  (a) aircraft
  (b) ships;
- logistics
  (a) Armed Forces
  (b) geographical: (i) developing countries;
      (ii) mission hospitals; (iii) expeditions.

In theory, oxygen concentrators could use as a power source any source of mechanical energy, since the only energy-consuming component is a compressor. All currently manufactured oxygen concentrators are electrically powered.

The principle of the oxygen concentrator depends on the property of an *artificial zeolite* (dust-free aluminium silicate and is sometimes referred to as a molecular sieve) to adsorb molecules of nitrogen onto the very large surface area presented, and to allow oxygen to pass through.

The component parts of the oxygen concentrator are shown in Fig. 3.6. The two chambers, A and B are identical and contain the zeolite. Initially, chamber A is charged with compressed air; the nitrogen is retained in the zeolite, while the remainder of the gas, comprising more than 92% oxygen, passes on to a reservoir and from there to the patient. When the zeolite in chamber A is calculated to have been fully charged with nitrogen, there is an automatic change-over to chamber B and a vacuum is applied to chamber A to remove the nitrogen and expel it to the atmosphere. The change-over is made usually on a time basis. The output provides at least 92% oxygen, the other gases being argon, other rare gases and a little nitrogen.

To these basic components of the oxygen concentrator are added an air filter which is especially important in dusty climates, a heat exchanger to cool the compressed air, which has gained heat by being compressed, and some form of output flow control and meter.

Small oxygen concentrators are in regular use for the treatment, in their own homes, of patients with

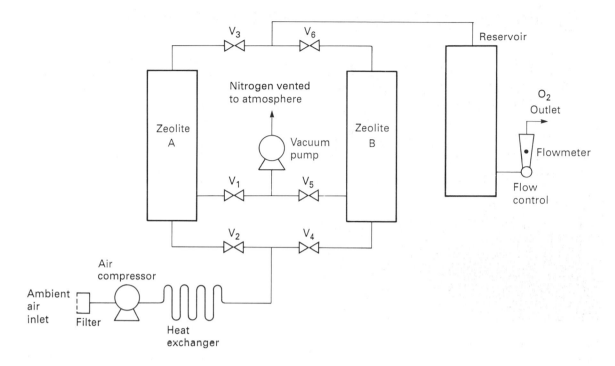

**Figure 3.6** An oxygen concentrator. To start, valves $V_1$, $V_4$ and $V_6$ are closed. Compressed air passes via $V_2$ into cylinder A, where the nitrogen is absorbed by the zeolite, and concentrated oxygen passes out via $V_3$. When the capacity of cylinder A is used up, valves $V_1$, $V_4$ and $V_6$ are opened and valves $V_2$, $V_3$ and $V_5$ are closed. Cylinder B then takes over the function, while nitrogen from cylinder A is discharged to the atmosphere via the vacuum pump.

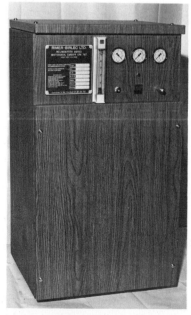

**Figure 3.7** A small domiciliary oxygen concentrator.

respiratory disease. The whole equipment is housed in a small cabinet (Fig. 3.7) no larger than the average television set and operates from standard mains electricity supply. Typically, the output might be 2–3 litres of oxygen per minute, which is the optimum for the patients for whom it is intended. Similar devices are used in military aircraft to enrich the atmosphere breathed by the crew at high altitudes.

Very much larger oxygen concentrators may be used to supply a hospital. Of these there are currently two varieties: those with two large chambers, such as that shown in Fig. 3.8; and plants with air compressors and concentrators, such as that shown in Fig. 3.9. Not only is the latter system by MGI fully automated, but it is also capable of supplying medical compressed air. A further refinement has been the addition of a facility for filling cylinders with this 'pressure swing gas'. These may be used in an emergency, when the load becomes excessive for the plant or when the plant needs to be shut down temporarily for service, maintenance or repair.

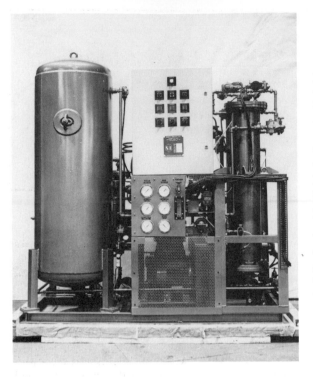

The use of oxygen concentrators in hospitals is likely to increase, especially in those areas where reliable deliveries of oxygen in cylinders or liquid form may be impossible to guarantee. There may be prejudice by some physicians against the delivery of a gas which is not pure oxygen; however, the use of mixtures containing more than 90% oxygen is seldom vital.

The financial economy resulting from the use of oxygen concentrators greatly depends on the cost of oxygen supplied by other means. It should be pointed out, however, that there may be a considerable saving in labour in the delivery and handling of cylinders, a task which is sometimes beyond the capabilities of domiciliary patients or their relatives. The domiciliary use of an oxygen concentrator for a period of over 1 year has been shown to produce financial economy, but as yet there is insufficient experience for evaluation of its use in hospitals.

**Figure 3.8** The Rimer-Birlec oxygen concentrator of sufficient capacity to supply a hospital.

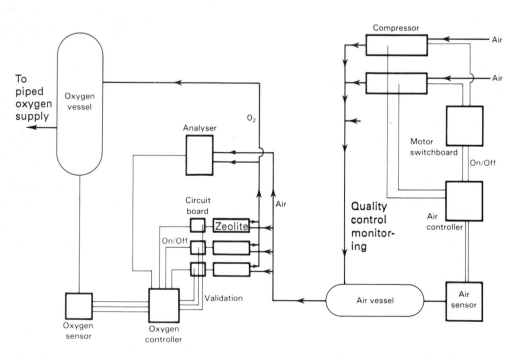

**Figure 3.9** The Oxymaster oxygen cascade concentrator. In this a number of compressors, either alone or in company with others, take the load in turn. Similarly, there are multiple absorption vessels. One advantage of this system is that it may also supply medical compressed air as required.

# 4 Piped Medical Gas and Vacuum Systems

## Introduction

The information given in this chapter refers mainly to the practice in the UK, though similar systems have been used for many years in other countries. In some of these other systems the nominal pressure is 310 kPa (45 psi) rather than the British Standard of 420 kPa (60 psi). In some systems a higher pressure is used for oxygen than for other services.

By virtue of the installation of a piped medical gas and vacuum (PMGV) system (Fig. 4.1) the need for provision of small 'duty' cylinders of oxygen and nitrous oxide on anaesthetic machines and similar items is obviated, and the number in 'reserve' may also be greatly diminished. However, in BS 4272 Part 3: 1987 (UK), the Standard requires that anaesthetic machines should have a reserve supply of oxygen. The advantages of piped gases are not only that there may be a reduction in the cost of the gases, but also that there is a saving of the cost of labour for transporting cylinders, a reduction in the introduction into the anaesthetic room and operating theatre of cylinders that may carry infection, and also a reduction of the incidence of accidents due to cylinders becoming exhausted. Much publicity has been given in recent years to the few accidents that have occurred in connection with piped medical gas supplies, but it is not easy to make a rational comparison between the incidence of accidents before and after the introduction of pipelines, owing to the great increase in the amount and complexity of work undertaken.

The PMGV services may be considered in five sections.

1. The bulk store or production plant.
2. The fixed distribution pipework.
3. The terminal outlets.
4. The flexible hoses, flowmeters and vacuum controllers, which are all detachable.
5. The connections between the flexible hoses and the anaesthetic machines.

Items 1 and 2 above may be considered as 'behind the wall' and it is usually felt that apart from broad strategy this is the province of the Engineering, Supplies and Pharmacy departments and the anaesthetist can take it on trust that the correct gases will be supplied. He cannot be held responsible for what goes on 'behind the wall'. In the case of items 4 and 5, the anaesthetist takes his share of responsibility to assure the maintenance of good standards, of checks and of tests and to prevent abuse. The terminal outlet is the interface between the two. The majority of the rare accidents that have occurred have been between the wall and the patient, and possibly these could be deemed to be the most preventable — though several deaths have occurred in the UK and elsewhere due to cross connections (called 'confusion') which have led to gases other than pure oxygen being delivered from the oxygen outlet. It should be stressed that nearly all accidents have been caused by alterations or faulty repairs made by incompetent and sometimes unauthorized people rather than because the installation was that of one manufacturer or another or of a more modern or an older model, such as the BOC Mk 1 or Mk 4. Little benefit is to be gained by ripping out an older type of installation and replacing it with a more modern one just because new developments have been made. Indeed, the confusion that this could cause might add to, rather than diminish, the dangers. It has been suggested that if oxygen only were supplied by pipeline, there would be no possibility of confusion.

In most instances the cost of medical gases is reduced when they are delivered in large containers,

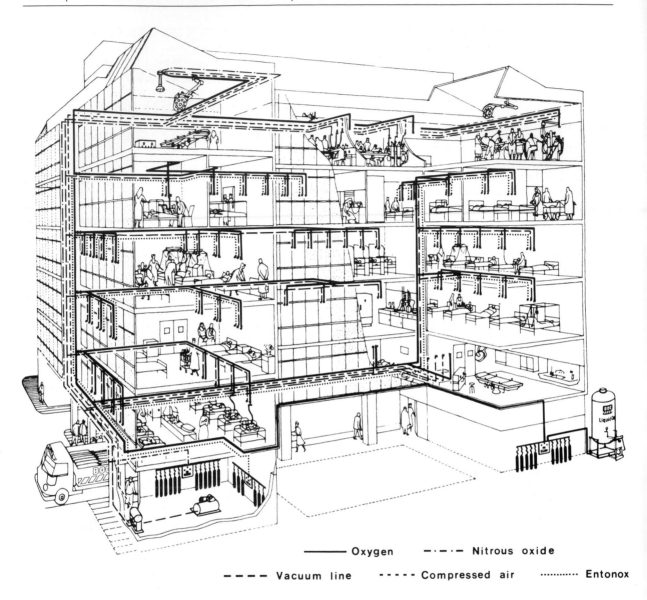

Oxygen ——————  Nitrous oxide —·—·—

Vacuum line —— —— ——  Compressed air ····  Entonox ··········

**Figure 4.1** A diagrammatic representation of piped medical gas system.

and particularly in the case of oxygen when it is supplied in the liquid state. It should be noted, however, that the economy achieved in this manner is to some extent offset by the wastage that occurs during the use of a piped medical gas system. This wastage occurs at two points: mainly at the terminal outlet, which may be leaking or may be left running after the need for the supply has ceased, but also during the delivery of liquid oxygen, when a considerable volume is required to cool the delivery tube between the tanker and the vacuum-insulated evaporator (VIE) to below the critical temperature for oxygen (− 118.4°C). Another small loss of oxygen from the liquid container occurs when there is little

or no demand. In order to maintain a sufficiently low temperature, between 0.5 and 1.0% of the volume of liquid oxygen needs to evaporate daily so that the requirement of the latent heat of vaporization may offset the gain in heat owing to the inefficiencies in the insulation: if this vaporized oxygen is not drawn off into the pipeline it is voided to the atmosphere.

The 'gases' that are commonly supplied by pipeline are oxygen, nitrous oxide, Entonox (a nitrous oxide/oxygen mixture), compressed air and vacuum. Other gases such as helium and hydrogen are supplied in piped services to pathology laboratories and the like, but are not frequently used in direct connection with patients. They will not, therefore, be considered in this book.

# Bulk Store

### Oxygen

In smaller installations oxygen is normally supplied and stored in cylinders as compressed gas. These are attached to *manifolds*, which consist of banks of several cylinders. There are usually two such banks, of which one is termed the 'duty' (or running) bank and the other the 'reserve' bank. The number of cylinders in each bank depends on the expected demand. The cylinders in each bank are all turned on and interconnected. However, the flow of oxygen from one cylinder to another is prevented by non-return valves. When the duty bank is almost exhausted the supply is automatically switched to the reserve bank. This now becomes the duty bank and an indication is given that this has occurred. The exhausted cylinders must now be replaced by full ones, and if this is not done before the second bank reaches a certain level of exhaustion, a compelling warning is given (see below). Figure 4.2 shows a typical modern, automatic manifold for nitrous oxide that operates in the same manner.

Figure 4.3 shows an emergency supply manifold, which may be used to continue the supply during periods of maintenance or repair, when the main manifold is out of action. Under these circumstances the pipeline is isolated from the main manifold by closing valve A and connected to the emergency manifold by opening valve B. Both of these latter operations are performed manually. Note that there is a pressure relief valve, which, like that on the main manifold, is vented to the outside rather than to an enclosed area where it might be dangerous. The valves on the cylinders of the emergency manifold may be kept open during periods of standby when valve B is closed, in order to show by means of the contents gauge on the pressure regulator that they are full, and by the regulated pressure gauge that the regulator is correctly set.

In many instances relatively small establishments such as dental clinics have piped gas installations with very few outlets. In the UK those employed by general dental practitioners are provided and owned by individual practitioners. However, these

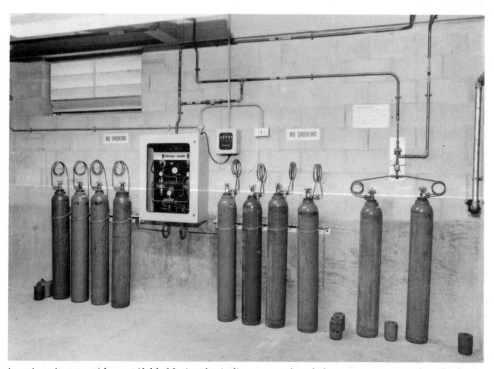

**Figure 4.2** A major nitrous oxide manifold. Notice the indicator panel and the emergency supply cylinders on the right-hand side. The coils in the tailpipes provide greater flexibility so as to prevent damage to the pipes during cylinder changes.

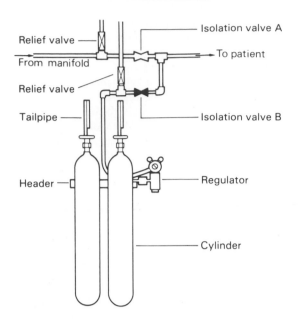

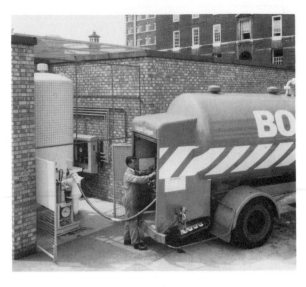

**Figure 4.4** A vacuum-insulated evaporator for storage of liquid oxygen.

**Figure 4.3** Emergency supply manifold. Note that valve A isolates the main manifold and valve B opens the emergency manifold.

installations are required to meet the appropriate standards in the UK (BSS 5682: 1984).

### Liquid oxygen

In the case of larger consumers it may be found more economical to have deliveries of oxygen in the liquid form. Since the critical temperature of oxygen is −118.4°C, if it is stored in liquid form it must be kept at an ever lower temperature. Liquid oxygen is transported in specially insulated tankers and is delivered into a VIE (Fig. 4.4). This consists of an inner shell of stainless steel, separated from an outer shell of carbon steel by a space in which is maintained the greatest degree of vacuum possible and which also contains perlite powder. The temperature within the inner chamber is around −183°C and since the container cannot be a perfect insulator arrangements are made to maintain this very low temperature (see below, Mode of operation). There may be four connections to the inner cylinder.

- The filling port, through which fresh supplies of liquid oxygen are introduced.
- A gaseous withdrawal line at the top of the cylinder, from which gaseous oxygen may pass via a restrictor plate and then a superheater (a

length of copper tubing about 2.5 cm in diameter on which are mounted metallic fins to conduct ambient heat), to the control system and distribution pipework. The purpose of the superheater is to raise the temperature of the gaseous oxygen to that of the ambient air, for otherwise dangerously cold oxygen might be delivered to the terminal outlets in those parts of the hospital close to the VIE.
- A liquid withdrawal line, which may withdraw liquid to enter the main flow downstream from the restrictor and upstream from the superheater.
- A second liquid withdrawal line, which may pass through an evaporator and then either into the distribution network or back into the gaseous compartment of the container.

In older models there may be only two connections: one to the lower part, for the introduction and withdrawal of liquid, and the other at the top, for the withdrawal or reintroduction of gas.

*Mode of operation of a liquid oxygen plant (Fig. 4.5).* Since no insulation can be perfect, the inner container is continually receiving heat from the exterior; the effects of this are offset by the evaporation of liquid oxygen, thus helping to keep the liquid at the appropriate temperature. If there is no demand for oxygen for a period of time, the pressure within the chamber may rise above normal (around 1055 kPa), and at a predetermined pressure

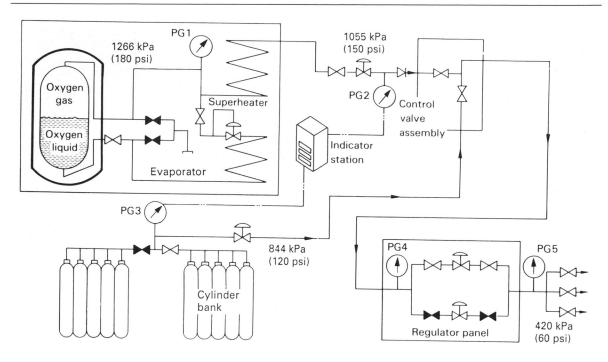

**Figure 4.5** Schematic diagram of a liquid oxygen plant (see text for details).

a safety valve opens to allow the escape of some gas. The loss of oxygen due to this venting is, as a rule, fairly small. Conversely, if the demand for oxygen is increased, there may be a fall of pressure within the vessel. In this case a control valve opens in the lower liquid withdrawal line and liquid passes through an evaporator and then either to the pipeline or to the gaseous compartment of the VIE until the pressure within it is restored to normal. In the event of an exceptionally high demand for oxygen, liquid may pass through the upper liquid withdrawal line directly to the superheater and via the control panel to the distribution system.

A cause of considerable waste is that during the delivery of fresh supplies of liquid, the hose between the tanker and the VIE needs to be cooled to below the critical temperature of oxygen before delivery can be effected. This is done by allowing liquid to escape from the tanker through the hose to the atmosphere. The oxygen delivered is metered at the tanker and on occasions it has been found that as much as one-quarter of the total delivery has been required for this pre-cooling.

The VIE rests on three legs, two of which are on hinged supports. The third rests on a simple steelyard weighing device with an appropriate counterweight. The contents of the VIE are expressed in weight and indicated on a dial.

The VIE is sited outside a building, within an enclosure which also houses two banks of reserve

cylinders in a manifold similar to that described above (Fig. 4.6). The reserve cylinders automatically take over the load if the output from the VIE falls below a predetermined level. Being in the open, the VIE is subject to adverse weather conditions and it was once found that the weighing mechanism was immersed in water which had subsequently frozen into a solid block of ice. The estimation of the contents may well have been erroneous in this case.

*Relative capacities of cylinders and the VIE.* The pressure within a full cylinder of oxygen is 13 700 kPa (1980 psi). Thus, when used on a pipeline, a cylinder can be expected to give approximately 130 times its capacity of oxygen at atmospheric pressure. Compared with this, one volume of liquid oxygen gives 842 times its volume of gas at 15°C and normal atmospheric pressure. Since the VIE has a very much greater capacity than a cylinder, it will be obvious that it can deliver a far greater volume of oxygen than a whole manifold of cylinders.

*Safety precautions.* The manifolds for oxygen, nitrous oxide, Entonox and compressed air should be housed in a well-ventilated room constructed of a fireproof material such as brick or concrete. The space within the room should be adequate for handling trolleys carrying cylinders and for the unimpeded changing of cylinders on the manifold. All oils, greases and flammable materials should be excluded from the room, as should pipes carrying

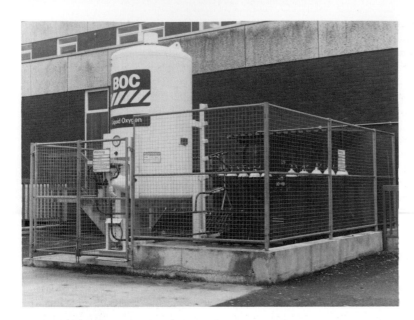

**Figure 4.6** Banks of reserve cylinders for a liquid oxygen plant.

town gas or oil. There should be no high voltage electric cables. The room should be well ventilated at high and low level and there should be no drains or gulleys in which gas could collect.

Cylinders of the gases used on the manifold may be stored in this room or in another location. They should preferably be sited where there is easy and close access from the delivery point by the supplier. The compressors and reservoir for the central vacuum plant and the plant for medical compressed air should not be housed in the manifold room. It should be impressed on all personnel that cylinders of compressed gas, particularly oxygen, can be dangerous if mishandled. Provisions should be made for securing the cylinders to the wall.

Liquid oxygen plants should not be housed within a building. They should be sited in the open, a minimum distance of 6 m from any combustible material; no smoking should be permitted within this space. The ground surface should be of concrete or similar non-combustible material — and certainly not tar or asphalt, since they both form explosive mixtures when in contact with liquid oxygen. The plant should be surrounded by a fence of non-combustible material and there should be adequate access for the delivery tanker. There should be no overhead wires, drains or trenches within the prescribed area.

## Nitrous oxide

As stated previously, nitrous oxide liquefies at room temperature when stored under pressure in a cylinder. It is therefore supplied to a piped medical gas system from a manifold of cylinders similar to those for oxygen, described above.

When considering the size and number of cylinders to be installed in each bank, thought must be given to the maximum demand that will be required. This is because nitrous oxide cools not only as it expands but also due to the latent heat required to vaporize the liquid. If a heavy demand is taken from a bank of small capacity, the gas may cool to such a low temperature that water vapour in the ambient atmosphere condenses, and may even freeze, on the surface of parts of the pipework and in particular the pressure regulators. In the days when nitrous oxide cylinders contained some water vapour, this used to freeze *within* the regulator, causing obstruction. For this reason a regulator heater, thermostatically controlled at 47°C may be fitted to warm the gas and prevent condensation. A typical nitrous oxide manifold is shown in Fig. 4.2. There is not yet a practical method for the local manufacture of nitrous oxide, though progress in this field is being made.

## Entonox (50% nitrous oxide + 50% oxygen)

This mixture is used for the administration of inhalational analgesia, principally in the obstetric department. The manifolds employed are essentially the same as those for nitrous oxide and oxygen, but additional safeguards are required in the handling of the cylinders. This is because the mixture has a pseudocritical temperature of approximately −6°C and if the cylinder were allowed to cool below this point, the nitrous oxide and oxygen might separate out by a process known as lamination.

The large cylinders for Entonox manifolds have pin index outlets as shown in Fig. 3.3 and, unlike smaller cylinders for this purpose, there is an internal tube from the valve block, leading down to within 10 cm of the bottom of the cylinder. The contents are supplied through this tube, the position of which would prevent the discharge of pure nitrous oxide if lamination had occurred. Excessive cooling of the cylinders is prevented by ensuring that there are a sufficient number of cylinders on the manifold and that all of them are turned on at the same time. No single cylinder should supply gas at a rate greater than 300 litres/min.

Cylinders of Entonox should be stored for 24 h after delivery before being connected to the manifold. There should be a special store for them and they should be kept in a horizontal position at a temperature between 10 and 38°C.

There does not yet seem to have been much interest shown in the problems of atmospheric pollution arising from the use of Entonox analgesia. However, efficient scavenging would be difficult to achieve and this may, in the future, lead to a reduction in the popularity of a piped supply of this mixture.

## Medical compressed air

Medical compressed air (CA) differs from industrial compressed air in that a greater degree of purity is required. Industrial CA may well contain not only water vapour but also an oil mist. Indeed, much industrial equipment operated by CA requires the addition of a lubricant. Medical CA may be administered to patients through both anaesthetic equipment and lung ventilators in the theatre and the Intensive Therapy Unit and it is also employed to power some surgical instruments. Whereas a pressure of 420 kPa (60 psi) is sufficient for the former, many surgical instruments require a higher pressure of about 700 kPa (105 psi). Although the CA driving surgical instruments is not intentionally administered to the patient, it would, if not clean, contaminate the operating field. At first sight it might be thought that a 700 kPa compressed air system would on its own be suitable to supply a hospital (this pressure being required for surgical instruments); however, it must be borne in mind that this might present difficulties in the Intensive Care Ward, where blenders are used for mixing

oxygen with medical compressed air to achieve the appropriate mixtures for administration to patients. Where the use of surgical instruments is expected to be relatively infrequent, it might be considered better to install a piped medical CA system at 420 kPa and to use separate cylinders with the appropriate pressure regulators for a 700 kPa supply. This would seem to be particularly appropriate since it is sometimes the practice of surgeons to vary the precise pressure of CA to suit the power tool in use and the speed at which it is required to run.

Piped medical CA may be supplied either from a manifold of cylinders, as described above for oxygen, nitrous oxide and Entonox, or by a compressor. A cylindered supply is relatively expensive, but the quality of the air can be assured. Since the cylinders of compressed air have the same right-hand thread on a bull-nosed outlet as oxygen, care must be taken in the storage of such cylinders to ensure that they are not accidentally interchanged. It is recommended that the storage bins be separated from each other, for example, by a wall or partition, and that they be clearly marked.

In a larger hospital it may well be economical to install a compressor. In this case the air has to be both dried and filtered at the outlet of the compressor in order to achieve adequate quality. A scheme for such a compressed air plant is shown in Fig. 4.7.

Too often in the past it has happened that when a hospital was being built an industrial CA plant was installed and the air was found to be unsuitable for medical purposes. In one such instance the author found that the pipe run to an outlet in the basement was completely filled with condensed water which had gravitated there from the rest of the distribution pipework.

As was shown above, a single plant may be used both to provide medical CA and to run an oxygen concentrator.

In some instances it has been considered appropriate to install a small local compressor for a particular department in order to save extensive pipework. If this is done, it is essential to ensure that there is adequate oil separation and filtration to suit the requirements of that department. This is often lacking in small compressors.

## Indicators and alarms

The gauges and indicators that are an integral part of a major manifold are shown in Fig. 4.2. A typical arrangement has one green indicator marked 'running' or 'duty' and one red indicator marked 'empty' for each bank of cylinders. Thus when the

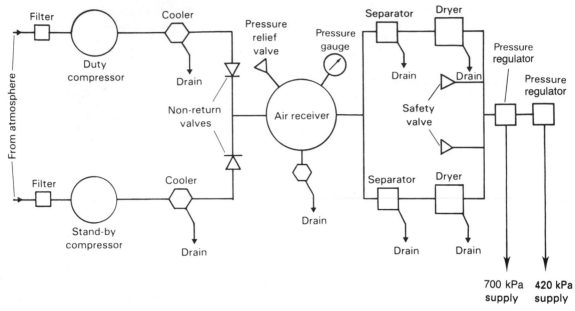

**Figure 4.7** Simplified diagram of a medical compressed air plant.

first bank of cylinders becomes exhausted, the green 'running' indicator on that side is extinguished and the red 'empty' indicator on that side is illuminated. At the same time the green indicator marked 'running' for the second bank will illuminate. The red indicator on the first bank stays lit until the cylinders have been replaced by full ones and have been turned on.

Since the manifolds are usually remote from the users and the members of staff responsible for changing the cylinders, repeater indicators may also be installed — for instance at the telephone switchboard or in the porters' lodge.

The above indicators may be expected to operate when the installation is running normally. Warning signals, which may consist of a red or orange flashing light, and an audible alarm are given when there is some impending failure — for example if one bank is empty and the pressure in the cylinders in the other bank falls to a predetermined level, i.e. if there has been a failure to heed the indication that one bank of cylinders needs replenishing. Another warning may be given if the pressure in the output of the manifold falls below a predetermined level.

On smaller installations such as the 'Minor' manifold (Fig. 4.8), on which the cylinders on one side are turned on manually, there are two indicator lamps per gas. A white one shows that the electric current is turned on and a red one that the cylinder pressure has fallen to a predetermined level.

The indicators for a liquid oxygen plant may show 'normal running', 'running from cylinders', 'first bank of cylinders empty' and 'low line pressure'.

## Piped medical vacuum

It is the author's view that this is the most advantageous of all the piped services. If the provision of vacuum is left to local suction machines throughout the hospital, there is too often a disastrous delay, either because a particular machine is faulty or because the electric supply is not within reach. The most important limitation of the use of piped medical vacuum is the availability of an outlet point in close proximity to the patient for whom it is needed. The prompt use of suction, for example to clear the gastric contents from a patient's air passages, is of great importance, and in the author's experience the failure to provide this from small local suction machines is far more common than, for example, the exhaustion of an oxygen cylinder. More consideration of this will be found in the next section, where the distribution of medical vacuum outlets is considered.

In the UK guidance on the design and installation of piped medical vacuum services is set out in BS 4957 of 1973 and Hospital Technical Memorandum (HTM) No. 22 as revised in 1977.

Figure 4.9 shows the layout of a typical vacuum

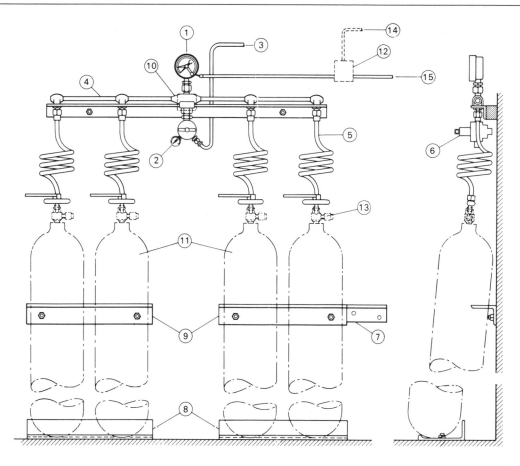

**Figure 4.8** The BOC Minor manifold. Changeover from one bank of cylinders to the other is performed manually. The near exhaustion of one bank of cylinders is indicated by a warning signal that is ideally situated within view of the anaesthetist. 1, High-pressure gauge with contacts for the warning light; 2, regulated pressure gauge; 3, supply pipe; 4, header assembly; 5, tail pipe; 6, pressure regulator; 7, tool rack; 8 and 9, frames to secure cylinders; 10, header connection; 11, cylinder banks; 12, fused switch; 13, cylinder valves; 14, electrical supply; 15, wiring to distant warning light.

plant. The precise details of this may vary according to the type of pump in use.

The distribution pipework may take the form of a 'ring main', the two ends of which each pass towards the pump through an isolating valve and then a drainage trap in which any aspirated liquid or condensed vapour, for example from body cavity drainage, may separate out and be removed. The pipes then pass through bacterial filters and from there to the vacuum reservoir. At the bottom of the reservoir is a drainage pipe, with a manual drain valve, to evacuate any liquid which may collect.

The connection between the reservoir and the vacuum pumps is made through flexible hoses in order to reduce vibration and the noise that this might transmit through the pipework. There are two pumps, each of which is adequate for the needs of the system. Thus one pump may be 'on duty', whilst the other is on standby or being serviced.

There are various types of vacuum pump, but particular mention should be made of those that are oil-lick lubricated. It has been suggested that if the vacuum system is employed for the purpose of scavenging waste anaesthetic gases, the vapour of halothane and other anaesthetic agents may be absorbed by the lubricating oil, and by reducing its efficiency may cause failure of the pump. Furthermore, the Department of Health in the United Kingdom does not recommend the use of medical suction systems for scavenging, because the high inflow of anaesthetic gases will reduce surgical suction below desired levels and because experience

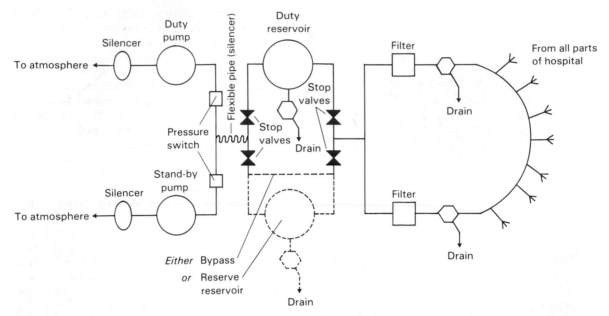

**Figure 4.9** A simplified diagram of a piped medical vacuum plant.

has shown that such high vacuum levels can injure the patient if safety devices fail.

The output of the pump passes through a silencer to be exhausted at a suitable point, such as above roof level where the gases may be vented to atmosphere without risk of polluting the air breathed by staff or patients.

*Performance levels and specifications for a medical vacuum*

For the UK the specifications for a piped vacuum are laid down in BS 4957 of 1973. A few of these are quoted below, but for more complete information the full specifications should be consulted.

A vacuum of at least 53 kPa (400 mmHg) below the standard atmospheric pressure of 101.3 kPa (760 mmHg) should be maintained at the outlets, each of which should be able to take a flow of free air of at least 40 litres/min; there should be at least two outlets per operating theatre, one per anaesthetic room and one per recovery bed.

The suction control units are described in Chapter 19 so that comparison may be made with other types of suction apparatus.

### Electrical supply to PMGV systems

The pumps for compressed air and vacuum should be powered by the 'non-interruptible' supply, which is backed up by the emergency generator. If possible, the manifold controls and warning lights

should also have their own emergency supply. Some manifolds are so constructed that if there is total power failure the indicators and warning lights will fail, but all the cylinders, of both banks, are switched on so as to continue the supply. Other manifold controls have a manual override that may be used to switch from one bank to the other.

# Distribution Pipework

For detailed information concerning the regulations and standards required for fixed distribution pipework, the regulations imposed by the appropriate Government or Health Ministries should be consulted. In the UK these are quoted in HTM 22 and its supplement, which refer to the 'permit to work' system laying down the procedures to be adopted when service maintenance, repair or alterations are to be undertaken.

In this chapter only a brief description can be given of the fixed pipework; since this part of the installation is 'behind the wall', it is more properly the concern of the hospital engineer rather than of the medical man. The anaesthetist should, however, be aware of the nature of the installation and should always be informed *and consulted* before any alterations to it are made.

The tubes used are copper, of a special degreased quality. Before they are delivered to the site, i.e.

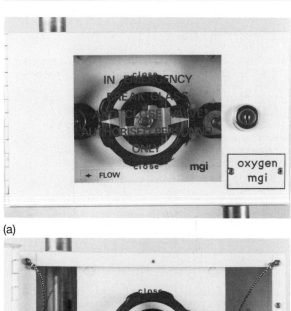

(a)

(b)

**Figure 4.10** An area valve box: (a) with the door in the normal closed position; (b) with the door open, showing the NIST (non-interchangeable screw thread) connections.

prior to installation, the ends are sealed so that there can be no ingress of dirt or other foreign material. The copper is also of a special alloy which prevents degradation of the gases. There is some relaxation of this in the case of the vacuum installation. The fittings are of degreased brass. Joints are made by brazing rather than with soft solder or compression fittings. Recently a system of brazing without the use of a flux has been developed and this results in a greatly reduced incidence of corrosion of both the surface and interior of the pipe and fittings. The diameter of pipe is determined by the demand that it will carry. Commonly it may start from the manifold with a diameter of 42 mm, but after branching to supply one or more areas pipes as narrow as 15 mm may be employed. Six millimetre pipework has been used for the final runs in many cases, but this is not now considered good practice for new work. In many instances a pipe of 6-mm diameter has been found to deliver gases at a

perfectly satisfactory rate, and there is no valid reason for replacing it with pipes of a larger bore simply to comply with a new standard.

Large installations may be divided into sections, supplying various departments. Each of these sections may be isolated by valves. Each department or ward, or section thereof, may be further isolated by a valve that is readily accessible to the staff, which may be used to turn off the gas supply in case of fire, fracture or other catastrophe. In earlier installations the isolating valves were often placed in a position that was not readily accessible or known to the staff working in the department.

Area valve and service units (Fig. 4.10) may be installed in such positions as to protect a number of departments or wards. These consist of a locked box containing an isolating valve, upstream and downstream of which are branches with the appropriate NIST (non-interchangeable screw thread) unions. These latter are normally closed with a blanked off NIST union. When the blanking nut is removed, a self-sealing valve within the union again closes it off. When the appropriate NIST connection is made (see page 95), the self-sealing valve is reopened. These branches may be used to purge pipelines or to introduce a local supply during alterations or breakdowns. The box also contains a 'spade', which may be used to ensure absolute closure of the pipeline, irrespective of the action of the valve.

Regional flowmeters may be incorporated in piped medical gas systems to detect the section in which an excessive leak or wastage of gas is occurring. Moisture traps may also be installed.

The actual pipework should be identified by labels placed upon it at regular intervals, in accordance with the identification code described in Fig. 4.11. Indeed, it is good practice for all pipework, whatever substances are carried, to be correctly labelled at regular intervals. The pipework may be hidden behind the wall or buried within the plaster, or alternatively it may be mounted on the surface. The latter arrangement is not only aesthetically less attractive, but also less satisfactory from the standpoint of general hygiene and cleanliness.

There are two exceptions to the method of jointing: (i) isolating valves may be screw-threaded in order to facilitate later replacement or alteration and to avoid damage during fitting; and (ii) a special type of compression joint, referred to as cold-jointing, may sometimes be used. A particular coupling manufactured by Hydroculpin is specified in HTM 22.

The pipework for medical gases and vacuum, and their fittings should be separated from other pipework so as to avoid confusion. The isolating valves

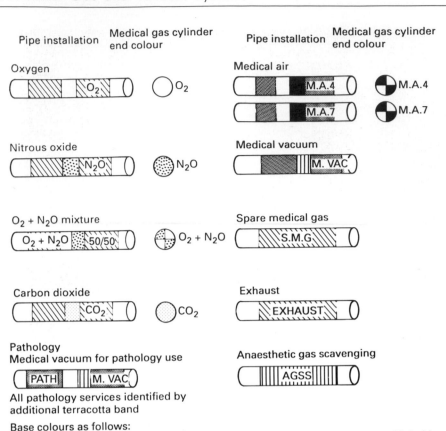

**Figure 4.11** Colour code for the identification of medical gases, vacuum and active gas scavenging pipeline installations in the UK. Flexible hoses must be colour-coded throughout their length, or by means of the coloured bands shown (in the form of a tubular sleeve), which must be securely fitted at both ends (BS 5682:1984). 'BS' refers to the appropriate British Standard (e.g. BS 4800:1972) defining the colours used. Each colour shade has a specific number — e.g. French blue is 20 D 45.

Note that medical air is supplied at two different pressures: MA4 refers to medical air at 420 kPa pressure (60 psi), which supplies respiratory equipment; MA7 is medical air supplied at 700 kPa (105 psi) primarily to power air-operated surgical equipment.

should be clearly labelled and positioned so that they may be closed by the retreating staff in the event of a fire.

## Terminal Outlets

The distribution pipework terminates in outlets that are in the form of self-closing sockets. Into each of these sockets one may introduce a probe attached either to a terminal unit such as a flowmeter or to a hose that is, in turn, connected to an anaesthetic machine. By design each terminal outlet will accept only the probe appropriate to the gas for which it is intended, as can be seen in Figs 4.12–4.15. This is therefore a non-interchangeable system. In the ideal situation, non-interchangeability would be continued right back to the bulk supply of the gas concerned. Unfortunately this ideal is not yet universally achieved, but in more recent practice steps are being taken to prevent a terminal outlet for one gas being attached to the base fittings for another.

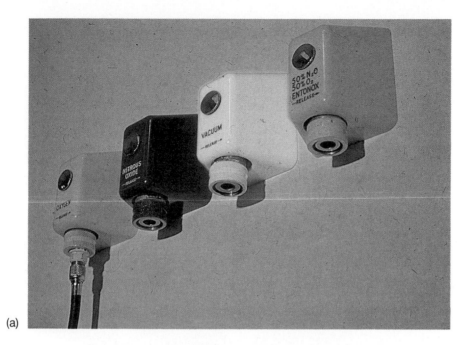

(a)

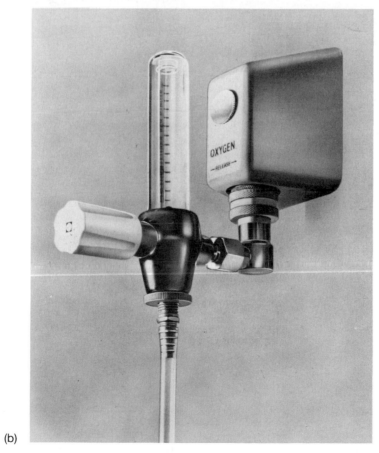

(b)

**Figure 4.12** (*Continued overleaf*).

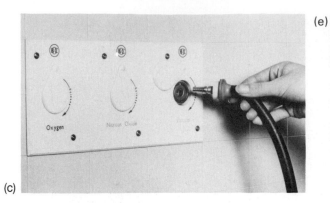

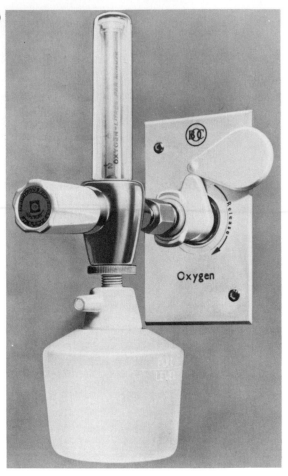

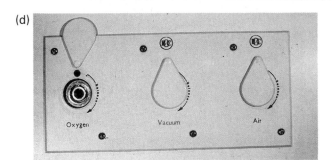

Figure 4.12 (a) BOC Mark 1 terminal outlets and probes. Note that there is a skirt (indexing collar) of different diameter for each gas. (b) A 'direct' probe attached to a flowmeter (BOC Mark 1). (c) BOC Mark 2 probe and outlet. (d) BOC Mark 2 terminal outlets. Note the difference in diameter of the recess for each skirt. (e) The same flowmeter as in (b), having been adapted for use with a Mark 2 probe and a humidifier.

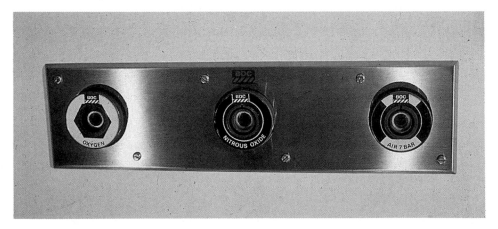

Figure 4.13 BOC Marks 3 and 4 terminal outlets.

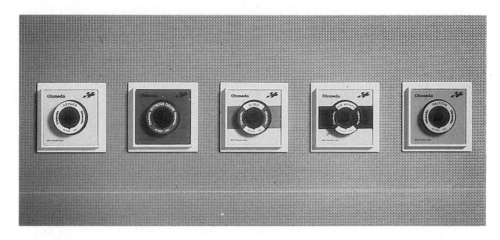

**Figure 4.14** The GEM IO terminal outlet, replacement for the Mark 4.

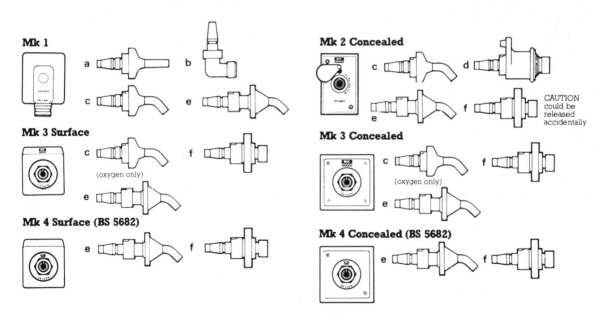

**Figure 4.15** Profiles of BOC Mark 1, 2, 3 and 4 terminal units and probes. Probes: (a) Mark 1 remote; (b) Mark 1 direct; (c) Mark 2 remote; (d) Mark 2 direct; (e) Mark 3 and Mark 4 remote (BS 5620), (f) Mark 3 and Mark 4 direct (BS 5682).

Several manufacturers have produced systems that have been used in the UK. These have included Dräger Medical Ltd, Puritan–Bennett Corporation and BOC (The British Oxygen Company, now marketed by Ohmeda). Each manufacturer's system for any specific gas was not compatible with another manufacturer's. In 1978 a British Standard was published (BS 5682, upgraded in 1984) that laid down a specification for the design of terminal units. This specifies a Schrader socket and probe collar indexing system for these units. Designs that currently conform to these specifications are the BOC Mark 4 (now replaced by the GEM 10 unit), the current Dräger unit (but not the original design) and the MGI TU2. BOC probes from Marks 1, 2 and 3 were of a Schrader design and could fit British Standard sockets.

The British Standard specifies that the terminal unit should consist of two sections. The first, a termination assembly, should be permanently attached to the appropriate pipeline. The second, the socket assembly, can be removed by a service engineer but must be designed so that it cannot be accidently connected to a different gas service. A termination assembly for a pressurized gas (but not a vacuum) must have an isolating valve so that work may be carried out on any terminal unit without shutting down all the terminal units for that gas in that area. It should be designed to operate automatically as soon as the socket assembly is removed. Furthermore, the identity of the gas for that terminal unit should be permanently displayed on the socket.

*Pipeline probe for the terminal outlet.* The design of the Schrader probe is such that it is the same size for all gases. To prevent connection to the wrong gas service, the probe for each gas supply has a protruding indexing collar (see Fig. 4.15). This collar has a unique diameter that fits only the matching recess fitted to the socket assembly for that gas. The British Standard also stipulates the following. (1) It must not be possible to twist the probe while it is connected to the unit. To this end, the collar is provided with a notch that fits over a rigid pin in the socket assembly. (2) It must be possible to insert or remove the probe simply and quickly using one hand only. The socket assembly has a spring-loaded outer ring, which when depressed releases the locking mechanism holding the probe, and causes the probe to be ejected. (3) The unit must seal off the flow of gas when the probe is withdrawn.

The BOC Mark 4 unit (see Figs 4.13 and 4.15) conforms to the above British standard. The socket assembly incorporates a pin indexing system to prevent it being attached by accident to a different gas service (see Fig. 4.16).

The replacement for the Mark 4, the GEM 10 (Fig. 4.14), is claimed to be more durable, surviving 10 000 probe insertions. Design improvements have incorporated all the 'O-ring' gas seals within the socket assembly into a single unit so as to reduce servicing time.

The BOC Mark 1 (Figs 4.12a and 4.15) was only supplied as a surface mounted unit with the probe being inserted vertically into its base. The probe was released from the terminal unit by twisting the outer ring of the socket.

The BOC Mark 2 (Figs 4.12d and 4.15) units were mounted flush with the wall and were provided with a removable cover. The probe was removed by twisting it. The socket assembly was fitted with an extra hole to take a locating pin fitted to some directly mounted equipment such as flowmeters. This prevented accidental disconnection (Fig. 4.12e).

The BOC Mark 3 (Figs 4.13 and 4.15) was the precursor to, and as such is similar in appearance to, the Mark 4. The socket was also pin indexed to

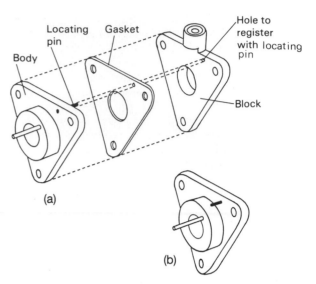

**Figure 4.16** (a) Locating pin on BOC Mark 4 conversion kit, showing the locating pin in a gas-specific location on the base plate, to prevent the accidental fitting of a socket for the wrong gas. (b) To show how, in the specimen tested by one of the authors, the pin could easily be displaced, thus rendering the system ineffectual.

prevent accidental connection to a terminal unit for a different gas, and the isolating valve was manually operated (using an Allen key). However, there have been occasions when the valve was left either partially or fully closed following a service! The socket has two locks with which it engages the probe. By depressing an outer ring on the socket (secondary lock), the probe is disengaged from the gas supply, but remains in the socket in a 'parked' position. The probe is then removed by twisting, which disengages the primary lock. The parked position was thought to be useful in that pipeline supplies could be isolated when not in use thus minimizing leaks, and at the same time the probes were stored in a convenient position. However, this occasionally led to the assumption that the probes were apparently properly inserted but with no gas supply.

# Flexible Hoses

The hosepipe connecting the terminal outlet of the fixed pipeline installation to the anaesthetic machine is the section of the system in which damage and wear are most likely to occur, and which is most accessible to well-meaning but uninformed members of staff who may attempt to make repairs or alterations. Originally the hosepipe for each gas was constructed of the same black reinforced rubber or neoprene tubing, identified only by a short length of coloured sheath at each end. This predisposed to accidents when, during repairs, cross-connections were made. More recently characteristically coloured tubing has been used for each gas. The development of such self-identifying tubing was unfortunately delayed by the difficulties involved in manufacturing it with the necessary antistatic (electrically conductive) properties.

Several accidents have been caused by the connection, or reconnection, of the probe for one gas at the upstream end of such a hose, but with the socket or union for another at the downstream end. On the commissioning of one hospital, the author found that a pair of hoses intended for the supply to an anaesthetic machine had been supplied, as new, by the manufacturer with the oxygen and nitrous oxide probes and sockets reversed.

The incidence of such accidents should be reduced by the current practice of most manufacturers to produce hoses, complete with the appropriate connections, in different factories or different areas of one factory. Furthermore, it is now a recommended practice that a damaged hose should not be repaired on site but should be returned in its entirety to the manufacturer in exchange for a factory-made service replacement.

The connections between the hose and fittings must be secure. Originally a fairly thin ferrule was used. This could be crimped on by a special pair of pliers or a purpose-made crimping clamp (Fig. 4.17). These ferrules could be removed without difficulty by using a pair of wire cutters. 'O' clips have also been used, but these are equally vulnerable to tampering. An improved ferrule (Fig. 4.18), manufactured by M & IE, is made of stainless steel and is of much greater thickness; it is applied by a 30-ton press and is sufficiently robust to defy all but the most determined attempts at removal.

Under no circumstances should one use devices such as the deservedly popular Jubilee clip which can be released and retightened easily and repeatedly.

The development of the attachment of the hose to the anaesthetic machine requires some consideration. When PMGV systems were originally installed they were commonly connected to anaesthetic machines designed to be supplied by cylinders. It was often required to retain the facility to return to a cylindered supply without difficulty. The hoses, therefore, terminated in a pin index block which resembled the valve block of a pin indexed cylinder. The block had either a tail (Fig. 4.19a) onto which

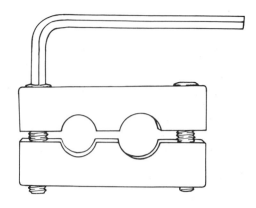

**Figure 4.17** A purpose-made crimping clamp.

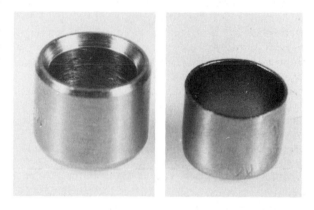

**Figure 4.18** An improved ferrule (left) manufactured by M & IE, with an old-type ferrule for comparison.

the hose could be directly attached (and secured by a ferrule), or a probe which fitted an appropriate terminal outlet, which in turn was attached to the end of the hose (Fig. 4.19b).

This system was safe so long as no one tampered with it. If it became damaged, it could be safely replaced by an entire assembly — provided that such an assembly was available. Lack of spare parts often led to 'on the spot' repairs, some of which turned out to be disastrous.

In 1973 the Department of Health (DOH, formerly DHSS) drew attention to the dangers, and among other recommendations advised that the connection of the hose to the anaesthetic machine be 'made permanent'. However, the varying interpretations of this gave rise to problems. If the hose were ferruled onto a spigot on the machine, this would encourage

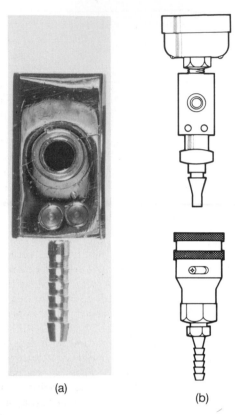

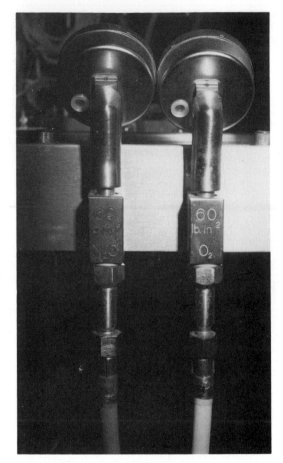

**Figure 4.19** (a) A pin index block with a tail for a flexible hose. (b) A pin index block fitted with a BOC Mark 1 spigot (top); a Mark 1 terminal fitted to the end of a flexible hose (bottom). Such systems are now discouraged owing to the increased risk of mistakes being made during repairs that could lead to the confusion of gases.

**Figure 4.21** Hosepipe union block.

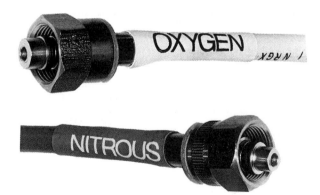

**Figure 4.20** Nut and probe (nipple) connection to an anaesthetic machine. Note the different sizes of shoulders of the male probes (nipples) for the different gases.

the very type of repair that it sought to prevent. A more satisfactory solution was the employment of a nut and probe (nipple) (Fig. 4.20) for a gas-specific non-interchangeable connection to a branch of the regulated pressure pipework of the machine extra to the usual complement of cylinder yokes. Provided that an appropriate spanner and an adequate stock of spare hose assemblies are to hand, such a system should be safe. To this end anaesthetic machines are now manufactured with the appropriate fittings (Fig. 4.21).

In addition to the above, and probably even more important, proper arrangements should be made for planned preventive maintenance by suitably qualified engineers, and one named member of the medical staff should be appointed to act in a supervisory and advisory capacity.

# Tests and Checks for PMGV Systems

The anaesthetist should be held responsible for checking only that part of the PMGV system between the terminal outlet and the patient. He should be able to take for granted the quality and unfailing supply of gases.

Quality control is usually considered to be the province of the hospital pharmacist, who should make, or have made, tests to confirm the identity of the gas, its purity and composition, and freedom from contaminants, including solid particulate matter. Compressed air should be examined for water vapour and oil mist. The pharmacist is usually responsible for maintaining adequate supplies of cylinders.

The engineering department is responsible for organizing both planned preventive maintenance and emergency repairs.

The portering staff are usually responsible for changing cylinders and holding a store of portable oxygen cylinders with flowmeters and suction equipment for use in emergencies or during shutdown for maintenance and alterations.

The anaesthetist is responsible for the correct insertion of his pipeline probes and any necessary adustments. A fuller description of 'cockpit drill' is to be found in Appendix IV, but at this point two simple tests may be recommended.

(1) *The single hose test*
  (a) Ensure that all cylinders connected to the anaesthesia machine, as well as flowmeters, are turned off.
  (b) Plug in the oxygen probe only and check that, on opening the oxygen flow control valve, oxygen flows only through the oxygen flowmeter and that no gas flows through any other flowmeter.
(2) When all probes are plugged in, give each a short, sharp tug to make sure they are properly engaged. It is possible, in older designs, for a probe to be retained in a socket 'park position' even vertically without proper connection having been made; no gas will flow.

The supplement to HTM 22, which should be consulted for further details, describes a 'permit to work' system. Essentially this is a code of practice in which the engineer discusses with the appropriate people the nature of the work to be done so that services such as oxygen and vacuum independent of the PMGV system may be made available as required. Only too often there has been a lack of communication between the medical, nursing and engineering staff, invariably because no one named person has been specified for responsibility in each discipline. The 'permit to work' document (Fig. 4.22) with no less than six parts to be completed (depending on the degree of hazard) may at first seem to be yet another proliferation of the already burdensome paperwork in hospitals. It does, however, increase safety and improve the relationships between departments.

HOSPITAL ...........................................                              PERMIT: 0789

**PERMIT TO WORK FOR PIPED MEDICAL GASES**

System to be isolated    OXYGEN:    N$_2$O:    VACUUM:    ENTONOX:    MEDICAL AIR: .......................
Delete as necessary.

**PART 1**  The piped medical gas system indicated above, supplying the following area,

...........................................................................................

may be taken out of service without hazard to patients
From ........................................    AM/PM on ................................................. date
until ........................................    AM/PM on ................................................. date
Signed ...........................................    Medical/Nursing Officer .................... date ................. time am/pm

**PART 2**  The piped medical gas system indicated above is isolated as follows at:-

The following work ONLY shall be carried out:-

Other associated Permits to Work in use are(a) Number ........................... issued to ........................... date ..............
(b) Number ........................... issued to ........................... date ..............

Signed Authorized Person ........................................... date ........................... time ........................... am/pm

**Figure 4.22** (*Continued overleaf*).

**PART 3** **I accept responsibility** for carrying out the work detailed in PART 2.

No attempt will be made by me or any person under my control to work on any other part of the installation. Should the work transpire to exceed that indicated in Part 2, I will advise the Authorized Person **IMMEDIATELY**.

Signed Competent Person .............................................. date ............................ time ............................. am/pm

**PART 4** I declare that:-
    * this permit to work is cancelled;
    * the work described in Part 2 has been completed;
    * all modifications have been incorporated on Drawing No. .................................................
* delete if inapplicable
    * the tests initialled overleaf have been carried out;
    * all valve keys have been returned;
    * the system is safe for use by patients

Signed Authorized Person .............................................. date ............................ time ............................. am/pm

**PART 5** I have been advised by the Authorized Person named in PART 4 that the system named above is now available for use.

Signed ............................................. Medical/Nursing Officer ................................. date .............. time .............. am/pm

I acknowledge receipt of the following valve keys:-

Signed Competent Person .............................................. date ............................ time ............................. am/pm

I acknowledge return of the following valve keys:-

Signed Authorized Person .............................................. date ............................ time ............................. am/pm

I declare that in conjunction with the work detailed in PART 2, the following tests and/or procedures were carried out:-

| Test | Initials | Date |
|---|---|---|
| Valve Tightness | | |
| Pipeline Pressure Tests | | |
| Anti-confusion Tests | | |
| Flow Rate Test | | |
| Delivery Pressure | | |
| Alarm Test | | |
| Cleaning Procedure | | |
| Purging Procedure | | |
| Purity Test | | |
| Manifold Changeover | | |
| Relief Valve Operation | | |

Signed Authorized Person .............................................. date ............................... time ............................. am/pm

**Figure 4.22** A 'permit to work' form.

# 5 Measurement of Gas Flow and Volume

## Introduction

The measurement of gas flow is a complex and fascinating subject. Knowledge of gas flow rate and measurement of inhaled and exhaled gas volumes are very important to the safe practice of anaesthesia. In view of the current and future development of electronic measurement and control of gas flow in anaesthesia, a broad survey of flow measurement will be presented.

Flow measurement techniques may be classified in several ways. Flowmeters may respond to gas velocity, volumetric flow, gas momentum or mass flow. *Velocity meters* measure the gas flow at a specific point in the cross section of the flow and in anaesthetic practice are calibrated to approximate to the total volume flowing. *Volumetric flowmeters* respond to the entire flow of gas whatever the velocity profile across the diameter of the tube. An example of a volumetric flowmeter is the positive-displacement meter used for measuring domestic gas consumption, also used in medicine to measure exhaled minute volume. *Differential pressure flowmeters* respond to the momentum of the moving gas. *Mass flowmeters* measure directly the total mass of gas passing during a period of time.

There are many thousands of designs of flow-metering devices but those relevant to gas flow in anaesthesia may be classified as follows: differential pressure, variable area, inferential, positive-displacement, anemometric, ultrasonic, and fluidic. The choice of flow measurement technique depends, in the main, upon the characteristics required, as shown in Table 5.1.

## Differential Pressure Flowmeters

The differential pressure flowmeter is very versatile

**Table 5.1** Characteristics required of flow and volume measurement in anaesthesia

1. Gas flow *into* breathing system
   Continuous flow
   Dry gas
   Resistance to flow irrelevant
   Slow response to change in flow rate
   Single or mixed gases

2. Gas flow and volume *within* breathing system*
   Intermittent flow
   Wide range of flow rates
   Rapid response
   Very low resistance to flow
   Mixed gas composition
   High humidity
   Integration of flow, breath-by-breath

* NB. *Exhaled* volumes should *always* be measured rather than inspiratory, as then the anaesthetist always has an indication that *at least this volume* has been exhaled and none of it lost through leaks.

and probably the most common flowmeter used for industrial flow measurement. It finds application in anaesthesia both for machine gas flow and respiratory gas flow measurement.

A constant resistance is applied to the total gas flow and the pressure drop across the resistance is measured with a pressure gauge, manometer or, for very rapid response to changes in flow rate, an electronic pressure transducer. The resistance may be tubular, when the flow rate is proportional to the differential pressure; an orifice, in which case the pressure drop is proportional to the square of the flow rate; or a venturi (Fig. 5.1).

The Fleisch pneumotachograph is a constant-orifice differential pressure flowmeter designed to have a very low resistance to flow and a fast response rate necessary for the measurement of

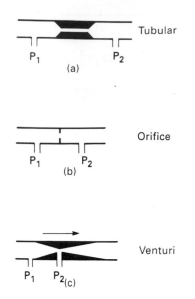

Figure 5.1 Differential pressure flowmeters.

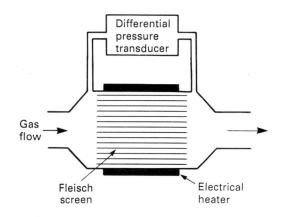

**Figure 5.2** Fleisch pneumotachograph.

# Variable-Area Constant Differential Pressure Flowmeters

In the variable-area constant differential pressure flowmeter the size of the orifice varies with flow rate. The variation in size of the orifice maintains a constant pressure differential, and gives the indication of the flow rate. The most common constant-pressure variable-area flowmeter in anaesthetic practice is the Rotameter. Strictly speaking, Rotameter is the trade name used by one manufacturer, Elliot Automation, but it has become synonymous with this type of flowmeter. The Rotameter is the final development in a line of earlier constant-pressure flowmeters (Coxeter, Heidbrink, McKesson, Connel) that have been used in anaesthesia.

The Rotameter (Fig. 5.3) consists of a vertical tapered metering tube and a float which is free to move up and down in it. For a given flow rate, the float remains stationary since the forces of differential pressure, gravity, viscosity, density and buoyancy are all balanced. When there is zero flow, the float rests at the bottom of the measuring tube where the maximum diameter of the float is the same as the bore of the tube. When gas enters the inlet at the base, the float rises, allowing gas to flow through the annular space between the float and the wall of the tube. The float moves up or down in proportion to the increase or decrease in the gas flow rate such that the pressure drop across the float remains constant, higher flows requiring a larger annular area than lower flows. At low flow rates, flow is a function of viscosity because the comparatively longer and narrower annulus behaves like a tube. With higher flow rates, the annulus is shorter and wider and behaves like an orifice and is therefore density dependent. The float has oblique notches cut in the rim so that it rotates freely in the middle of the gas stream and should normally not touch the walls of the tube. There is therefore no tendency for it to stick unless the Rotameter is out of the vertical plane. The taper of the bore of the Rotameter tube may be constructed so that it varies in order to elongate part of the scale as shown in Fig. 5.4. This has the advantage that, even with a short tube, low flows may be measured accurately, while high flows are also indicated.

respiratory gas flows (Fig. 5.2). A linear flow resistance is provided by a bundle of small-bore parallel tubes in the gas pathway. Its accuracy, sensitivity and response rate are dependent on the quality of the differential pressure transducer. The Fleisch screen is electrically heated to prevent water condensation affecting the calibration.

In the venturi flowmeter, the gas is passed through a narrowed portion of tubing. The gas accelerates in that portion and the pressure is less than in the broader part of the tube. The pressure difference is approximately proportional to the square of the flow rate and thus may be used to indicate flow.

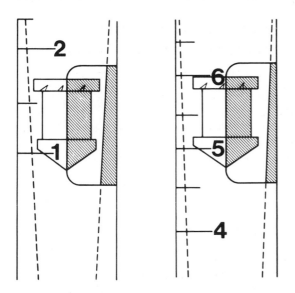

**Figure 5.3** The Rotameter. In each case a portion of the tube has been cut away to show that the gap, or annulus, varies with the flow rate. The calibration should be read from the top of the float (e.g. in the right-hand diagram the flow rate is 6 litres/min).

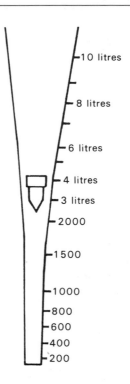

**Figure 5.4** A flowmeter tube with varying taper to give an elongated scale at lower flow rates but allowing calibration for high flow rates also.

## Calibration of Rotameters

Rotameters may be calibrated with great accuracy. Flowmeter tubes are calibrated individually, with their floats, at a specific pressure and temperature. Should there be any back pressure, for example when a minute volume divider ventilator is used, the density of the gas is increased and therefore the calibrations become inaccurate. In some old anaesthetic machines, particularly in the USA, the flow control valves are fitted downstream of the flowmeters. This results in the flowmeters being pressurized at the regulated pressure and they need to be calibrated for these conditions. This prevents variations in back pressure. Figure 5.5 demonstrates the principle of a pressure-compensated flowmeter.

Changes in temperature, except when extreme, cause inaccuracies which are insignificant in clinical practice.

Flowmeters should be read from the top of the float. They are not calibrated from zero to the top of the scale, but from the lowest accurate point, and this is the lowest mark on the scale. Readings by extrapolation below this mark should not be attempted. A typical tube may be calibrated from 100 to 8000 ml/min, with the lower part of the scale elongated by a more gradual taper.

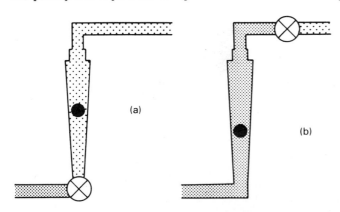

**Figure 5.5** A pressure-compensated flowmeter. In (a) the flow control valve is upstream from the flowmeter tube. Any output resistance, as for example when minute volume divider ventilators are being used, will result in compression of the gas, leading to a false reading. In (b) the flow control valve is downstream from the flowmeter tube. The flowmeter tube is therefore constantly pressurized (pressure compensated) at the supply pressure, at which the tube must be calibrated.

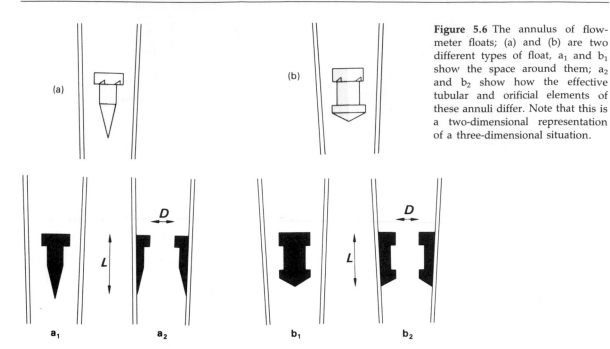

**Figure 5.6** The annulus of flowmeter floats; (a) and (b) are two different types of float, $a_1$ and $b_1$ show the space around them; $a_2$ and $b_2$ show how the effective tubular and orificial elements of these annuli differ. Note that this is a two-dimensional representation of a three-dimensional situation.

### Causes of inaccuracy in Rotameters

*Tube not vertical.* The orifice between the float and the tube is an annulus of complex shape (Fig. 5.6). If the tube is not vertical, the shape of the annulus becomes asymmetrical and at certain flow rates there is a significant variation in the proportion of the orifice and tubular elements of the resistance, and therefore inaccuracies occur. If the flowmeter is grossly out of the vertical position, then the float may come into contact with the wall of the tube and the resulting friction will cause even greater inaccuracy.

*Static electricity.* The float may also stick to the side of the tube as a result of static electricity, particularly in very dry atmospheres. Moist air can discharge static from the outside of the tube. The effects of static may be reduced by spraying the outside of the tube with an antistatic agent. Improvements may also be made by coating the inside of the tube with a transparently thin layer of a conductor such as gold.

*Dirt.* Dirt on the tube or float may also cause sticking, especially in the case of nitrous oxide. Even if they do not cause sticking, particles of dirt either on the float or on the inner wall of the tube can change the effective diameter of the annulus and therefore cause an inaccurate reading. In some older machines, the wire stop at the upper limit of the Rotameter was shaped in such a way that the float could become impaled upon it. When the gas supply is turned off or fails, the float may remain at the top of the tube and give the impression that there is still a high rate of flow. Some flowmeters of the Rotameter type are so constructed that the top of the tube is hidden behind the bezel, so that accidental high flow rates of carbon dioxide may not be observed.

### Causes of failure of Rotameters

On a number of occasions patients have suffered oxygen deprivation due to leakage from a cracked or broken flowmeter tube in a flowmeter block arranged so that the oxygen is at the upstream end. If, for example, the carbon dioxide tube is broken, the force of the nitrous oxide flow will tend to cause a much higher proportion of oxygen than nitrous oxide to leak out of the fractured tube. This is prevented by making sure that the oxygen is the last gas to enter the mixed gas flow (Fig. 5.7). In fact, ISO 5358 requires that '. . . the oxygen shall be delivered downstream of all other gases . . .'.

## Inferential Flowmeters

The commonest example of the inferential type of flowmeter in anaesthetic practice is the Wright's respirometer (Fig. 5.8) which is, in fact, an *integrating* flowmeter since it indicates volume rather than flow rate.

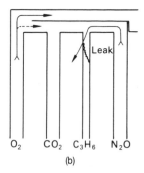
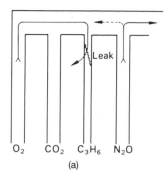

(a)

(b)

**Figure 5.7** Diagram to show the effect of a leak from one of the Rotameter tubes. (a) A leak from the cyclopropane tube in the traditional form of flowmeter block would result in back pressure from the nitrous oxide, causing oxygen to escape through the leak. The patient would therefore receive an anoxic mixture. (b) A rearrangement whereby the oxygen is the last gas to enter the mixed gas flow and nitrous oxide rather than oxygen would be expelled through a leak. This would not lead to the patient receiving an anoxic mixture.

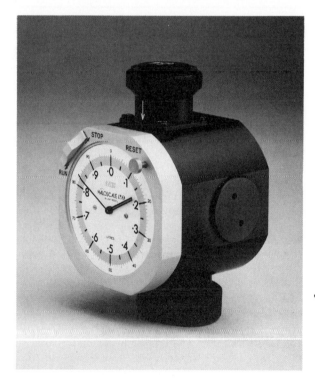

**Figure 5.8** Inferential type of flowmeter, colloquially referred to as the Wright's respirometer.

The Wright's respirometer is a turbine flowmeter, the principle of which is shown in Fig. 5.9. Exhaled gas is induced to flow around the stator, which has a series of tangential slits that cause a circular motion of the gas flow that produces rotation of the vane. In the mechanical version, the rate of rotation of the vane is reduced by a gear-train so that a single revolution of the appropriate hand on the dial

(a)

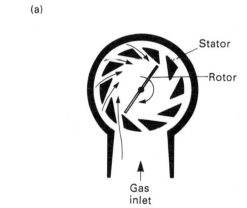

(b)

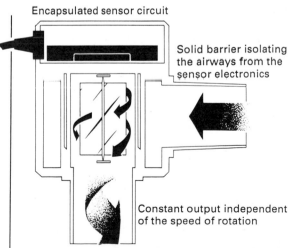

**Figure 5.9** (a) Plan view of the Wright's respirometer; (b) side view of electronic version of Wright's respirometer.

indicates one litre of gas having passed through the device. One of the problems of measuring exhaled gases is that they contain water vapour, which condenses on the internal parts of the respirometer. The mechanical version of the Wright's respirometer has a mercury seal interposed between the turbine and the gear-train to prevent water vapour condensing and the gears becoming corroded. It is also constructed so that only gases entering by the radial port cause movement of the vane, so that if it were mounted in a to-and-fro part of the breathing system, as when attached to a catheter mount, only gases passing in one direction would be measured.

Modern versions of the Wright's respirometer (Fig. 5.9b) overcome the water vapour and other problems by doing away with the gear-train and mechanical display and replacing them by detection of the rotation of the vane by means of a light source and photodetector or a Hall effect detector. The Hall effect detector is a semiconductor device which responds to very small changes in a magnetic field. These pulses are then converted electronically into indications of tidal and minute volume. Another advantage of these electronic versions is that alarms for minimum volumes and respiratory rate may be incorporated.

## Positive-Displacement Flowmeters

Positive-displacement flowmeters are mechanical meters that measure total volumetric flow over the entire diameter of the pipe through which the gas is flowing. Two types of positive displacement flowmeters are commonly used in anaesthesia, namely the intermeshing figure-of-eight rotors type and the

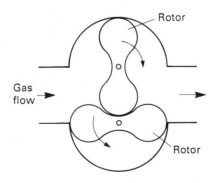

**Figure 5.10** Principle of the Dräger volumeter.

diaphragm meter.

The Dräger *volumeter* (Fig. 5.10) consists of a pair of intermeshing rotors connected via a gear-train to an analogue scale as is the case with the Wright's respirometer. Again, its accuracy and susceptibility to water vapour are improved by using an electronic transducer rather than the gear-train.

The diaphragm or bellows flowmeter is a simple, inexpensive and reliable meter of moderate accuracy, widely used as a domestic gas meter. It will not be described in detail here as it finds application mainly in physiological research for measuring minute volume.

## Anemometry

Anemometers measure gas *velocity* at a given *point*, and do not necessarily give the actual total flow rate along the tube. For this reason they are sometimes referred to as insertion meters, especially when the point of velocity measurement is very small compared with the total cross-section of the tube. The hot-wire anemometer is the only type of anemometer used in anaesthetic practice and has only recently been introduced. This is because it is too dangerous to use them in the presence of flammable anaesthetic agents. An electrically heated element in the form of a very fine resistance wire, a thin metallic film or a thermistor, is placed within the stream of gas. The passing gas tends to cool the element, and the higher the flow rate the greater the cooling; the change in temperature causes a change in electrical resistance. If a constant current is used to heat the element, then the voltage across the element will vary inversely with flow rate. The finer the element, the faster the response time. A hot-wire anemometer transducer is very small, lightweight and easy to sterilize or make disposable. It has a very low resistance to gas flow. However, the wire may be very delicate and there is a need for fairly frequent calibration.

## Fluidic Flowmeters

Fluidic flowmeters rely on some dynamic instability in the gas which generates an oscillation whose frequency is proportional to the flow rate.

Ohmeda uses a flowmeter in its current machines

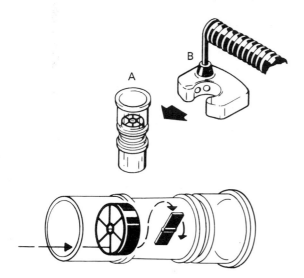

**Figure 5.11** Sensor components for the Ohmeda respiratory volume monitor. This sensor assembly is composed of two parts: A, cartridge and B, optical sensor clip.

that uses a series of fixed vanes to induce a swirl that is detected by causing the rotation of a single vane, as shown in Fig. 5.11. The rotation of the vane is sensed optically.

The vortex-shedding flowmeter has a very low resistance to gas flow and no moving parts. A laminar flow of gas is passed along a smooth-bore tube that has a bluff body causing a very small obstruction. Vortices are generated when the gas hits the bluff body (Fig. 5.12). The frequency of shedding is linearly proportional to the flow rate. In anaesthetic practice, the vortices are detected by their interruption of a narrow ultrasonic beam.

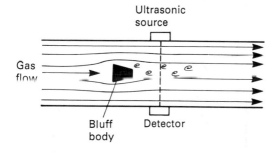

**Figure 5.12** Vortex shedding flow transducer.

# Ultrasonic Flowmeters

The term *ultrasonic* indicates that 'sound' above the reception capability of the human ear is the physical principle of operation. Frequencies used are usually over 1 MHz. There are two ways of measuring flow ultrasonically. The Doppler principle is not applicable to respiratory gas flow measurement as the technique requires particulate impurities to be present in the gas to reflect the 'sound'; doppler flowmetering is very successful in measuring liquid flow as most liquids contain minute bubbles and blood contains cells. Ultrasound can be used to measure gas flow by using the 'time-of-flight' or 'transit time' principle. Sound takes a finite time to travel through a gaseous medium. If short pulses of ultrasound are injected into a gas flow and then detected at a fixed distance from the source, the time taken will be altered proportionately with the rate of gas flow. This type of flowmeter has a low resistance to flow, very fast response, and is easily sterilized. However, it is very expensive.

# Spirometers

*Spirometer* is a term used to describe devices that are used to measure exhaled tidal volumes and flow rates.

The commonest single-breath spirometer in clinical use is that manufactured by the Vitalograph company and is shown in Fig. 5.13. Exhaled gas from the patient causes a lightweight bellows to be filled, causing a stylus to move across a chart at the same time as the chart is moved at a constant speed at right angles to the stylus movement. Thus a chart of exhaled volume against time is plotted from which volumes and flow rates may be deduced.

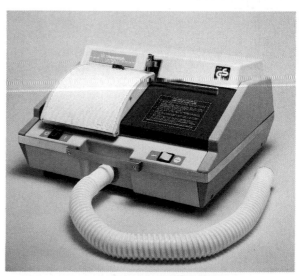

**Figure 5.13** Vitalograph single-breath spirometer.

There are now available a number of inexpensive, pocket-sized 'spirometers' that use microprocessor techniques to measure FEV (Forced Expiratory Volume), $FEV_1$ (Forced Expiratory Volume in 1 s) and VC (Vital Capacity), using differential pressure flow transducers.

Calibrated bellows may also be used to measure exhaled gas volume. Very lightweight bellows are inflated against gravity by the gas exhaled from the patient. These are usually part of the ventilator and may be inaccurate because of leaks in the breathing attachment or around the endotracheal cuff, and also because of the comparatively enormous compliant volume in the expiratory circuit of some ventilators.

# 6　Vaporizers

## Introduction

Many inhalational anaesthetic agents are liquids under normal conditions and need to be vaporized before they can be administered to a patient. They are not used as pure vapours but are diluted by a carrier gas such as air or pure oxygen or by a gaseous mixture of nitrous oxide and oxygen. The various anaesthetic inhalational agents have widely differing properties and hence require vaporizers constructed specifically for each agent. Very potent agents (halothane, enflurane and isoflurane) require vaporizers that can accurately control the concentration of vapour leaving the vaporizer. However, agents such as diethyl ether, with a lower potency, may be used safely with simpler apparatus (if necessary) in which the vapour concentration is not accurately known, since there is less risk of overdosage.

## Vaporization of Liquid Anaesthetic Agents

In constructing a suitable vaporizing system to provide clinically effective vapour concentrations, the following principles need to be considered. The ease with which sufficient quantity of anaesthetic vapour can be produced depends on:

- the ease with which molecules of the agent leave the liquid phase to become a vapour above that liquid (i.e. its volatility) (see Table 6.1);
- the temperature of the liquid (the warmer it is, the more easily it vaporizes);
- the temperature of the carrier gas flowing over the liquid;
- the rate at which carrier gas flows across the surface of the liquid to be vaporized;

**Table 6.1** Volatile inhalation anaesthetic drugs

|  | Potency MAC* value (vol. %) | Vapour pressure (mmHg; 20°C) | Boiling point (°C; 760 mmHg) | Induction time | Induction (%) | Maintenance (%) | Recovery time | Analgesic property | Colour |
|---|---|---|---|---|---|---|---|---|---|
| Diethyl ether | 1.92 | 450 | 35 | Moderate | 10–30 | 5–15 | Moderate | Yes | Clear |
| Trichloroethylene | 0.20 | 60 | 87 | Slow | 2.5 | 1–1.5 | Slow | Yes | Blue |
| Halothane | 0.76 | 243 | 51 | Rapid | 3–5 | 0.5–2 | Rapid | None | Clear |
| Methoxyflurane | 0.16 | 22.5 | 104 | Slow | 3 (+) | 0.25–1 | Slow | Yes | Clear |
| Enflurane | 1.68 | 180 | 56 | Rapid | 3–5 | 1.5–3 | Rapid | Yes? None claimed | Clear |
| Isoflurane | 1.15 | 238 | 48 | Rapid | 1.5–3 | 1–2.5 | Rapid | None claimed | Clear |

*MAC = Minimum alveolar concentration (vol. %) at 1 atm, which produces immobility in 50% of subjects exposed to noxious stimuli.

- the surface area of contact between carrier gas and liquid;
- the shape and volume of the vaporizing system containing the liquid. Chapter 1 explains the laws governing vaporization in more detail.

# Vaporizing Systems (Draw-over Systems)

## Open drop method

The earliest method of vaporizing anaesthetic agents such as ether and chloroform was to pour the liquid drop by drop into a napkin that was placed close to the patient's mouth and nose. The spread of the liquid over the napkin increased the surface area for vaporization and the vapour concentration was gradually raised by increasing the number of drops per minute. The napkin was later replaced by devices such as the Schimmelbusch mask (Fig. 6.1) There are several varieties of the mask, but in essence it consists of a metal frame over which gauze or lint is spread. In the case of ether, the liquid is dropped evenly over the whole area of the gauze, whereas with chloroform it is restricted to one half of it, in order to ensure that the air may be freely inhaled without too high a concentration of the vapour. For ether 16 thin layers of gauze are put on the mask, whereas for ethyl chloride or chloroform 12 layers of gauze or one of lint are used. When ether is being used its high rate of vaporization requires so much latent heat that the mask becomes cool and water vapour from the exhaled air may condense on it and eventually freeze. This not only causes increased resistance to the air passing through the gauze, but also reduces the rate of vaporization. For this reason a second mask, or a fresh supply of gauze, is required during a long administration. When using the Schimmelbusch mask it is customary to cover the patient's face with a piece of gamgee about 25 × 20 cm and to cut (or tear) in this a central hole to expose the patient's nose and mouth (Fig. 6.2). The gamgee is used primarily in order to prevent vapour or liquid from entering the patient's eyes, but it also reduces the amount of air drawn in by the patient between the mask and his face. Sometimes a similar piece of gamgee is used to cover up the mask. Open drop administration has little place in modern anaesthesia, and anaesthetic vapours are usually introduced into breathing systems by vaporizers sited away from the patient's face.

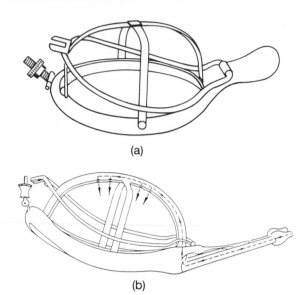

(a)

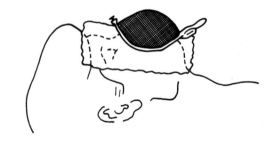

(b)

**Figure 6.1** (a) The Chadbourne modification of the Schimmelbusch mask. (b) Another modification, in which oxygen or anaesthetic gases may be delivered via the two perforated tubes.

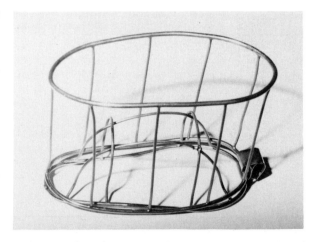

**Figure 6.2** A layer of gamgee over the patient's face protects his eyes during open-drop administration.

**Figure 6.3** Ogston's inhaler.

## Semi-open drop method

In this technique a mask somewhat similar to the Schimmelbusch was used, but this mask, the Ogston's inhaler, was surmounted by a wire frame round which a napkin or some gauze could be erected in order to 'keep the ether in' (see Fig. 6.3). These early vaporizers inherited the name 'draw-over' because the carrier gas was drawn over the surface of the vaporizing liquid by the patient's own inspiratory effort. However, this system provided unknown quantities of anaesthetic vapour because the vaporizer (the cloth) rapidly cooled, providing very variable vaporizing temperatures; the flow rate of carrier gas varied both with inspiration and depth of anaesthesia; and the vaporizing surface area diminished as ice crystals formed in the cloth.

## Modern draw-over systems

These systems employ a number of compensating devices (see Fig. 6.4). These include:
- a heat source (or heat sink). This normally takes the form of a waterbath or metal jacket that surrounds the vaporizing liquid in order to keep it from cooling too rapidly;
- a flow-splitting valve to vary the proportion of carrier gas either entering or bypassing the vaporizer. This device exerts some control over the quantity of vapour leaving the vaporizer;
- a temperature-compensating device (in this case a bimetallic strip) to compensate for the inevitable fall in vaporizing temperature (albeit buffered by

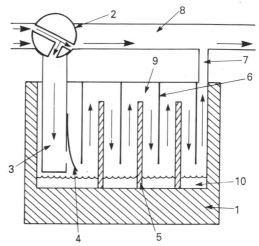

1  Heat sink
2  Flow-splitting valve
3  Inlet
4  Bi-metallic strip
5  Wick
6  Baffles
7  Outlet
8  By-pass
9  Vaporizing chamber
10 Liquid level

**Figure 6.4** The tap controls the proportion of the carrier gas flow that passes through the vaporization chamber, as compared with that which passes through the bypass and does not come into contact with the liquid anaesthetic agent. In the 'off' position the whole of the fresh gas flow passes through the bypass.

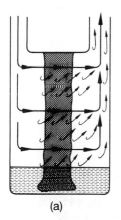
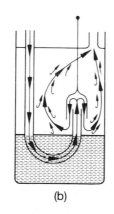
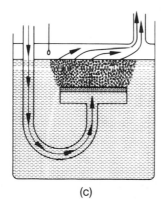
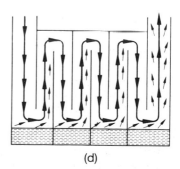

(a)　　　　(b)　　　　(c)　　　　(d)

**Figure 6.5** Methods of increasing the vaporization rate in a vaporizer. (a) The liquid anaesthetic agent is drawn up a wick, thus presenting a greater surface area for vaporization. (b) The mixed gas flow is directed onto the surface of the liquid anaesthetic agent by a cowl. (c) The mixed gases are broken up into a large number of bubbles, which pass through the liquid anaesthetic agent, thus presenting the maximum possible surface area to the liquid. (d) A series of baffles repeatedly redirect the mixed gas flow onto the surface of the liquid anaesthetic agent.

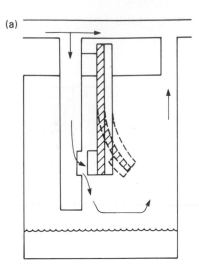

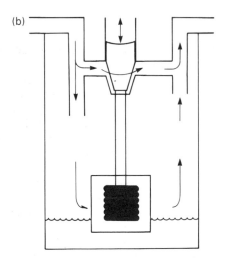

**Figure 6.6** (a) Bimetallic strip, as used in the TEC range of vaporizers. (b) Ether-filled bellows, as used in Penlon vaporizers.

the heat sink) and subsequent fall in vapour concentration during prolonged use;
- the use of wicks and other devices (Fig. 6.5) to increase the surface area for vaporization.

*Heat sink.* When a liquid releases its vapour, it is the molecules with most energy that leave the liquid to form this vapour, i.e. the 'hottest' molecules. The remaining liquid becomes cooler, having lost its hottest molecules. If it is surrounded by a heat reservoir (heat sink), this heat will be transferred to the liquid, reducing the rate at which its temperature drops. Thus a vaporizer with a heat sink will

sustain a lower fall in operating temperature and a more controlled vapour output than one without such a device.

*Flow-splitting valves.* There are rotary valves incorporated within the vaporizer inlet. They proportion the flow of carrier gas between the vaporizing chamber and the vaporizer bypass system, thus controlling the final vapour composition (i.e. the more gas going through the vaporizer chamber, the greater the amount of vapour leaving the vaporizer). The flow-splitting valve is calibrated in percentage of the vapour in the final gas/vapour composition. However, this valve is accurate only if the vaporizer is temperature-compensated (see below).

*Temperature-compensating devices (see Fig. 6.6a, b).* As the vaporizing liquid cools, a greater proportion of carrier gas is required to pass through the vaporizing chamber in order to collect the same number of vapour molecules required to maintain the expected output of the vaporizer. This is achieved by using devices that sense temperature changes and which then alter the flow through the vaporizer.

Two types are commonly used. The first (Fig. 6.6a), consists of two dissimilar metals or alloys placed back to back (i.e. a bimetallic strip). As the two metals have different rates of expansion and contraction with temperature, the device has the ability to 'bend'. It can therefore be used to vary the degree of occlusion in the aperture of the gas channel into the vaporizer chamber and thus alter the flow of carrier gases through it.

A second arrangement (Fig. 6.6b) uses the expansion and contraction properties of an ether-filled copper bellows for the same purpose. The bellows produces movement changes in one plane and hence produces a linear change in gas flow resistance (making calibration easier). The resistance produced by a bimetallic strip is nonlinear.

As both the temperature-compensating mechanism and the flow-splitting valve work by altering resistance through the vaporizer chamber, the devices are dependent on each other. Therefore, each vaporizer should be individually calibrated at the factory (see below) at a specific temperature and flow rate of carrier gas. Ideally, it should also be calibrated at a specific barometric pressure. Strictly speaking, as a saturated vapour is only altered by temperature, one might expect the calibration of a vaporizer to be independent of barometric pressure. However changes in barometric pressure will affect the carrier gas composition passing through the vaporizer, which in turn will affect the concentration of vapour in the mixture leaving it. For example, when the barometric pressure is reduced (at altitude) the number of molecules of carrier gas flowing through the vaporizer is reduced. However the number of vapour molecules collected by the gas in the vaporizing chamber remains unchanged, although these now represent a higher percentage of the total number of molecules leaving the vaporizer. This effect, however, is so small under the normal operating conditions, that it is inconsequential.

Despite use of the measures mentioned above, vapour output is still sensitive to the variable flow rate caused by the intermittent demand from either a patient- or a bellows-operated breathing system (see below). Furthermore, a draw-over vaporizer requires a very low-resistance pathway through it in order not to embarrass the respiratory efforts of a spontaneously breathing patient. This restricts the design of the vaporizer components, especially the flow splitting valve (see below).

# Vaporizers for Use with Gases under Pressure and in Continuous Flow Anaesthetic Equipment (Plenum Vaporizers)

Draw-over systems are subjected to very variable flow rates, i.e. from 0 to 60 litres/minute (the peak inspiratory flow rate in a hyperventilating adult). At these higher flow rates the carrier gas produces a more rapid dilution of the available vapour in a vaporizing system, resulting in a reduced concentration leaving that vaporizer. A vaporizing system in which a smaller constant flow of gas flowing through the system is known, would allow the vaporizer to be calibrated more accurately. Plenum vaporizers are designed to work with carrier gases at more stable flow rates. In common with a modern draw-over vaporizer, a Plenum vaporizer has a heat sink (to compensate for the cooling effect caused by vaporization), a flow splitting valve, wicks or other devices to increase the surface area of vaporization and a temperature-compensating device. The major difference between it and a draw-over vaporizer is the increased resistance to flow, particularly at the flow-splitting valve (see below), which requires the carrier gases to be passed through the vaporizer under pressure.

# Other Factors Affecting Vapour Concentration

## Extremes of temperature

It is obvious that a temperature-compensating mechanism can operate only within a reasonable temperature range. At too low a temperature, vaporization will be low, and it may be uncontrollably high when it is too hot. In the case of the Emotril obstetric analgesia apparatus, for example, the temperature is indicated on a dial which shows whether the ambient temperature is within safe limits.

## Pumping effect

When gas-driven ventilators of the 'minute volume divider' type such as the Manley are employed, or even when manually assisted or controlled ventilation is used, there is a 'back pressure' exerted on the vaporizer. This back pressure is intermittent or variable and causes an oscillating flow of carrier gas in the vaporization chamber, increasing the vapour pick-up. Furthermore, a sufficient surge in back pressure can force saturated vapour back through the vaporizer and into the bypass circuit. This further increases the vapour concentration, especially at low fresh gas flows when the gas destined to go through the bypass will be increasingly contaminated by saturated vapour.

This effect is now minimized by the fitting of internal compensating mechanisms. It may be achieved either by increasing the resistance to flow through the vaporizer and bypass, which in turn reduces the amount of back-flow of saturated gas. This requires the carrier gas to develop a higher pressure in order to pass through the vaporizer, hence the rationale for calling these vaporizers 'Plenum' (forcing gas in and out). The pumping effect may also be minimized by building an elongated flow passage into either the inlet or outlet of the vaporizer to prevent saturated vapour entering the bypass circuit. Some vaporizer designs employ both mechanisms.

Furthermore anaesthetic machines now incorporate a non return valve on the end of the back bar so that these back pressure surges on the vaporizer are reduced. However, pressure still builds up to some extent in the back bar when the non return valve closes due to high downstream pressure. Prior to this, some older anaesthetic machines were modified to take a flow restrictor on the end of the back bar as a stop gap measure to restrict these back pressure surges. Paradoxically, the flow restrictor itself caused a pressure to build up in the back bar and within the vaporizer. The pressure increase due to vaporizer design should be as small as possible, as these pressures are transmitted back to the flowmeters, which are calibrated for use at atmospheric pressure.

### Flow-splitting valves

It is very difficult to design a flow-splitting valve that will work accurately over a wide range of flow rates, i.e. 1–60 litres/min. In a draw-over vaporizer, the valve must possess a low flow resistance so that at flows of 60 litres/min (the peak flow in a patient breathing spontaneously) no respiratory embarrassment is caused. However, if the flow across this valve drops to about 4 litres/min, the resistance through the valve will be so low that carrier gas will preferentially pass across the bypass channel rather than through the vaporizing chamber where it has to mix with and then push the 'heavy' vapour out into the attached breathing system. At this flow and below, there is therefore bound to be a marked fall in vaporizer performance.

A Plenum vaporizer may be required to work accurately with carrier gas flows as low as 1 litre/min. In order to divert sufficient carrier gas into the vaporizer at these low flows, the flow-splitting valve is constructed with smaller, high-resistance gas channels. Furthermore, the gas pathway through the vaporizer itself is constructed so as to cause an appreciable resistance to flow. These two factors allow the sufficient build up of pressure within the vaporizer required to push the relatively heavy vapour out. The typical flow resistance (2 kPa (22 cm $H_2O$) at 5 litres/min) found in plenum vaporizers renders them unsuitable for use as draw-over vaporizers.

The final design of a Plenum vaporizer therefore, develops from a compromise between the high carrier gas pressures required for accurate vapour delivery, and the low pressures required to maintain the accuracy of the flowmeters.

### Gas direction

With some vaporizers, a higher concentration of vapour is given if, by misconnection, the gas is made to pass in the reverse direction.

### Liquid levels

The liquid level within the vaporizing chamber may affect performance. If the vaporizer is overfilled, insufficient exposed surface area of wick may cause a drop in output concentration of vapour. On the other hand, overfilling may result in dangerously high concentrations, due to spilling of liquid agent into the bypass.

### Halothane

The anaesthetic agent halothane contains a stabilizing agent, thymol. This is a waxy substance which, if left in the vaporizer, clogs the wick, reducing the potential surface area for vaporization. This then reduces the vaporizer performance. Thymol may also 'gum up' the vaporizer making the control knob difficult to adjust, as well as compromising the internal mechanism. The manufacturers therefore advise that the liquid agent be drained off and replenished at intervals of two weeks. This advice should be tempered by consideration of economy and the frequency with which the vaporizer is employed.

### Carrier gas composition

Vaporizer output may be affected when the carrier gas composition is changed. This is due to changes in viscosity and density which alter the performance of the flow-splitting valve. Increasing the concentration of nitrous oxide reduces the vapour concentration. However, this is of little importance in clinical practice. There is also a further but temporary decrease in vaporizer output when nitrous oxide concentrations are increased: nitrous oxide dissolves in volatile agents, so that the effective total gas flow through the vaporizer is temporarily reduced.

### Stability

Many vaporizers, if tilted, may allow the liquid agent to contaminate the bypass. A fatal outcome has occurred when a vaporizer was accidentally overturned. Liquid halothane was thought to have run into the bypass and into the patient's lungs. Even if the spilled agent found in the breathing system did not reach the patient as a liquid, the vapour concentration could be so high as to have fatal results.

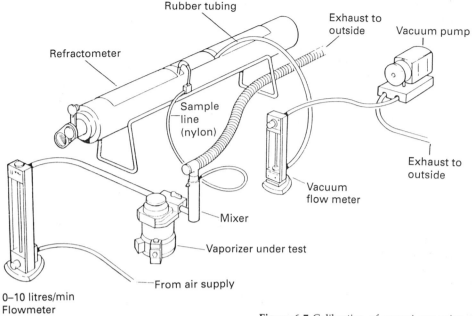

Rubber tubing

Exhaust to outside

Vacuum pump

Refractometer

Sample line (nylon)

Exhaust to outside

Vacuum flow meter

Mixer

Vaporizer under test

From air supply

0–10 litres/min Flowmeter (air)

**Figure 6.7** Calibration of vaporizers using a refractometer: general arrangement for room temperature (22°C) test.

## Summary of Vaporizer Performance

Vaporizer performance can thus be affected by:

- temperature (unless the vaporizer includes some compensatory device that minimizes the effect of temperature, such as a heat sink and/or temperature compensator);
- flow (all vaporizers are affected to some degree by flow (see performance data supplied with the various vaporizers described). Plenum vaporizers perform better than draw-over vaporizers;
- barometric pressure (minimal effect in clinical practice);
- variable vaporizer working pressures (back pressure surges);
- liquid levels within the vaporizer;
- movement and tilting of vaporizers (see under specific vaporizers below);
- carrier gas composition;
- stabilizers in the inhalational agent (e.g. thymol).

## Calibration of Vaporizers

Figure 6.7 illustrates how vaporizers are tested for calibration accuracy at the factory, both during

initial assembly and following servicing (see also pages 263–269). The output of the vaporizer is initially checked using a refractometer at room temperature (22°C) over a wide range of flow rates (1–10 litres/min).

## Filling of Vaporizers

In early systems (Boyle's bottles) the vaporizer jar was simply unscrewed, filled and reconnected. The TEC Marks 1 and 2 had a funnel-shaped filling port sealed by a screw-threaded stopper on the side of the vaporizer just above the maximum filling level. However, both systems were criticized in the late 1970s because neither system eliminated the potential for filling the vaporizer with the wrong agent. Agent-specific filling devices (Fraser Sweatman pin safety system; Fig. 6.8) were introduced by Cyprane (now Ohmeda) in the early 1980s in which the distal end was keyed to fit a specific vaporizer and the proximal end keyed to fit the neck of the bottle of the inhalational agent. Although this device goes some way to reducing the potential for filling vaporizers with the wrong agent, it is by no means foolproof. Some countries take supplies of agent in large bottles and then subsequently decant into smaller bottles. Early supplies of isoflurane into the UK could be fitted (prior to 1984) to enflurane-keyed fillers.

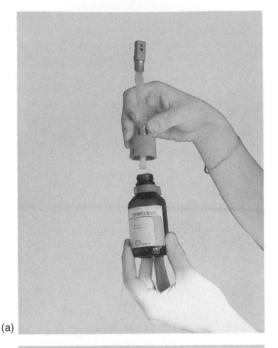

(a)

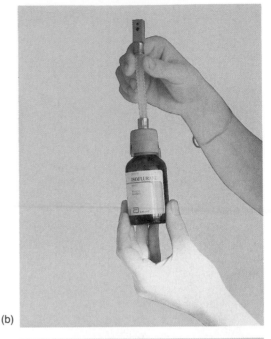

(b)

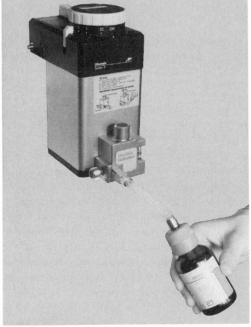

(c)

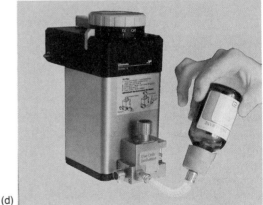

(d)

**Figure 6.8** The Fraser Sweatman pin safety system. The vaporizer filling parts are pin indexed to match the grooves on the filler nozzles. The bottle for each agent is fitted with a collar which only fits the relevant filler caps (a & b). (c) Insertion of the filler nozzle prior to filling or emptying. (d) Filling a vaporizer.

# Examples of Vaporizers

## The Boyle's vaporizer

This is a Plenum-type vaporizer (designed for continuous flow of carrier gases through it). It is not temperature compensated. The Boyle's vaporizer (Fig. 6.9) and similar types of 'bottle' were commonly used to vaporize ether, methoxyflurane (Penthrane) and trichloroethylene (Trilene), although none of these vapours is manufactured in the UK any longer. It is neither calibrated nor temperature or level compensated.

When the control lever is in the 'off' position, the mixed gas flow passes entirely through the bypass, as shown in Fig. 6.10. As the lever is turned progressively towards the 'on' position, a steadily

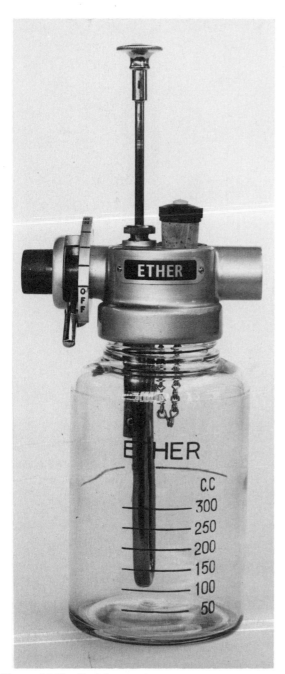

**Figure 6.9** The Boyle's vaporizer.

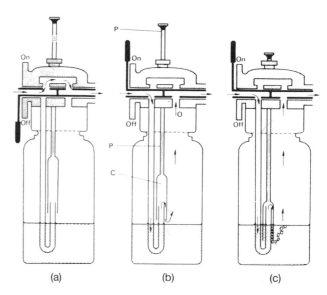

**Figure 6.10** Three schematics of the Boyle's vaporizer showing (a) the control lever in the 'off' position; (b) the control lever fully 'on' and the cowl C lowered so as to cause the gas to impinge on the surface of the liquid; (c) the cowl further lowered so as to cause the gas to bubble through the liquid.

6.10c, they are forced to bubble through the liquid, thus producing the maximum rate of vaporization. The position of the cowl is adjusted by the plunger P, which passes through a gland to maintain a gas-tight seal. The working parts of this vaporizer are best seen in an exploded diagram (Fig. 6.11). The control drum rotates inside the body of the vaporizer, and is positioned laterally by the adjusting and locking rings at each end. Special grease is used to maintain a seal and yet allow free rotation; there is spare grease in the grease injector cap and by turning this it can be fed into the seating of the drum. As gases and vapours pass through the vaporizer, even when it is turned off, the grease tends to be slowly washed away and this results in stiffness if extra grease is not added. In order to remove the drum for cleaning, the actuating lever is first unscrewed and then the locking and adjusting rings are removed from the inlet end. If the drum is so tight that it cannot be easily withdrawn, it can be pushed through by screwing inwards the adjusting ring at the other end. Note that in some instances the drum is conical and can be withdrawn only from one end. This operation is usually carried out by a service engineer.

### Problems with the Boyle's vaporizer

After long service the plunger may become loose and tend to fall down on its own. This can be

increasing proportion of gases is passed through the bottle. In the fully 'on' position all the gases pass through the bottle. The 'natural' path the gases would take is straight from the end of the U-tube to the outlet O. They may be diverted, however, by lowering the cowl C over the end of the U-tube, so that they impinge on the surface of the agent, as shown in Fig. 6.10b. With the cowl fully down, Fig.

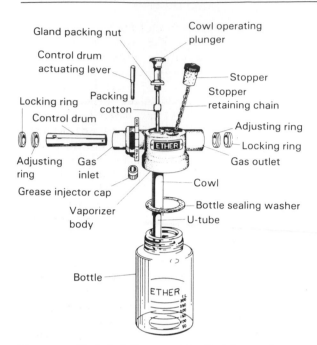

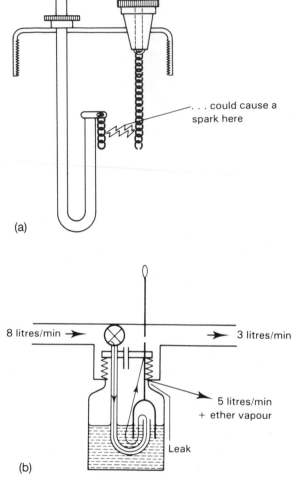

**Figure 6.11** Exploded diagram of the Boyle's vaporizer.

(a)

(b)

**Figure 6.12** Potential problems with the Boyle's vaporizer. (a) If the chain that retains the cork should break and the metal stud on top of the cork connect with it, it could act as a sparking-plug if touched by someone carrying static electricity. (b) A leak from the jar could result in the loss of much of the carrier gas and all of the ether vapour.

corrected by tightening the gland nut. Eventually the packing in the gland will need to be replaced. This usually consists of cotton, but in some of the more modern vaporizers the cotton is replaced by neoprene or nylon, which should not wear out. The cork stopper in the filling orifice should be a good fit, and is normally retained by a small chain. In some vaporizers the metal anchor for this chain passes through the cork. Should the chain be broken, this metal core to the cork could act as a sparking-plug if somebody who was charged with static electricity were to touch the metal cap (see Fig. 6.12a). For this reason it is important that the chain is intact. Sometimes the top of the cork is insulated so as to prevent this hazard.

The bottle sealing washer is usually made of cork, sometimes with a canvas or metal insert. It often becomes brittle and damaged and may fall out. This allows a leak of anaesthetic gases and vapour. There may also be a leak if the top of the bottle is chipped. This leak can assume considerable proportions and may lead to a situation where the gas flow reaching the reservoir bag is very much less than that indicated by the flowmeters and much of the volatile agent escapes (Fig. 6.12b). Rebreathing by the patient ensues, and this leads to difficulties during the induction and maintenance of inhalation anaesthesia.

It will be noticed that in some vaporizers the metal parts within the bottle are not plated but are left as bare copper. The reason for this is that copper

is an anticatalyst that prevents the decomposition of ether. Some bottles are made of dark glass, either brown or green, to prevent the decomposition of anaesthetic agents by light. Two sizes of bottle are commonly used, a broad one for ether and a narrow one for other volatile agents. In the case of chloroform and trichloroethylene a sufficient concentration is produced by turning the control lever fully on without depressing the plunger at all. Indeed, by doing so a dangerously high concentration would be produced. The concentration of vapour depends on the temperature (which drops as vaporization proceeds), the level of the liquid anaesthetic agent in the bottle and the rate of gas flow.

### Practical use of the Boyle's vaporizer

The graduations for the control lever are entirely arbitrary and as a rule the vaporizer begins to operate when the lever is at about the second mark. When using ether the lever should be turned on very slowly. A common practice is to advance it one-quarter of a division after each four consecutive regular breaths.

The bottle may be charged with as much as 270 ml (10 fl oz) of ether, which fills the bottle to nearly half full. In the case of trichloroethylene and chloroform only about 1-cm depth of the anaesthetic agent is used. Note that the Boyle's vaporizer is not particularly suitable for methoxyflurane because of the difficulty of producing a sufficiently high concentration of this agent for the induction of anaesthesia.

Because ether is so volatile, vapour pressure tends to build up in the bottle when it is turned off, especially if the anaesthetic machine is kept in a warm environment. If this has happened, there is a surge of high-concentration ether vapour when the vaporizer is turned on. This undesirable effect can be prevented by turning the vaporizer on and running a small quantity of mixed gases through it immediately prior to the anaesthetic being commenced, or simply by removing the stopper from the filler orifice for an instant.

Volatile anaesthetic agents used in the Boyle's vaporizer should be removed from the bottle after use, and preferably be discarded in order to prevent a risk of their being poured back into the wrong bottle. It is desirable that all agents should be characteristically coloured, but such an ideal has yet to be realized.

### Temperature-compensated vaporizers

From the foregoing it will be appreciated that the output concentration of a simple vaporizer may alter considerably from time to time, depending on flow rates, the length of time the vaporizer has been in use and the type of anaesthetic agent used. With some agents it is important that the vapour concentration be kept constant. Examples of how this may be achieved are shown in Figs 6.13 et seq.

*TEC 2 (Ohmeda).* Although obsolete this vaporizer is still in use in many parts of the world and is a good example of the principles of a temperature-compensated vaporizer. The Fluotec version is described in Fig. 6.13. In this vaporizer the gases pass through the vaporizer by two channels, one leading through a bypass and the other through the vaporization chamber. The proportion of gases passing through the bypass is determined by the calibrated control knob M, which operates the portions F and G of the valve, which are individually adjusted both by the manufacturer and during servicing. The fraction of gas passing through the vaporization chamber is varied not only by the position of this valve but also by a bimetallic thermostatic valve H, inside the vaporization chamber, where a series of wicks, saturated with halothane, present a very large area from which the agent evaporates. This ensures that the gases passing through the vaporization chamber are saturated with vapour. The percentage of halothane vapour at the outlet depends on the amount of vapour-laden gases that is mixed with the fresh gases passing through the bypass. As the temperature within the vaporization chamber falls (and therefore the vapour concentration in the gases passing through it also falls), the thermostatically operated valve opens wider and a greater proportion of the total gas flow passes through the chamber; by this means the vapour concentration in the output is kept constant.

*TEC 3 (Ohmeda).* Figure 6.14 shows a Fluotec version of the TEC 3 which operates in much the same way as the Mark 2 but incorporates several refinements. Note the improvement in accuracy of delivered vapour concentration at the lower carrier gas flow rates (Fig. 6.14c).

The *TEC 4* and *TEC 5* are shown in Figs 6.15 and 6.16 respectively. See captions for working principles. Table 6.2 highlights the differences between TECs 3, 4 and 5.

*Dräger 'Vapor' vaporizers.* Figure 6.17 shows an early model of the 'Vapor' range which did not have automatic temperature compensation. However, a thermometer is provided, together with a concentration adjustment control for compensation of variations in temperature. Figure 6.18 shows a recent model with automatic compensation.

*Penlon vaporizers.* This company utilizes stainless-steel wicks rather than cloth so that the vaporization chamber and wicks require less maintenance (Figs 6.19 and 6.20).

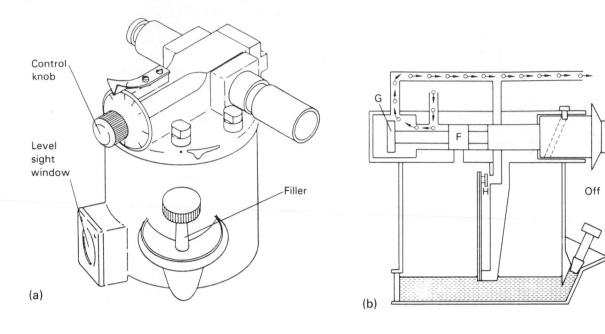

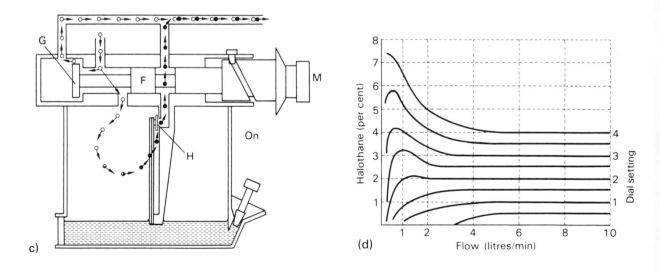

**Figure 6.13** (a) The TEC 2 vaporizer. (b) Schematic diagram showing how in the 'off' position all the gases are channelled through the bypass. (c) Schematic diagram showing how in the 'on' position a carefully metered proportion of the gases passes through the vaporization chamber. (d) Performance characteristics. NB. This vaporizer is now obsolete, but it is included here because so many are still in use.

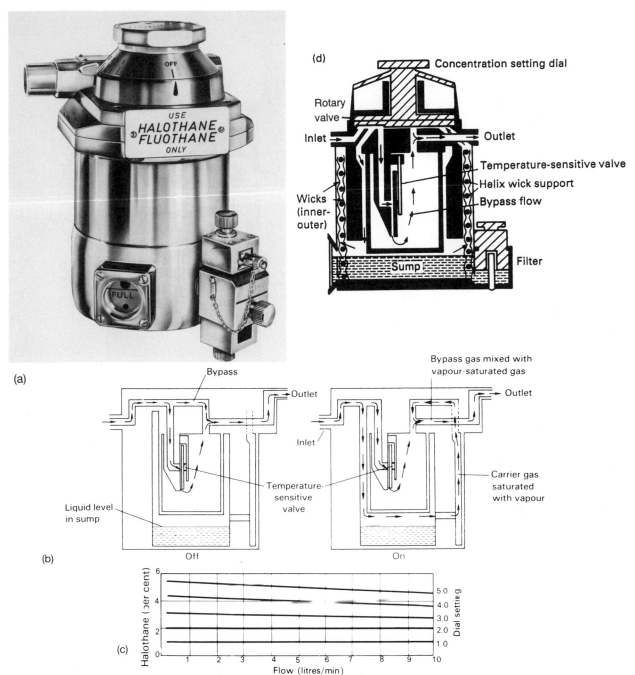

**Figure 6.14** (a) The TEC 3 vaporizer, which operates in much the same way as the Mark 2 but incorporates several refinements. (b) Working principles. For simplicity the control valve has been omitted. In the 'off' position the carrier gases pass through two passages, a simple bypass and a second bypass in which the flow is regulated by a temperature-sensitive valve. In the 'on' position the first bypass is closed but the second remains open, and the gases also pass through a passage leading to the vaporization chamber, the valve for which is opened to a degree according to the vapour concentration required. Note that in this vaporizer the carrier gases passing through the vaporization chamber are fully saturated owing to the large area of wicks from which the fluid evaporates. The pathway by which the vapour-laden gases leave the vaporization chamber may be in the form of a relatively long tube to help overcome the 'pumping effect'. (c) Performance characteristics. (d) Schematic diagram showing the rotary flow-splitting valve, inner and outer wicks, and helical copper separator.

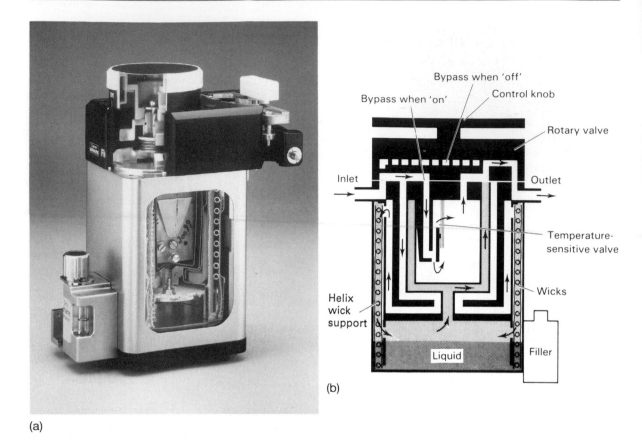

(a)

(b)

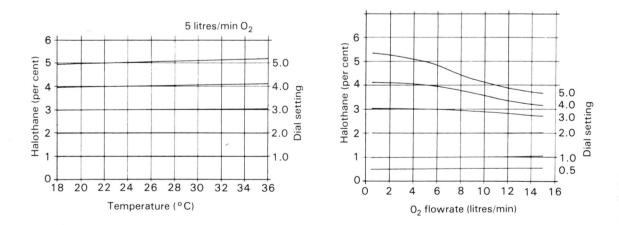

(c)

**Figure 6.15** (a) The TEC 4 vaporizer. (b) Working principles. Although this vaporizer is in a different housing from the Mark 3, it contains many of the features of the latter and functions in much the same way. Added features are that if it is accidentally inverted, the liquid agent will not spill into the by-pass and that, in one model, if two vaporizers are mounted side by side on the appropriate back bar a push-rod mechanism prevents their both being turned on at the same time. (c) Performance characteristics.

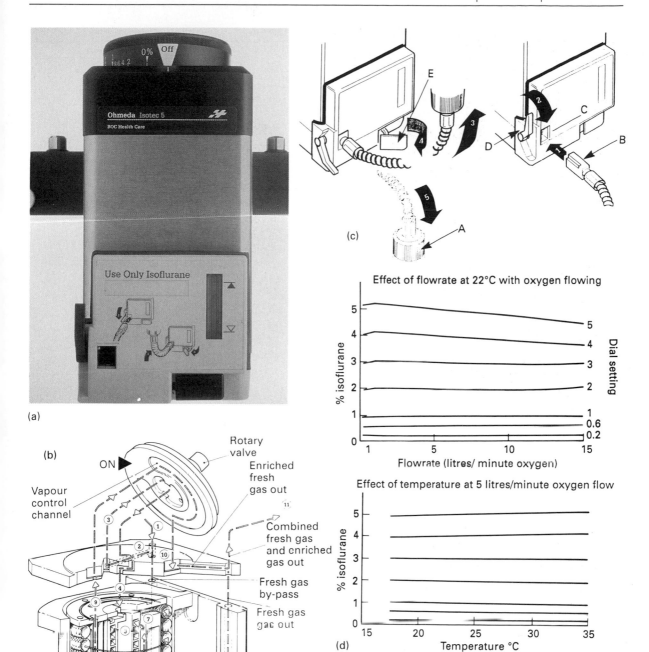

(a)

(b)

ON ▶

Rotary valve

Enriched fresh gas out

Vapour control channel

Combined fresh gas and enriched gas out

Fresh gas by-pass

Fresh gas gas out

ck sembly

porizing amber

Thermostat

(c)

**Effect of flowrate at 22°C with oxygen flowing**

% isoflurane

Flowrate (litres/ minute oxygen)

Dial setting

5
4
3
2
1
0.6
0.2

**Effect of temperature at 5 litres/minute oxygen flow**

% isoflurane

Temperature °C

(d)

**Figure 6.16** (a, b) TEC 5. This recently introduced vaporizer is claimed to have a number of advantages over its predecessor, the 4. The wick assembly is constituted using a hollow cloth tube that is held open by a stainless-steel wire spiral. The wick is subsequently wound into a helix within the vaporizer. This arrangement greatly improves the surface area available for vaporization as compared to the previous TEC models. Two additional features are the improved keyed filling action (c) and an easier mechanism for switching on the rotary valve and lock (now a single-handed action). (d) Performance characteristics.

**Table 6.2** Comparison of TEC vaporizers (using halothane)

| Element | Vaporizer | | | Element | Vaporizer | | |
|---|---|---|---|---|---|---|---|
| | Cyprane TEC 3 | Cyprane TEC 4 | Ohmeda TEC 5 | | Cyprane TEC 3 | Cyprane TEC 4 | Ohmeda TEC 5 |
| Nominal working range | | | | Keyed filler option | Yes | Yes | Yes |
| Flow (litres/min) | 0.25–15 | 0.25–15 | 0.25–15 | Selectatec | | | |
| Ambient temperature (°C) | 18–35 | 18–35 | 18–35 | mounting option | Yes | Standard | Standard |
| Capacity | | | | Non-spill | No | Yes | Yes |
| With dry wicks (cm³) | 135 | 135 | 300 | Allowable tilt | 90° | 180° | 180° |
| With wet wicks (cm³) | 100 | 100 | 225 | Integral interlock | No | Yes | Yes |
| Graduations | | | | Safety 'lock-on' facility | No | Yes | Yes |
| % Halothane v/v | | | | Safety 'off/ isolation' facility | No | Yes | Yes |
| Range | 0–5.0 | 0–5.0 | 0.5 | Resistance to gas flow | | | |
| Increments | 0.5 | 0.25 (0–0.5) | 0.2 (0–1) | Vaporizer 'off' | | | |
| | | 0.5 (0.5–5.0) | 0.5 (1–5) | (kPa) | 0.49 | Not applicable for TECs 4 & 5 | |
| Weight (kg) | 6.3 | 7.2 | 7.0 | (cmH₂O) | 5 | Not applicable for TECs 4 & 5 | |
| Dimensions | | | | Vaporizer 'on' | | | |
| Width (mm) | 135 | 105 | 114 | Carrier gas O₂ @ | | | |
| Depth (mm) | 145 | 145 | 197 | 5 litres/min @ 21°C | | | |
| Height (mm) | 205 | 225 | 237 | (kPa) | 2.06–2.84 | 2.06–2.84 | 1.47–1.96 |
| Temperature-compensated (Ambient and cooling effect) | Yes | Yes | Yes | (cmH₂O) | 21–29 | 21–29 | 15–20 |
| Pressure-compensated | Yes | Yes | Yes | | | | |

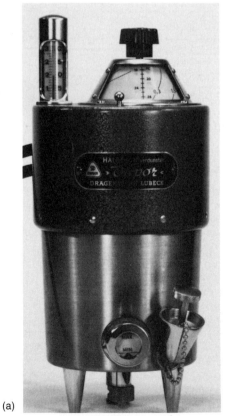

(a)

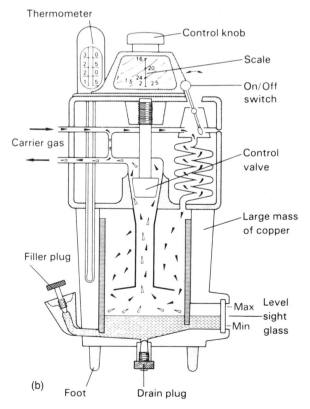

(b)

**Figure 6.17** An early model of the Dräger Vapor temperature-indicated level-compensated vaporizer. Note the enormous copper heat sink. (b) Working principles.

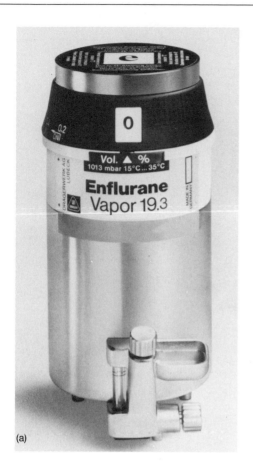

(a)

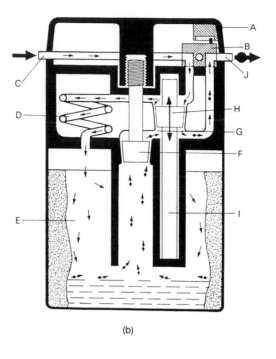

(b)

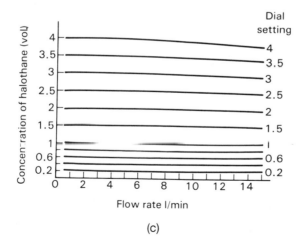

(c)

**Figure 6.18** A recent model of the Dräger Vapor vaporizer, which is now both temperature- and level-compensated. (b) Working principles. A, vapour concentration control; B, on/off switch (actuated by A); C, inlet; D, pressure compensator; E, vaporization chamber; F, control valve; G, mixing chamber; H, vaporization chamber bypass valve, which is operated by I, expansion element of temperature-compensation sensor; J, outlet. (c) Performance characteristics.

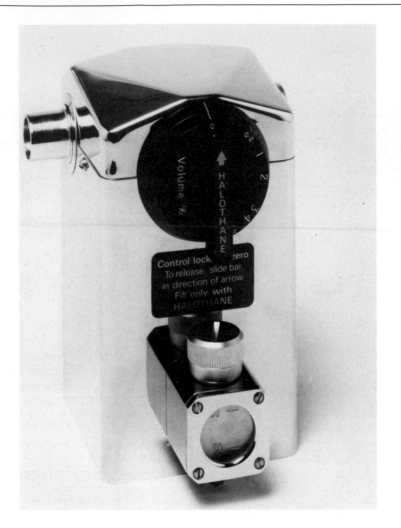

(a)

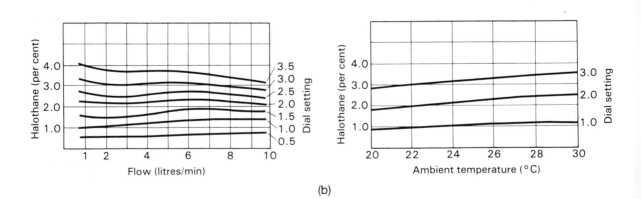

(b)

**Figure 6.19** (a) The Penlon Abingdon vaporizer. (b) Performance characteristics. The wicks and vaporization chamber of this vaporizer may be cleaned by the owner. Space does not permit full details here, but well-illustrated instructions may be obtained from Penlon.

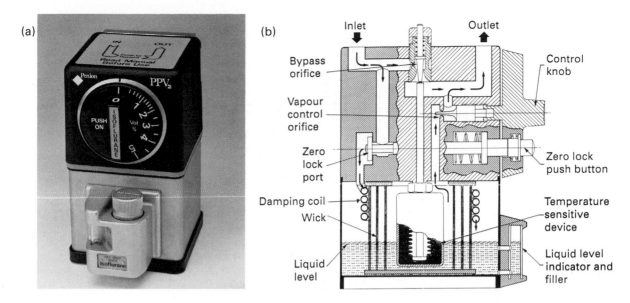

**Figure 6.20** (a) The Penlon PPV Sigma. (b) Working principles.

*The Penlon PPV Sigma* shown in Fig. 6.20 is the latest development of the Abingdon vaporizer and includes all the features of a modern Plenum vaporizer. The carrier gases pass through a helical damping coil that prevents saturated vapour contaminating gas in the back bar via the 'pumping effect'. The wick is novel in that it is made of stainless steel mesh (1 m long) that is welded to a backing plate. The two are then coiled into a spiral, the top and bottom of which are made gas-tight. The carrier gases then have to pass around the spiral, coming into contact with the whole surface area of the wick so that they become saturated. The wick assembly is designed as a cartridge for ease of removal and cleaning, and being steel has a long service life.

As another example of a temperature-compensated vaporizer, Fig. 6.21 shows the working principles and temperature-compensating valve operation of the *Vapamasta 5 (M&IE)*.

## The 'copper kettle' vaporizer

This type of vaporizer (Fig. 6.22) depends on maximum vaporization of the anaesthetic agent in a small volume of the carrier gas. A separate supply of oxygen from an extra flowmeter passes through the vaporizer. The oxygen is broken up into a large number of very small bubbles by a diffuser made of 'Porex' or sintered bronze. These bubbles are so small that they present an enormous surface area as they pass through the liquid anaesthetic agent and are totally saturated with its vapour. For halothane

at 20°C this saturation is about 33%. As its name implies, the vaporizer contains a large mass of copper which, in conjunction with its attachment to the anaesthetic machine as a whole, provides a sufficient reservoir of heat to prevent a great fall in temperature as the halothane is vaporized.

The oxygen, now saturated with the anaesthetic agent, is added to the fresh gas flow via a mixing chamber. A calculation is necessary to determine the required flow rate of oxygen through the vaporizer, as compared with that of the main mixed gas flow, to achieve the desired concentration of anaesthetic agent in the final mixture.

The *Halox* vaporizer, shown in Fig. 6.23, has been developed from the 'copper kettle'. In this the diffuser is made of sintered glass, and the large mass of copper is replaced by a glass container (for simplicity and to enable the level of halothane liquid to be observed). Since the vapour concentration of halothane required for anaesthesia is low, and therefore only a relatively small amount of liquid halothane needs to be vaporized, the fall in temperature is much less than is the case when ether is vaporized in the original 'copper kettle'.

At the outlet of the vaporizer there is a non-return gravity disc valve, which prevents halothane vapour entering the gaseous pathway of the back bar when the Halox is turned off, and also prevents the pumping action due to back pressure when positive-pressure ventilation is employed. There is a thermometer in the vaporizer, and a slide-rule is provided for the necessary calculations.

A danger of both the 'copper kettle' and Halox

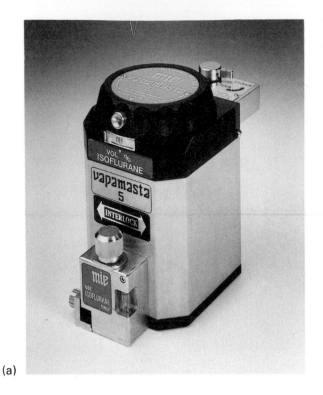

(a)

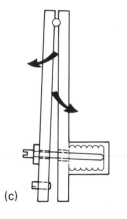

Temperature HIGH
bellows expand
valve decreases gas flow

Temperature LOW
bellows contract
valve increases gas flow

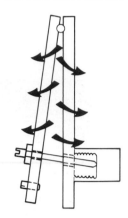

(c)

OFF            ON

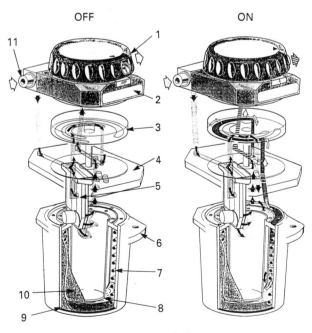

11

10

9

1 Control knob
2 Top housing
3 Rotary valve
4 Rotary valve plate
5 Temp. comp. valve
6 Outer canister

7 Coil
8 Inner canister
9 Outer wick
10 Inner wick
11 Inlet taper

(b)

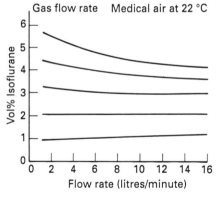

Gas flow rate    Medical air at 22 °C

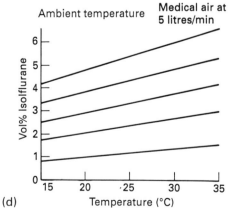

Ambient temperature    Medical air at 5 litres/min

(d)

**Figure 6.21** (a) The M&IE Vapamasta 5 temperature-compensated vaporizer. (b) Internal gas circuit. (c) Operation of temperature-compensating valve. (d) Performance characteristics for isoflurane.

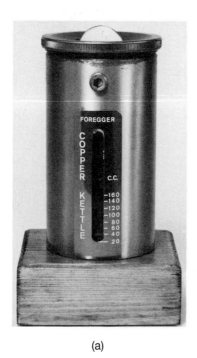

(a)

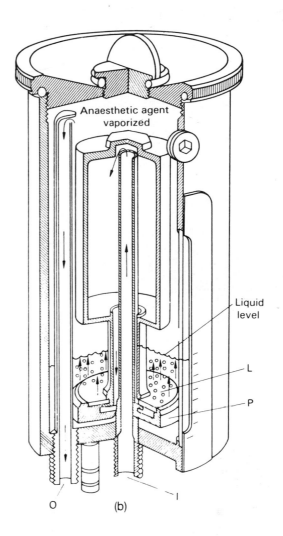

Anaesthetic agent
vaporized

Liquid
level

L

P

O          (b)          I

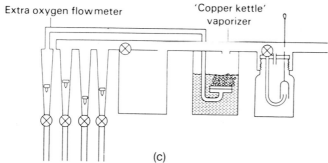

Extra oxygen flowmeter          'Copper kettle'
                                vaporizer

(c)

**Figure 6.22** (a) The 'copper kettle' vaporizer. (b) The carrier gas (oxygen) enters via the inlet I, is broken up into very small bubbles by the Porex diffuser P, and passes through the liquid agent L, becoming saturated with the vapour. It then passes out via the outlet O to join the main fresh gas flow. (c) The position of a 'copper kettle' vaporizer in the back bar. Note the extra oxygen flowmeter, the gas from which is saturated with the anaesthetic agent before being added to the mixed gas flow.

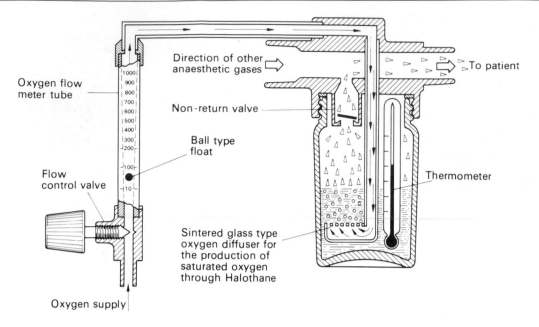

**Figure 6.23** The Halox vaporizer.

vaporizers is that, should the total gas flow be diminished (for example if the nitrous oxide cylinder runs out), a high and possibly dangerous concentration of halothane vapour will be delivered to the patient in a situation where, owing to a reduced fresh gas flow rate, rebreathing, hypoxia and hypercarbia may occur. To new users of the 'copper kettle' or Halox, the necessary calculations must seem to be a disadvantage. However, those anaesthetists who have used it routinely do not find them an undue burden.

The *Heidbrink Kinet-O-meter* unit contains a number of flowmeters of the Rotameter type, and a separate 'copper kettle' type of vaporizer for each volatile agent. The vaporizers are fitted with electric heating coils and thermostats, and their temperature is maintained at about 24°C. The maintenance of a constant temperature has the advantage of eliminating the need for calculations of temperature drop, and also gives an adequate vapour concentration of agents, such as methoxyflurane (Penthrane), (now no longer in use) which cannot easily be achieved at lower temperatures. There are two oxygen flowmeters (one for low and the other for high flow rates), and from these the oxygen passes to a special 'bypass' valve, which diverts part of the flow to the vaporizer. The amount of oxygen diverted to each vaporizer is controlled by a fine adjustment valve and is indicated on a flowmeter labelled for the particular volatile agent in question. The flowmeter

is calibrated in actual flow rate of *vapour* per minute, and does not include the oxygen passing through the vaporizer. The accuracy of this calibration depends on the vaporizer being at the correct operating temperature, which is indicated by a thermometer and also by the illumination of only one of two pilot lights in the heating circuit for the vaporizer. The vapour-laden oxygen and the main oxygen stream from the bypass valve both join the mixed gas flow.

The concentration of the anaesthetic vapour may be determined by the following formula:

$$\text{Vapour concentration} = \frac{\text{ml vapour/min} \times 100}{\text{total gas and vapour flow/min}} \%$$

For example, with the following flow rates:

| Oxygen | = 1880 ml/min |
|---|---|
| Nitrous oxide | = 2000 ml/min |
| Oxygen to halothane vaporizer | = 120 ml/min |

The vapour concentration would be:

$$\frac{120 \times 100}{1880 + 2000 + 120} = \frac{12\,000}{4000} = 3\%$$

The original 'copper kettle' vaporizer included two important features.

- A small, carefully measured fraction of the oxygen flow is saturated with anaesthetic vapour, so that a predetermined *amount* of the latter is added to the system per minute — a different concept from a mixed gas flow containing a specific *percentage* of vapour regardless of absolute quantity. The 'copper kettle' is therefore rather more applicable to circle systems with low fresh gas flow and where reduction of pollution and economy are important.
- The provision of a large 'heat sink', by virtue of the great mass of copper, minimizes the fall in temperature by supplying sufficient heat to replenish that lost by the latent heat of vaporization. This is of particular importance when ether is being used.

It is regrettable that the term 'copper kettle' is associated with both these otherwise unrelated principles.

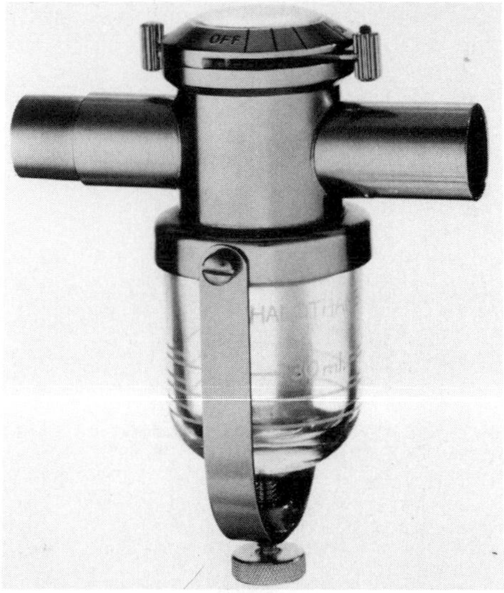

Figure 6.24 The Goldman halothane vaporizer.

## Draw-over vaporizers

All the Plenum vaporizers described above offer resistance to the gas flow. For this reason the gases have to be driven through them and it is not, therefore, possible to install them in a breathing system. However, pressurized gas sources are not always available in some countries or in certain situations. Draw-over vaporizers, with their low-resistance gas pathways are therefore a useful alternative to Plenum systems despite not being as accurate.

Typical examples of draw-over vaporizers are described below.

*The Goldman halothane vaporizer* (Fig. 6.24) is a small, simple and inexpensive vaporizer which is used for halothane in relatively low concentrations, when it is introduced as an adjuvant to nitrous oxide and oxygen anaesthesia; it is commonly used in dental anaesthesia. It is neither temperature nor level compensated and its output is somewhat influenced by the gas flow rate. Typical performance figures are shown in Table 6.3. Since the resistance to gas flow is small, this vaporizer may be used within the breathing system.

*The McKesson and Rowbotham vaporizers* are somewhat similar, the latter having a wire-gauze wick (see Figs 6.25 and 6.26 and Tables 6.4 and 6.5).

**Table 6.3** The Goldman vaporizer

| Drum position* | Gas flow rate (litres/min) | | |
|---|---|---|---|
| | 2 | 8 | 30 |
| Halothane | | | |
| 1 | 0.03 | 0.03 | 0.03 |
| 2 | 0.41 | 0.74 | 0.92 |
| 3 | 0.73 | 2.21 | 1.31 |
| On | 0.74 | 2.08 | 1.21 |
| Trichloroethylene | | | |
| 1 | 0.01 | nil | 0.01 |
| 2 | 0.16 | 0.44 | 0.35 |
| 3 | 0.47 | 0.68 | 0.52 |
| On | 0.45 | 0.70 | 0.45 |

* Halothane and trichloroethylene percentages by volume, liquid levels 20 ml at 21°C after 1 min.

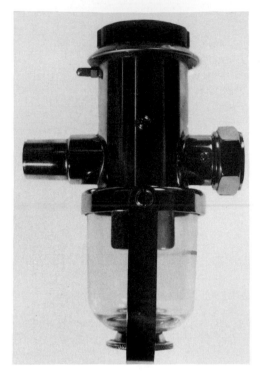

Figure 6.25 The McKesson vaporizer.

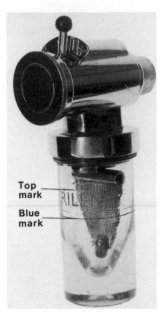

Figure 6.26 The Rowbotham vaporizer. Note that there is a wick made of wire gauze.

**Table 6.4** The McKesson vaporizer

| Dial reading | Halothane (%) |
| --- | --- |
| 1 | 0.05 |
| 2 | 1.05 |
| 3 | 1.84 |
| On | 2.80 |

These are performances on a particular occasion with the halothane at 20°C, gas flow at 8 litres/min and a pressure of 5 mmHg.

**Table 6.5** The Rowbotham vaporizer

| Setting* | Gas flow rate (litres/min) | |
| --- | --- | --- |
| | 4 | 8 |
| Top mark | | |
| Full on | 3.10 | 2.50 |
| ¾ | 2.10 | 1.95 |
| ½ | 1.40 | 1.55 |
| ¼ | 0.60 | 0.65 |
| Blue mark | | |
| Full on | 1.10 | 1.40 |
| ¾ | 0.65 | 1.00 |
| ½ | 0.40 | 0.65 |
| ¼ | 0.30 | 0.25 |

* Halothane percentages by volume at 20°C.

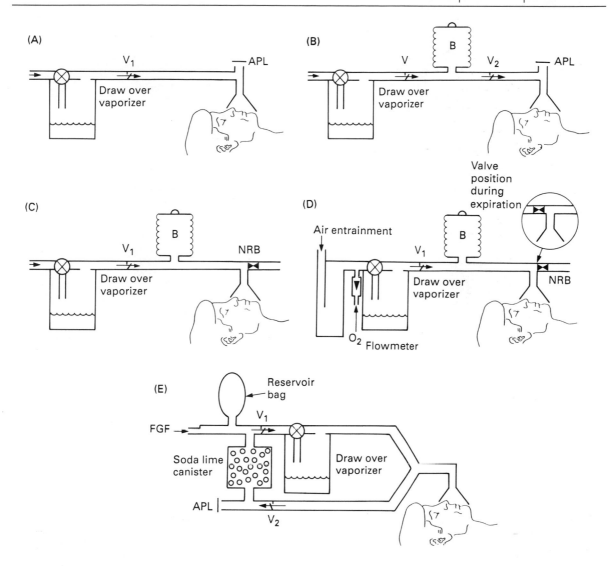

**Figure 6.27** Draw-over anaesthetic systems. Note that they all contain non return valves to prevent reverse flow through the vaporizer. System A is used for spontaneous respiration. System B incorporates a bellows and therefore requires a second non return valve ($V_2$). If this is used for controlled ventilation (system C), a non return valve is often substituted for the APL valve. If the former is of a design which has a tendency to jam, the second valve $V_2$ is either removed, or in the case of the Oxford Inflating Bellows, held open by a magnet. In system D an oxygen flowmeter has been added. During the expiratory phase, the continuing supply of oxygen flows into the reservoir and is stored for use in subsequent breaths. In system E the vaporizer has been placed in a circle breathing system. A vaporizer in this position is often referred to as a VIC (vaporizer in circle).

As seen in Fig. 6.27 there are various breathing systems in which such a vaporizer may be installed.

In systems A to D, exhaled gases are vented to the atmosphere (suitably scavenged where appropriate). However in system E, the patient's exhaled gases are recirculated through the vaporizer. This is of importance since not only will the concentration of volatile agents be increased by the repeated passage of the gases through the vaporizer, but the vaporizer must be of a type that has cloth wicks, since these could become saturated with water condensed from the expired air.

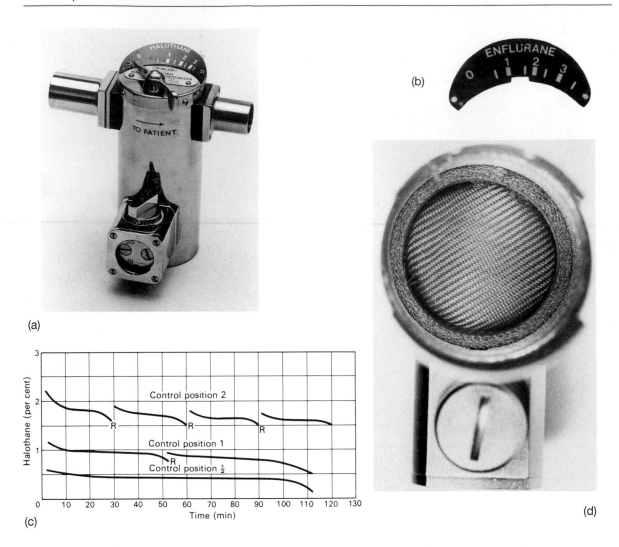

(a)

(b)

(c)

(d)

**Figure 6.28** (a) The Oxford Miniature vaporizer. Note that the direction of flow is indicated. On some models the flow to the patient is from right to left. Note also that the scale is fixed by two screws and is detachable. It may be replaced by scales for other agents, shown in (b). (c) Performance characteristics. Note that there is no temperature compensation, but a mass of water in the base of the vaporizer acts as a heat sink and reduces temperature changes during use. The letter R indicates refilling of the vaporizer. (d) The wick within the vaporizer is constructed of wire gauze and may therefore be cleaned by rinsing the vaporizer with ether, draining it, and then blowing air or other gases through it until all the ether has been eluted.

*The Oxford Miniature vaporizer* (Fig 6.28) is primarily used with portable anaesthetic equipment and has the advantage that it may be drained of one anaesthetic agent and charged with another. Detachable scales are available for several agents. It is very simple to use and needs little in the way of servicing.

It is not temperature compensated, but there is a sealed compartment, filled with water plus antifreeze, which acts as a heat sink to minimize changes of temperature. The triservice version is described in Chapter 22

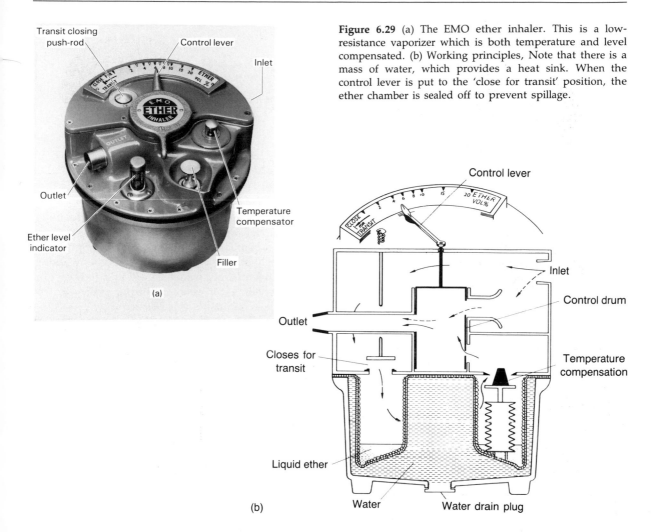

**Figure 6.29** (a) The EMO ether inhaler. This is a low-resistance vaporizer which is both temperature and level compensated. (b) Working principles, Note that there is a mass of water, which provides a heat sink. When the control lever is put to the 'close for transit' position, the ether chamber is sealed off to prevent spillage.

*The EMO (Epstein, Macintosh, Oxford) vaporizer, or EMO Ether Inhaler* (Fig. 6.29). This has been deservedly the most popular draw-over vaporizer for the administration of ether, and is still widely used throughout the world. For spontaneous respiration it is often used in conjunction with the OMV (Oxford Miniature Vaporizer). The latter is usually filled with halothane to provide smooth and rapid induction of anaesthesia which is then continued by ether from the EMO. Both vaporizers may be used in conjunction with a self inflating bellows for techniques employing controlled ventilation.

# 7 The Continuous Flow Anaesthetic Machine

## Introduction

Inhalational anaesthesia is still the most commonly used technique worldwide. Where compressed gases are available this is usually achieved by the use of the continuous flow anaesthetic machine (Fig. 7.1).

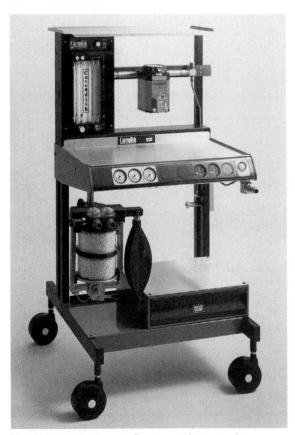

**Figure 7.1** A continuous flow anaesthetic machine.

A typical machine would consist of:

- a rigid metal box framework on wheels. Attached to this is a source of compressed gas consisting of a pipeline system and/or metal cylinders containing the relevant gases;
- pressure regulators for reducing the high pressures in the attached cylinders to machine working pressures of approximately 420 kPa (60 psi)* or 310 kPa (45 psi) in some countries;
- secondary regulators (see below);
- pressure gauges to show pipeline and cylinder pressures;
- a method of metering (flowmeters), using adjustable valves for proportioning and mixing the various gases;
- a system for attaching vaporizing chambers (vaporizers) to the anaesthetic machine for the addition of volatile anaesthetic agents to the gas mixture;
- a safety mechanism to warn of the failure of the oxygen supply and to prevent hypoxic mixtures of gas/vapour reaching the patient (oxygen failure warning device);
- a safety mechanism for releasing high pressure build-up of gases (back bar pressure relief valve) should a fault occur in the machine;
- a flowmeter bypass system for the administration of a high flow of pure oxygen in an emergency;
- a single outlet for delivering the gases and vapours into an attached breathing system (the common gas outlet).

## Machine Framework

The machine framework consists of box-shaped sections of either welded steel or aluminium that provides both strength and ease of assembly. The machine is usually mounted on wheels with anti-

---

* The British Standard stipulates 420 kPa which is 61.3 psi. For convenience this has been rounded off to 60 psi.

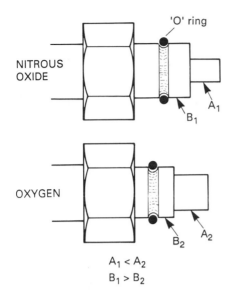

NITROUS OXIDE

OXYGEN

'O' ring

$A_1$

$B_1$

$B_2$

$A_2$

$A_1 < A_2$
$B_1 > B_2$

Dimensions of male NIST fittings

|  | Foreward shaft (A) | Second shaft (B) |
|---|---|---|
| Nitrous oxide | 9.5 mm | 15.5 mm |
| Oxygen | 11.5 mm | 13.5 mm |
| Vacuum | 12.5 mm | 12.5 mm |
| Air | 9.0 mm | 16.0 mm |

**Figure 7.2** Male section of NIST pipeline union.

static tyres. These conduct away any static electricity which may affect flowmeter performance and which also presents a risk of ignition of flammable anaesthetic agents (where these are still used).

The compressed gas attachments (for pipelines and cylinders) may be sited at the sides, as well as at the back of the machine (see Chapter 4). Each pipeline source is attached to the machine via a gas specific connection, comprising of a body (attached to the machine), and a nipple and screw threaded nut (attached to the machine end of the pipeline hose). In the UK this is called a 'NIST' (non-interchangeable, screw threaded) connection. The non-interchangeability of this connection is effected by the nipple (Fig. 7.2), which is stepped to produce two different diameters along its shaft and which includes a slot for a rubber sealing washer ('O' ring). The two diameters are specific to each gas service and should fit only the equivalent female recesses in the body. The nipple is inserted into its matching body and the connection is made gas tight by securing the nut on the thread provided on the

outer surface of the body. The nut is the same size and uses the same thread diameter for all 'NIST' connections. Hence, the term non-interchangeable, screw threaded connection is somewhat misleading, as it implies that the screw threads for each connection are different, which is not the case. The incompatability is created by the individual shape of the body and nipple for each gas.

In the USA a similar system is employed called 'DISS' (diameter indexed safety system). However the diameters of the nipples and bodies for the various connections are smaller and not compatible with the 'NIST' system. Also, there are further differences in the oxygen and vacuum systems. The oxygen nipple has a small single diameter shaft and a smaller than standard securing nut. The vacuum nipple also has a single (large) diameter nipple, but a standard diameter securing nut which is longer than the others.

The pipeline union block usually contains a metal gauze filter and also a one-way spring loaded check valve to prevent retrograde gas leaks should the relevant system be disconnected.

The cylinders are clamped on to the machine by a yoke arrangement and secured tightly using a wing-nut or tommy-bar (Fig. 7.3).

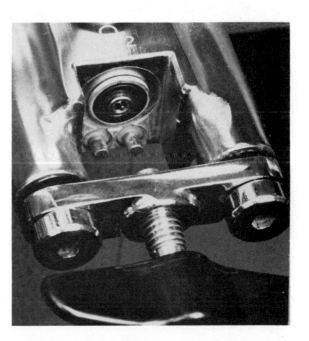

**Figure 7.3** Anaesthetic machine cylinder yoke showing a wing-nut.

# Pin Index System for Gas Cylinders

The cylinder heads are coded with appropriately positioned holes which match pins on the machine yoke (see Chapter 3). This prevents installation of the wrong gas cylinder to a yoke (ISO 2407). The yokes are permanently and legibly marked (BS 1319 in UK) for the appropriate gas. A thin neoprene and aluminium washer (Bodok seal) or other non-combustible washer is interposed between the cylinder head and yoke to provide a gas-tight seal when the two are clamped together. Cylinder yokes are also fitted with filters and one-way spring loaded non-return (check) valves (Fig. 7.4). These one-way valves prevent retrograde leaks where two cylinder yokes are connected in parallel and one does not have a cylinder attached. A leak of not more than 15 ml/min through an open yoke is acceptable in new machines. However in older machines the non return valve is not as efficient owing either to the design (valve not spring loaded) or to wear and tear, and could result in greater than acceptable back pressure leaks. These leaks, when occurring unexpectedly, have been shown to alter the composition of the gas leaving the flowmeter block and have resulted in the delivery of a hypoxic gas mixture to an attached breathing system (see section on flowmeters). Blanking plugs (dummy cylinder heads) are available to be inserted into empty yokes to overcome this problem.

Prior to the introduction of NIST fittings, pipeline hoses could be connected to the anaesthetic machine via the cylinder yoke using a pin indexed block on the end of a hose (Fig. 7.5). This was connected to a redundant yoke which was modified by removing the wing-nut or tommy bar (designed for hand operated use) and replacing it with an Allen screw that requires a special key (hexagon wrench) to release or tighten it. This practice was a temporary solution for the conversion of older machines and is now no longer acceptable in the UK (see page 55).

# Other Types of Gas-Tight Connections Within the Machine

The various components within the anaesthetic machine are joined to each other by a series of pipes of either metal or synthetic material.

### Permanent joints in metal tubing

Permanent joints are usually brazed or hard soldered. After making such a joint it is important that all traces of flux are removed. More recently a system of brazing copper pipes and brass fittings without flux has been evolved. This is used particularly for medical gas pipeline installations. In the case where provision has to be made for the subsequent disconnection and reconnection of the joint, a *union* is used. This consists of two parts which are held together in a gas-tight manner, usually by a nut or *cap*, which screws onto a parallel male thread. Figure 7.6 shows a *ball and cone* or *cone seated* union, in which the seating is by direct metal to metal contact. A *flange* or *flat seated* union (Fig. 7.7) requires a washer to complete the seal. With pipes carrying oxygen, this washer should be of non-flammable material.

Figure 7.8 shows a screwed high pressure joint such as that where a pressure gauge is fitted to a regulator or block. It will be noticed that a parallel

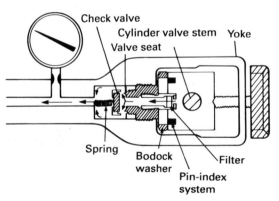

**Figure 7.4** Position of valves and gauge when one oxygen cylinder is turned on in a double-yoke assembly.

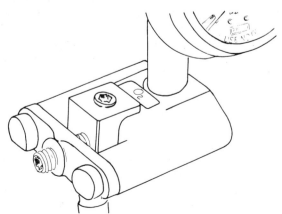

**Figure 7.5** The tommy-bar removed from the yoke and replaced by an Allen screw.

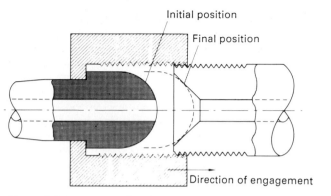

Initial position
Final position
Direction of engagement

**Figure 7.6** A cone-seated union.

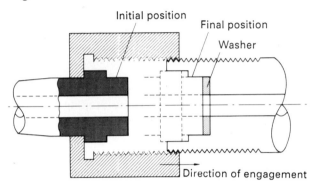

Initial position
Final position
Washer
Direction of engagement

**Figure 7.7** A flange- (or flat-) seated union.

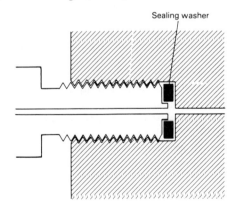

Sealing washer

**Figure 7.8** The joint such as that between an oxygen regulator and a pressure gauge. Note that the threads are parallel and that a sealing washer is required.

thread is used and the actual seal is made by a non-flammable washer. For some other purposes tapered threads (Fig. 7.9) may be used and the seal made either by screwing them down extremely tightly or by interposing a sealing compound such as PTFE (polytetrafluoroethylene or Teflon) in the form of a tape. The joint between the valve block and the body of the cylinder is sealed by a metal foil between two tapered threads.

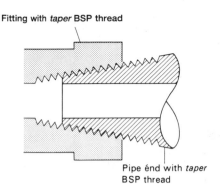

Fitting with *taper* BSP thread

Pipe énd with *taper* BSP thread

**Figure 7.9** A correct joint between two tapered threads.

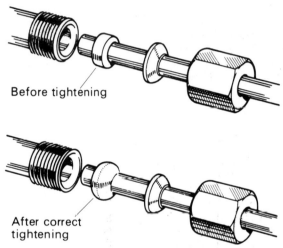

Before tightening

After correct tightening

**Figure 7.10** The Simplifix union.

For low pressure tubing, compression fittings are commonly used. Figure 7.10 shows a compression fitting, known as the 'Simplifix' connection which is used by several manufacturers. These joints are made by squeezing a soft ring, known as an 'olive', of metal or suitable plastic between the pipe and the parts of the union, thus making a mechanically strong gas-tight joint.

## Glands (stuffing boxes)

Where a valve spindle passes from an area of high pressure to one of low pressure, provision must be made to prevent the leak of gases along the line of the spindle. This is achieved by means of a *gland* or, as is colloquially known, a 'stuffing box' (Fig. 7.11). In Fig 7.12 the contents of the cylinder flow through the valve in the valve block and out through the

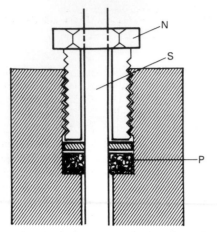

**Figure 7.11** A gland (stuffing box). The packing P is compressed by screwing down the nut N until it is applied sufficiently tightly round the spindle S to prevent the gas from leaking.

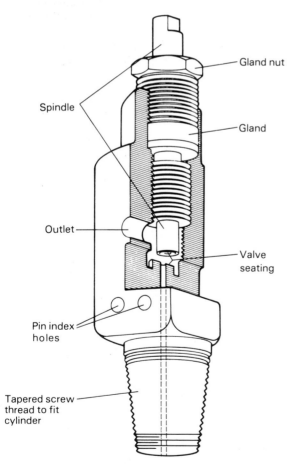

**Figure 7.12** A section through a pin-index cylinder valve block.

outlet. If the valve is turned fully clockwise (down)\*, the valve is closed. If it is turned counter-clockwise, to open the valve, the gas is permitted to escape from the cylinder and could do so by one of two routes — either through the outlet as intended or along the line of the spindle and past the nut N (Fig. 7.11). However, the latter course is prevented by the packing, or stuffing, P in the stuffing box. The nut N must be screwed down sufficiently tightly to ensure that the packing is applied so closely to the spindle that no gas can escape by this route. There is provision for the nut to be tightened down further so as to prevent leaks as the packing wears.

The principle can be used for a high-pressure gland such as that of an oxygen cylinder (as shown in Fig. 7.12) or in a low-pressure gland such as that in a flow-control (fine adjustment) valve (see Fig. 7.16). In the case of high-pressure valves, a special type of leather or long fibre asbestos was at one time used for the packing, but modern stuffing boxes are filled with specially shaped nylon. Stuffing boxes in low pressure flow control valves may be filled with rubber, nylon, neoprene or cotton.

## O-rings

In certain circumstances the packing of a stuffing box may be replaced by an O-ring (Fig. 7.13a). This consists of a simple ring made to a fine tolerance out of a material such as neoprene. If the spindle S and the casing C are suitably designed, an O-ring is all that is required to prevent leakage at this point. O-rings can withstand remarkably high pressures and yet cause very little friction between the spindle and the casing. One recent innovation is the use of an O-ring in the bull-nose oxygen cylinder coupling. Whereas a spanner was previously required to tighten the union sufficiently to prevent leaks, the O-ring now makes such an efficient joint that the nut needs to be turned down only hand tight to prevent a leak.

Metal pipes in the low pressure pipework (420 kPa (60 psi)) of an anaesthetic machine have always been joined by one of the methods described above. However, more recently, high density nylon tubing, connected by metal junctions, has been used to convey gas through the low pressure pipework. The joint is made gas-tight by a device which incorporates an O-ring (see Fig. 7.13b).

---

\* Note that it is a code of practice with nearly all valves, taps and control knobs, that they are closed by clockwise rotation and opened counter-clockwise.

(a)

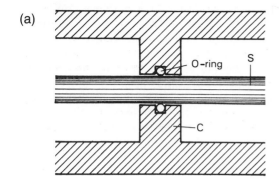

(b)

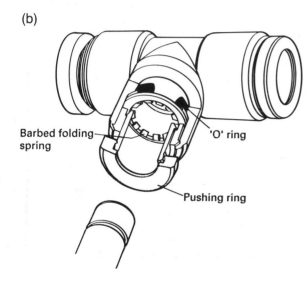

# Pressure (Contents) Gauges

The pressure in cylinders and pipelines is measured by Bourdon-type gauges. These are usually fitted adjacent to the yokes and the pipeline connections. (In modern machines a single cast brass block is often used to house the NIST/DISS pipeline connection, cylinder yoke, pressure regulator and housings for the pressure gauges in order to minimize the number of connections and potential leaks (see Fig. 7.14).) The gas entry to the pressure gauge has a constriction so as to smooth out surges in pressure that could damage the gauge, as well as to prevent total and rapid loss of gas should a gauge rupture. The gauges are labelled and colour coded (BS 1319C, UK) for the gases to which they refer, according to the standards for each country. They are also calibrated for each gas used on the machine. The scale on the gauge should extend to a pressure at least 33% greater than either the filling pressure of the cylinder or pipeline pressure as well as the 'full' indicated position at a temperature of 20°C. Each cylinder yoke should be fitted with a gauge, although this has not always been the case in the past.

**Figure 7.13** (a) A typical application of an O-ring. Leakage between the spindle S and the block C is completely prevented. (b) A high density nylon tube joined to a metal junction using an O-ring and a retractable barbed spring.

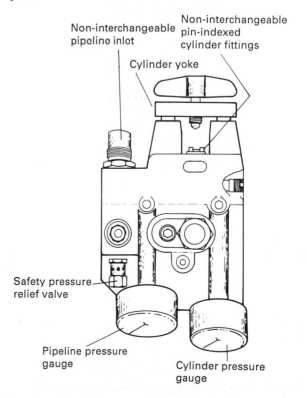

**Figure 7.14** Single-cast gas block.

The nylon tube is pushed firmly into the junction where it is gripped by an O-ring and a folding spring. The folding spring has backward pointing barbs which grip the tube preventing its removal. When removal of the tube is required (for maintenance purposes), the barbs of the spring can be retracted by applying pressure to the pushing ring situated on the inlet of the junction. This pushes a bush (leading bush) against the barbs forcing them away from the nylon tube.

# Pressure Regulators (Reducing Valves)

These are more fully described on pages 11–15. Modern anaesthetic machines have a number of pressure regulators (primary and secondary). Primary regulators are used mainly to reduce high cylinder pressures (potentially dangerous) to lower machine working pressure (typically 420 kPa (60 psi)). Table 7.1 shows the range of pressures employed within the anaesthetic machine and the variation between manufacturers and different countries. Some manufacturers adjust their cylinder regulators to just below 420 kPa (60 psi) (i.e. 375 kPa (45 psi)). This allows the anaesthetic machine to use pipeline gas preferentially when the reserve cylinders have been accidently left turned on, so reducing the potential for premature emptying of these cylinders. However, even with this differential many regulators are known to 'weep', i.e. gradually empty their contents through the pressure regulator. Reserve cylinders should therefore always be turned off after testing until required. Pressure regulators used to be labelled and coded for specific gases. This is because a special alloy was required in the valve seating for some gases (nitrous oxide) in order to prevent corrosion. However, modern regulators are designed to be compatible with all anaesthetic gases. This is achieved by using materials such as PTFE coatings on the diaphragms and Nitrile valve seats and chrome plated brass for the regulator body.

## Secondary pressure regulators

A number of factors cause the machine working pressure (420 kPa in the UK) to fluctuate by up to 20%. For example at times of peak demand in a hospital, pipeline pressures may well drop by this amount. Similarly, if an auxiliary outlet on the anaesthetic machine is used to drive a ventilator with a very high sudden gas demand, a similar pressure drop will intermittently occur before the pipeline or cylinder is able to restore the supply. These pressure fluctuations will produce parallel fluctuations in flowmeter performance. A second (secondary) regulator set below the anticipated pressure drop will smooth out the supply to the appropriate flowmeter minimizing these fluctuations. This is important in machines incorporating mechanically linked anti-hypoxia systems attached to the flowmeter bank (see below) as these systems assume that the oxygen supply pressure is constant in order to achieve an accurate flow of gas. A mechanically linked system would not be able to detect altered gas flow rates due to changing pressures. Furthermore, secondary regulators also prolong the accurate supply of oxygen to the flowmeter if there is a gradual failure of the oxygen supply (i.e. cylinder emptying) prior to the oxygen failure warning device being activated.

Regulators have to meet stringent criteria prior to being installed. They are required to withstand pressure of 30 MPa (megapascals) without disruption and their output should not vary more than 10% across a wide flow range (100 ml/min to 12 litres/min). They should also be fitted with a

**Table 7.1**   Pressures of the various gases within the anaesthetic machine

| Cylinder pressures[1] | | | Pipeline | | Manufacturer | | 1st stage regulator | | | 2nd stage regulator | | | Back bar pressure relief valve activated at: | Oxygen failure Alarm activation pressure | Flow from: |
|---|---|---|---|---|---|---|---|---|---|---|---|---|---|---|---|
| $O_2$ | $N_2O$[2] | $CO_2$[2] | $O_2$ | $N_2O$ | | | $O_2$ | $N_2O$ | $CO_2$ | $O_2$ | $N_2O$ | $CO_2$ | | | |
| 13700 kPa/1980 psi | 4400 kPa/640 psi | 4980 kPa/723 psi | 420 kPa/60 psi (approx.) | 310 kPa/45 psi (approx.) | M & IE Ltd | UK | 410 kPa/60 psi | | | Not fitted | | | 42 kPa/6 psi | 240 kPa/35 psi | 35 litres/min minimum |
| 15170 kPa/2200 psi | 5690 kPa/825 psi | 5690 kPa/825 psi | 345 kPa/50 psi (approx.) | | | USA | 310/45 psi | | | | | | | 205 kPa/30 psi | |
| | | | | | Ohmeda | UK | 410 kPa/60 psi | 140 kPa 16 psi | 265 kPa 30 psi | 265 kPa 30 psi | 265 kPa 30 psi 1 | | 42 kPa/6 psi | 172 kPa/25 psi | 35–75 litres/min |
| | | | | | | USA | 310 kPa/45 psi | | | | | | | | |
| UK  USA | UK  USA  UK  USA | UK  USA | UK  USA | France | Penlon Ltd | UK | 375 kPa/55 psi | 270 kPa 40 psi | | Not-fitted | | | 30 kPa/4.5 psi | 205 kPa/30 psi | 30–70 litres/min |
| | | | | | | USA | 310 kPa/45 psi | 250 kPa 37 psi | | | | | | | |
| | | | | | | France | 270 kPa/40 psi | | | | | | | | |

\* Not a standard fitting.
[1] Nitrous oxide and carbon dioxide are stored in cylinders as liquids under pressure. Therefore cylinder pressures only reflect their saturated vapour pressure at the temperature at which the cylinders are filled and not their content.
[2] Some slight discrepancies in converting kPa to psi are due to the rounding off of psi values.

pressure relief valve that opens at a pressure not exceeding 800 kPa (UK).

As mentioned above, primary regulators can be incorporated into single block castings of cylinder yokes and NIST/DISS connections (e.g. Ohmeda). However, older machines needed to employ heavy-duty metal pipework to connect the cylinder yokes to the regulators so as to cope with potential high pressure surges when cylinders are turned on. The metal joints in this pipework have to be either cap and liner unions or brazed (rather than soft soldered).

# Flowmeters (Rotameters)

A medical gas, on leaving its cylinder regulator, is connected to its matching pipeline gas. It is passed through a flowmeter which accurately controls the flow of that gas through the anaesthetic machine. The anaesthetic machine conventionally has a bank of flowmeters for the various gases used (Fig. 7.15). Flowmeters will be described briefly here, but more detailed information can be found in Chapter 5. A typical flowmeter assembly (Fig. 7.16) consists of a needle valve, valve seat, and a conically tapered and calibrated gas sight tube which contains a bobbin. Gas entering the sight tube pushes the bobbin up it in proportion to the gas flow. The bobbin floats and rotates inside the sight tube, without touching the sides, giving an accurate indication of the gas flow. The sight tube is made leak-proof at the top and bottom of the flowmeter block either by 'O' rings or neoprene sockets or by washers. The glass sight tubes are individually calibrated (in litres/min) at a

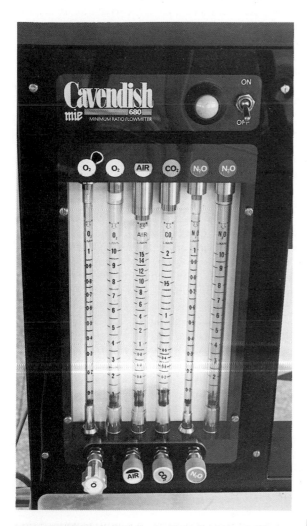

**Figure 7.15** A flowmeter bank. Note the 'cascade' flowmeters for oxygen and nitrous oxide, the protrusion of the oxygen flow control valve and the on/off master switch.

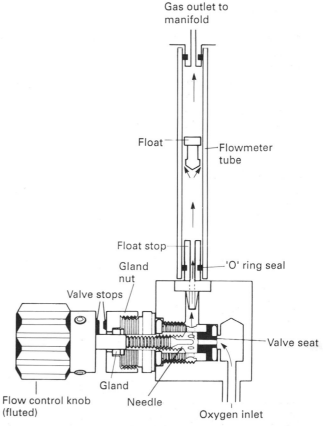

**Figure 7.16** The internal mechanics of an oxygen flowmeter and flow control valve.

temperature of 20°C and an ambient pressure of 101.3 kPa for their specific gases and should be non-interchangeable). Misconnection is made physically impossible by those manufacturers who construct the glass sight tubes of different diameters and/or lengths or by using a pin-index system at each end of them.

Flow control valves in the UK have to meet standards set down BS 4272 which relate to the following:

1.  That the torque (twisting force) required to operate them must be high enough to minimize accidental readjustment (this torque can be adjusted by the manufacturer by varying the degree of tightness of the gland nut, although these may work loose during frequent use).
2.  Values must be accurate to within 10% of the indicated flow (between 10 and 80% of the maximum indicated flow).
3.  When axial push or pull forces are applied to the valve spindle without rotation (at a flow rate 25% of the maximum indicated flow), the maximum flow change must not be greater than 10% or 10 ml/min, whichever is the greater. (A number of older machines have spindles that do not meet this requirement. Axial pressures at a flow rate of 1 litre/min have been shown to change the flow rate by 50% in these machines, with resultant hypoxic mixtures being delivered to the patient, when used with a low-flow anaesthetic breathing system.)
4.  Each flow control valve must be permanently and legibly marked indicating the gas it controls (using the name or chemical symbol).
5.  As well as conforming to (4), the oxygen flow control knob (Fig. 7.17) must have an individual octagonal profile. When the valve is closed the knob must project at least 2 mm beyond the knobs controlling other gases at all flow rates. Its diameter must also be greater than the maximum diameter of the flow control knobs for other gases.

### The flowmeter block

In the UK and many other countries, the flowmeters are traditionally arranged in a block with the oxygen flowmeter on the extreme left and the nitrous oxide on the extreme right. However some machines such as those manufactured by Ohmeda and Acoma incorporate a system that delivers a minimum concentration of oxygen such as 25%, and requires the oxygen and nitrous oxide flow control valves to be adjacent, as they are linked by a sprocket and chain. The flowmeters are mounted vertically, and

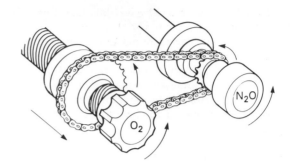

**Figure 7.17** The Ohmeda Link 25 antihypoxia system.

usually next to each other, in such a way that their upper (downstream) ends discharge into a manifold. In traditional models this was arranged in such a way so that if there were a leak in say the central tube, oxygen would be lost rather than nitrous oxide and as a result a hypoxic mixture might be delivered to the patient (see Fig. 5.7a). In most modern machines, oxygen is the last gas to flow into the manifold so that a leak would not lead to such a hypoxic mixture (see Fig. 5.7b). In some countries such as the US and Canada, the order of the flowmeters in the block has been reversed, with oxygen on the right, as a solution to the same problem. But this too has led to patients being given a hypoxic mixture owing to the fact that the anaesthetist was not aware of the transposition.

The practice of removing carbon dioxide and cyclopropane cylinders from their yokes has exposed a further hazard in older machines. Oxygen can be lost via a retrograde leak through a cyclopropane or carbon dioxide flowmeter, even when intact, if the corresponding needle valves are inadvertently left open. Gas can track back from the manifold via the flowmeter and open needle valve to the unblocked cylinder yoke and escape. The one-way (check) valves fitted to cylinder yokes in older machines were never intended to provide a perfect gas-tight seal under all conditions (see above). They were not spring loaded since they were designed to work against high back-pressures rather than the relatively low back-pressures produced in the retrograde leak mentioned. This leak may be increased by adding an extra resistance to flow downstream of the flowmeter block (i.e. some types of minute volume divider ventilator or high resistance vaporizer), which effectively increase the gas pressure in the flowmeter block.

Recent increased interest in low flow anaesthesia systems has created a demand for flowmeters that can more accurately measure flows below 1 litre/min. This is achieved by the use of two flowmeter tubes for the same gas. The first is a long thin tube accurate for flows from 0 to 1000 ml/min to complement the second conventional flowmeter tube calibrated for higher flows (1–10 litres/min or more). Both are activated from the same flow control valve. These 'cascade' flowmeter tubes for a specific gas are arranged sequentially so that when the flow control valve is opened the low-flow tube is seen to register first.

## Carbon dioxide flowmeters

The provision of carbon dioxide on anaesthetic machines is somewhat controversial, as a number of deaths have occurred owing to the inadvertent and excessive use of the gas. Typically, the flowmeter valve had been left fully open, either during a check procedure, or at the end of a previous case and the bobbin was not readily noticed at the top of the flowmeter tube. The next patient then received in excess of 2 litres/min of carbon dioxide.

Manufacturers have responded by producing flowmeters calibrated either for maximum flows of 600 ml/min, or by introducing a flow restrictor which limits the flow into a standard flowmeter to 600 ml/min. Also, flowmeters have been introduced that do not have a bezel at the top of the tube which can hide the flowmeter bobbin.

## Cyclopropane flowmeters

When cyclopropane is used on an anaesthetic machine, not only must full antistatic precautions be taken but also all mains electricity-operated equipment should be removed from the 'zone of risk' (see Chapter 22, pages 333–334). Any electrical sockets that are an integral part of the machine must be disconnected from the mains supply. All these risk factors have persuaded manufacturers to discontinue the inclusion of cyclopropane flowmeters on current anaesthetic machines. Cyclopropane yokes complete with flowmeters could until recently be purchased separately with a 'Selectatec' fitting so that they could be mounted on the back bar. Cyclopropane is now no longer produced in the UK.

## Anti-hypoxia devices

Several manufacturers have progressed one stage further in minimizing the availability of potentially hypoxic gas mixtures, by designing systems whereby it is physically impossible to set the nitrous oxide and oxygen flow rates in which an oxygen concentration can be less than 25%.

### 'Link 25' system (Ohmeda) (see Fig. 7.17)

This device incorporates a chain that links the flow control valves for nitrous oxide and oxygen. There is a fixed sprocket (cog) on the nitrous oxide spindle that relays its movement to a larger cog on the oxygen flowmeter spindle via a 'bicycle chain'. The oxygen cog moves along a static, hollow worm gear, through which the oxygen flowmeter spindle passes. As the nitrous oxide flowmeter control is turned counter-clockwise (increasing the nitrous oxide flow), the chain link moves this larger cog nearer to the oxygen flowmeter control so that, when a 25% oxygen mixture is reached, it locks on to the oxygen control knob and moves it synchronously with any further increase in nitrous oxide flow. The oxygen flow control can of course be independently opened further but cannot be closed below a setting, which, if nitrous oxide is flowing, will produce less than 25% oxygen in the mixture. This type of mechanical link, (a) takes no account of other gases in the flowmeter block (air and carbon dioxide) that could potentially dilute the mixture below a 25% oxygen concentration, and (b), on its own will not recognize and compensate for variations in gas supply pressure which affect flowmeter performance. However the Link 25 system does include secondary pressure regulators in both the oxygen and nitrous oxide systems, the purpose of which is to prevent variations in gas supply pressure from affecting flowmeter performance.

A further safety feature of this system includes a mechanical stop fitted to the oxygen flowmeter control valve, ensuring that a minimum standing flow of 175–250 ml/min of oxygen is maintained even when the valve is fully closed. This flow, of course, can occur only when the machine master switch for all the gases is switched on.

### 'Minimum ratio' gas system (M&IE)

This system relies on a ratio mixer valve (Fig. 7.18) to ensure that the oxygen concentration leaving the flowmeter block never drops below 25% of the nitrous oxide concentration. When the machine master switch is turned on, a basal flow rate of 200–300 ml/min of oxygen is established. This is independent of, and bypasses, the ratio mixer valve. Oxygen supplied to the ratio mixer valve exerts a pressure on one side of a diaphragm, which is opposed by the pressure of the nitrous oxide supplied on the other side. Any increase in the flow of nitrous oxide results in an increase in pressure on that side of the diaphragm, causing the latter to move towards the compartment containing oxygen. This increases the pressure on the oxygen contained

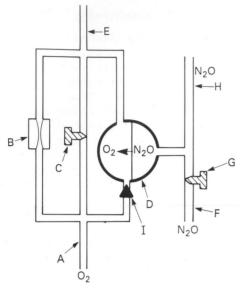

A = Oxygen supply
B = Flow restrictor
C = Oxygen flowmeter valve
D = Minimum ratio mixer valve
E = Oxygen flowmeter
F = Nitrous oxide supply
G = Nitrous oxide flowmeter valve
H = Nitrous oxide flowmeter
 I = One way valve

**Figure 7.18** Minimum ratio gas system.

in its compartment and therefore increases the flow rate of oxygen through the ratio mixer valve to the flowmeter tube. The diaphragm is so constructed that it will increase the oxygen flow rate by a ratio of 25% of any increase in the nitrous oxide flow rate. This increased oxygen flow is independent of the main oxygen flow control valve that bypasses the ratio mixer valve and, of course, can be adjusted independently. The ratio mixer valve ingeniously does not work in reverse; that is, if the nitrous oxide flow rates are reduced, the oxygen flows remain as set. This is because the nitrous oxide side of the ratio mixer valve diaphragm is connected downstream of the nitrous oxide flow control valve and does not have access to an unrestricted flow of gas (nitrous oxide) as the oxygen delivery system does.

### Electronically controlled anti-hypoxia device (Penlon Ltd)

Penlon use a Servomex paramagnetic oxygen analyser to sample the mixture of gases leaving the flowmeter bank. If the oxygen concentration in these gases falls below 25%, a battery-powered electronic device sounds an audible alarm and the nitrous

oxide supply is cut off. This results in an increase in the oxygen concentration and, as a result, the nitrous oxide supply is temporarily restored. If the oxygen flow rate has not been increased, the nitrous oxide disabling system is reactivated and the alarm will again sound. The whole process is repeated, thus providing an intermittent oxygen failure alarm and at the same time assuring a breathing mixture with more than 25% oxygen (although the total flow rate will be lower than intended).

If the oxygen supply fails completely, there is a continuous audible alarm. The power is provided by a maintenance-free lead-acid battery which is kept charged by the mains electricity supply while the machine is in use and will continue to operate in the absence of a mains supply for 1.5 hours. If the audible alarm is activated during this period it will sound for 20 minutes after which a visual and audible 'low battery' warning is given. If for some reason the lead-acid battery is not adequately charged at the beginning of an anaesthetic session, the nitrous oxide supply (as well as medical air in US versions) is disabled and cannot be used. However, under no circumstances is the oxygen supply interrupted. This alarm is in addition to the standard oxygen failure warning device (Ritchie Whistle, see below)

## The Back Bar

Strictly speaking, the term 'back bar' describes the horizontal part of the frame of the machine, which supports the flowmeter block, the vaporizers and some other components, but it is often used loosely to include also those components and the gaseous pathways interconnecting them. In fact, in modern machines the latter are often housed within the framework. The vaporizers are mounted, either singly or in series, along the back bar, downstream from the flowmeter block. Traditionally they were bolted on to the back bar and linked to each other by tapered fittings. The various manufacturers employed different sizes of tapers (see Table 9.2) and also mounting positions (Fig 7.19), but these have been superseded by the provisions of BS 3849 UK which recommends 23 mm 'Cagemount' tapers. The term cagemount originally refers to a type of tapered connection with a small wire cage fitted to the inlet of a reservoir or rebreathing bag. This prevents the neck of the bag from being obstructed, when the latter is empty and collapsed.

The most modern trend is towards vaporizers that may easily be removed and replaced by those for

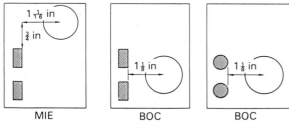

**Figure 7.19** Dimensions of the back bar. Notice in the case of M & IE fittings that the gas passages of the components are higher than the back bar, while in BOC fittings they are at the same level.

another agent. Thus, the back bar provides mounting blocks as described below. Figure 7.20 (a–c) shows some examples.

### The Penlon 'off-line' system (Fig.7.20a)

This uses a modified cagemount arrangement of flexible back bar hoses with tapered connections that can be separated and connected to a vaporizer to include it within the back bar. The system may allow partial or complete disconnection of a vaporizer (resulting in a major gas leak) to occur without being recognized in certain circumstances, rendering the machine inoperable.

### The Penlon 'back entry' system (Fig 7.20b)

This largely overcomes the problem of inadvertent gas leakage. The vaporizer is attached to the back bar by a fixing bolt protruding through the rear panel of the machine. Protruding pegs and seals on the back bar automatically locate and seal the inlet and outlet connections to the vaporizer. The fixing bolt is tightened using a gas cylinder key to produce a leak-proof seal. Three entry systems can be mounted in series along the back bar. Each system incorporates a cover which, when closed, shuts two valves in the back bar, effectively sealing the inlet and outlet ports on that back bar entry position and diverting the gases across that portion of the back bar. However, if the cover is inadvertently lifted without a vaporizer present, a leak will occur, and therefore the fitment of a blanking plate to effect a gas-tight seal is essential.

### The Ohmeda 'Selectatec' system (Fig. 7.20c)

The Selectatec system has, built in to the upper face of the back bar, two vertically mounted male valve ports (inlet and outlet) between which is a locking device. The matching vaporizer assembly has two female ports between which there is a key for the

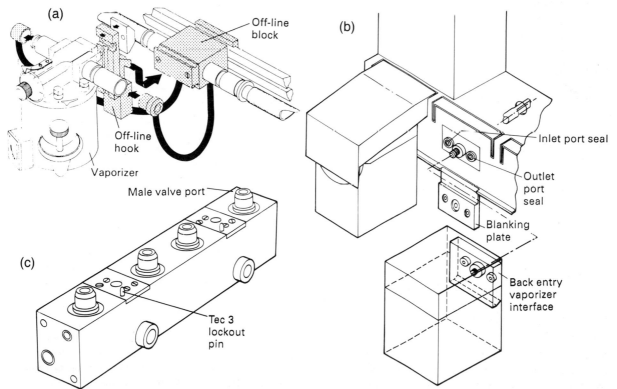

**Figure 7.20** (a) The Penlon 'off-line' block. (b) The Penlon back-entry system. (c) Selectatec block showing lock out pin to include TEC 3 vaporizers.

Selectatec lock. The vaporizer is lowered on to the male valve ports and the key is turned to lock it on to the back bar. 'O' rings on the male valve ports ensure a gas-tight fit. The two female ports on the vaporizer have recessed spindles, (TEC 4 and 5) that, when the vaporizer is switched on, protrude through the gas-tight seals of the male valve ports on the back bar. The ball valves (that provide the seals) in the male ports are displaced downwards occluding the back bar and gas from the back bar diverted into the vaporizer (see Fig. 7.20c). TEC 3 vaporizers have fixed spindles that automatically depress the ball valves in the male valve ports when the vaporizer is lowered on to the back bar assembly. Gas, therefore, passes through the head of the vaporizer even when it is not switched on nor even locked on. This arrangement obviously increases the potential for a gas leak and has been modified by the recessable spindle assembly on the TEC 4 and 5. The latter two models also incorporate a 'safety interlock'. This consists of a stout pin which protrudes sideways from a vaporizer which is turned on, and enters the vaporizer beside it, preventing the latter from being used by locking the control system. More recently, versions of the Selectatec back bar have been fitted with an accessory pin sited between the male valve ports at each vaporizer station to prevent TEC 3 vaporizers from being attached. The latter have no safety interlock mechanism (see below) and so cannot inactivate other vaporizers mounted on the back bar which are not in use. The absence of this mechanism allows two vaporizers to be used simultaneously (which is generally thought to be inadvisable).

Systems in which vaporizers may be detached are generally regarded as an advance over the permanent cagemount system. Ease of removal has resulted in a greater flexibility in the choice and use of vaporizers (especially with newer agents becoming available), and also ensure that anaesthetic machines do not have to be taken out of use to allow the servicing of the vaporizers.

Removable vaporizer systems, however, do generate their own specific problems. As mentioned above there is a greater potential for leaks. Also, in countries where trichloroethylene is still used, a vaporizer containing this agent may accidently be attached to a back bar station in a position that results in the vapour being passed into a breathing system containing soda lime. Trichloroethylene is known to react with warm soda lime to produce substances that are neurotoxic if inhaled.

On some older machines, the trichloroethylene vaporizer, where fitted, was always permanently

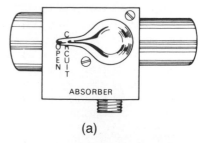

(a)

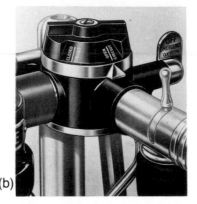

(b)

**Figure 7.21** (a) The trichloroethylene (trilene) safety bypass control of M & IE. (b) The (BOC) trilene safety interlock combined with a tap to direct the fresh gas flow to either a Mapleson breathing system or the absorber. There is also an oxygen emergency flush control.

sited downstream of a tap on the back bar. This diverted gas to a specific outlet to which the breathing system containing soda lime could be connected without trichloroethylene contamination (Fig. 7.21).

Newer systems now incorporate devices (safety interlock mechanisms) which prevent vaporizers, placed in series on a back bar, from being used simultaneously. If this were allowed to occur, the downstream vaporizer would become contaminated with vapour from the one upstream, and this may be administered inadvertently to a patient during a subsequent use of the machine. At one time it was recommended that the vaporizer for the more volatile agent in use should be mounted upstream. Later, when the danger of halothane contaminating a vaporizer for trichloroethylene was pointed out, it was considered prudent to mount the vaporizer for the more volatile agent downstream. The rationale for this is that if an upstream vaporizer for halothane were turned 'on' at the same time as a downstream one for trichloroethylene (prior to TEC 4 and 5, which have safety interlock systems), halothane could be dissolved in (or absorbed by) the liquid trichloroethylene. When the trichloroethylene vaporizer was next used a high concentration of halothane could be given off, the saturated concentration of halothane being 30% at room temperature. Bearing in mind the advent of other agents, perhaps one should consider the ratio between the saturated and the highest clinically safe vapour concentrations and mount the vaporizer for the agent with the lowest ratio upstream and that with the highest ratio, downstream. As mentioned previously, this situation is now remedied with newer vaporizer systems which have interlocking devices which disable all other vaporizers not intended to be in use on the back bar.

### Back bar working pressures

The flowmeter tubes in the flowmeter bank have as a rule been calibrated for gas flows assuming no downstream resistance. In a traditional back bar (23-mm internal diameter system) with the vaporizers switched off, the wide bore of the gas passages offers minimal flow resistance and so the back bar pressure developed at conventional flow rates (5–10 litres/min) is marginally above atmospheric pressure. However many modern back bars have narrow bore (8-mm) gas passages which increase flow resistance and thus back pressure on the flowmeters.

The addition of high resistance vaporizers and minute volume divider ventilators further increases back bar pressures. Table 7.2 below shows typical back bar pressures developed and percentage changes in flowmeter settings with the 'Selectatec' back bar

with and without a high resistance vaporizer fitted. It should be noted that the small decreases in the flowmeter indications produced does not mean a decrease in the flow of gas to a patient. It is merely that the gas is compressed at the higher pressures and subsequently re-expands downstream when the various resistances have been overcome. Readjustment of the flowmeters to the original settings following an induced pressure rise would therefore be inappropriate.

## Safety Features

A number of safety features are installed either on or downstream of the back bar. Intermittent back pressure surges from certain minute volume divider ventilators can adversely affect vaporizer performance, and so most machines employ a spring-loaded non-return valve (Fig. 7.22) in the system to

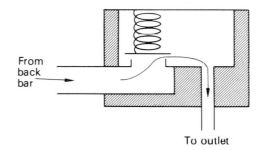

**Figure 7.22** Non-return valve in the back bar.

**Table 7.2**  Selectatec back bar working pressures

| Recorded Gas Pressures in a two station back bar | | Nominal flow rates at atmospheric pressure | | *Percentage change in flowmeter sight readings at | |
|---|---|---|---|---|---|
| | | 5 litres | 10 litres | 5 litres | 10 litres |
| Beginning of back bar (no vaporizers in situ) | | 1.18 kPa (12 cmH₂O) | 4.2 kPa (43 cmH₂O) | None | Minimal |
| At 2nd vaporizer station (no vaporizers in situ) | | 0.78 kPa (8 cmH₂O) | 2.45 kPa (25 cmH₂O) | None | Minimal |
| Beginning of back bar with TEC 4 vaporizer at 2nd station delivering different concentrations | 0% | 1.18 kPa (12 cmH₂O) | 4.2 kPa (43 cmH₂O) | None | Minimal |
| | 1% | 3.23 kPa (33 cmH₂O) | 8.5 kPa (87 cmH₂O) | None | <5% |
| | 5% | 2.74 kPa (28 cmH₂O) | 7.74 kPa (79 cmH₂O) | None | <5% |
| Total occlusion of common gas outlet | | 30.5 kPa (312 cmH₂O) | | 20% | 20% |

* This column shows the percentage change in sight readings, in a flowmeter initially calibrated at atmospheric pressure caused by the various resistances to flow seen in a 'Selectatec' back bar and TEC 4 vaporizer.

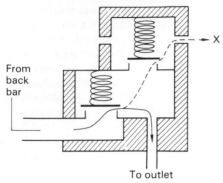

**Figure 7.23** Combined non-return and pressure-relief valve at the end of the back bar. If the outlet is obstructed, the gases escape at X, so protecting the back bar from overpressure. A low-pressure relief valve is also available to protect the patient.

prevent these surges reaching the vaporizers. Since high pressure build-up in the back bar can damage flowmeter and vaporizer components, a pressure relief valve (commonly set at 30–40 kPa) is fitted (Fig. 7.23). This is often fitted in the same housing as the non return valve.

## Emergency oxygen

A flowmeter bypass valve for an emergency oxygen supply is now fitted as standard (BS 4272, UK) near the common gas outlet so that, when activated, it preferentially supplies oxygen at a rate of not less than 30 litres/min into an attached breathing system. In earlier anaesthetic machines this bypass for oxygen was fitted near the flowmeter block. When it was operated, this resulted in an initial surge of gas and vapour to the patient prior to the pure oxygen being delivered. This valve should no longer have a locking facility since this is regarded as dangerous and has resulted in cases of barotrauma when it has been switched on accidently. Furthermore, cases of awareness during anaesthesia have occurred when the locking facility was in use and unnoticed, resulting in a substantial dilution of anaesthetic agents. The valve knob should also be recessed to minimize the chances of its inadvertent operation.

## Oxygen failure warning devices

These were first introduced in the late 1950s as a response to the problems of unobserved emptying of oxygen cylinders.

*The Bosun.* The first commercially manufactured design was the 'Bosun' (Fig 7.24). In this device

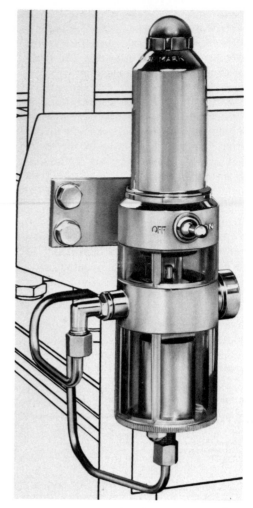

**Figure 7.24** The Bosun oxygen failure warning device.

nitrous oxide at regulated pressure is tapped from the supply on the anaesthetic machine and connected to the base of a piston sited within a sealed chamber. A similarly obtained supply of oxygen, also at regulated pressure, is fed into the sealed chamber above the piston, and prevents any movement of the piston. In the event of an oxygen supply failure, the piston is driven upwards by the pressure of the nitrous oxide and completes an electrical circuit which lights up a battery-powered red lamp. Nitrous oxide is diverted via an audible whistle to the atmosphere. The disadvantage of this device is that if the nitrous oxide supply to it is turned off, and this may be done on some models by simply turning off a tap adjacent to the device, the audible warning is not given. Similarly, the battery may be exhausted, and in any case it also can be switched off.

*The Ritchie whistle.* The Ritchie whistle was introduced in the mid-1960s and now forms the basis for most current alarms. It was the first device to rely exclusively on the failing oxygen supply for its power. Figure 7.25 shows an oxygen failure warning device incorporating a Ritchie whistle marketed at one time by Ohmeda.

The alarm is powered by an oxygen supply at a pressure of 420 kPa (60 psi) in the UK, which is tapped from the oxygen pipework upstream of the flowmeter block. This enters the alarm inlet valve and pressurizes the rolling diaphragm, opening the anaesthetic cut-off valve, and closing the air inspiratory valve and the port to the oxygen failure whistle. Anaesthetic gases may then pass freely through this device which is now at standby.

When the oxygen pressure supplying the flowmeter block drops below 260 kPa (38 psi), a spring causes the anaesthetic gases cut off valve to begin to close and the oxygen failure whistle valve to open, permitting a flow of oxygen, (via the restrictor) to operate the oxygen failure whistle. The whistle sounds continuously until the oxygen pressure has fallen to approximately 40.5 kPa (6 psi).

At a pressure of approximately 200 kPa (30 psi) the force of the magnet keeper return spring and the magnet causes the anaesthetic gases cut-off valve to be closed, cutting off the supply of anaesthetic gases. At the same time the spring load on the air inspiratory valve is released, allowing the patient to inspire room air. Whenever the patient inhales, the inspiratory air whistle sounds.

With the anaesthetic gases cut-off valve closed, the now potentially hypoxic gas from the flowmeter block vents through the pressure-relief valve on the back bar.

### Current oxygen failure warning devices

British Standard 4272 Part 3 specifies the criteria required for oxygen failure warning devices fitted to current anaesthetic machines.

1. The alarm shall be auditory, shall be of at least 7 s duration and shall have a noise level of at least 60 dB measured at 1 metre from the front of the anaesthetic machine.
2. The energy required to operate the alarm shall be derived solely from the oxygen supply pressure in the machine gas piping and the alarm shall be activated when this pressure falls to approximately 200 kPa.
3. The alarm shall be of a design that cannot be switched off or reset without initially restoring the oxygen supply pressure.
4. The alarm shall be linked to a gas shut-off device that performs at least *one* of the following functions.

- It shall cut off the supply of all gases other than oxygen (and air, where fitted) to the common gas outlet.
- It shall progressively reduce the flow of all other gases while maintaining the pre-set oxygen flow or proportion of oxygen until the supply of oxygen finally fails, at which point the supply of all other gases shall be shut off.
- Where an air supply is fitted, it shall progressively reduce the flow of all other gases except air while maintaining the pre-set oxygen flow or proportion of oxygen until the supply of oxygen fails, at which point the supply of all other gases, except air, shall be shut off.
- It shall establish a pathway between the machine

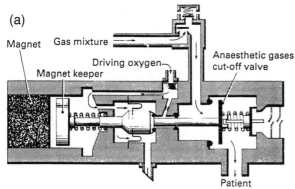

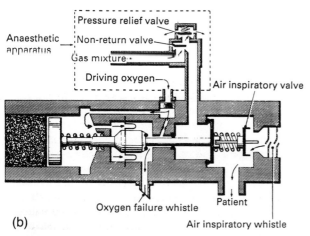

**Figure 7.25** Oxygen failure warning device: (a) normal operation; (b) operation during oxygen failure.

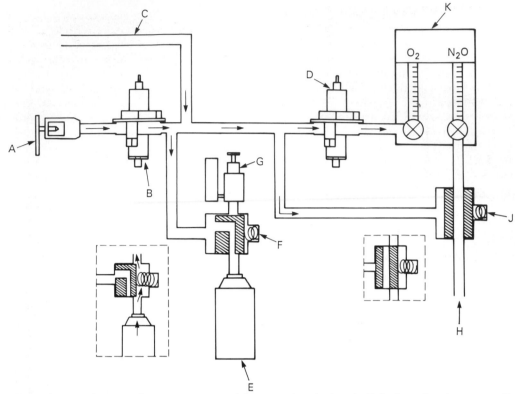

**Figure 7.26** A schematic diagram of a current oxygen failure warning device. A, Cylinder yokes for oxygen; B, Primary regulator for oxygen (137 000 kPa → 420 kPa); C, Pipeline oxygen supply; D, Secondary regulator for oxygen (420 kPa → 140 kPa (Ohmeda)); E, Reservoir of oxygen required to power the Ritchie Whistle for a minimum of 6 secs; F, Spring loaded regulator. When oxygen supply pressure drops to 200 kPa reservoir E is connected to Ritchie Whistle; G, Ritchie Whistle; H, Nitrous oxide supply; J, Spring loaded shut-off valve to nitrous oxide supply activated when oxygen supply pressure drops below 200 kPa; K, Flowmeter bank.

gas delivery system and the atmosphere.

- The gas cut-off device shall not be activated before the oxygen failure alarm is activated.
- It shall not be possible to re-set the gas cut-off device without prior restoration of the oxygen supply pressure to above the pressure of approximately 200 kPa.

A schematic diagram of such a device is shown in Fig. 7.26.

## The Common Gas Outlet

The various medical gases and vapours exit the machine via a 22 mm male/15 mm female conically tapered outlet (BS 3849 UK). This common gas outlet may be fixed, or swivelled through 90° (Cardiff Swivel), and should be strong enough to withstand a bending moment of force of up to 10 Nm applied to its axis, since heavy equipment is often attached.

BS 4272 UK, recommends that this outlet is fitted with an anti-disconnect device. The M & IE outlet includes a male thread for securing heavy devices such as a fuel cell oxygen analyser or other equipment. Older systems with two common gas outlets, (those fitted with a back bar switch which could divert gas to a separate outlet for the circle absorber system) are now discouraged since these can promote confusion to the unfamiliar user as to which outlet is operational.

## Auxiliary Gas Sockets

Anaesthetic machines may now be fitted with mini Schrader gas sockets (Fig. 7.27), but only for air or oxygen. These are used to power a number of devices such as ventilators for low-flow anaesthesia systems, venturi systems for bronchoscopy, and suction units. The sockets should be permanently

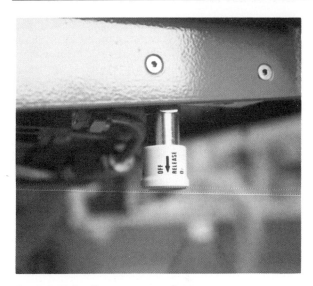

**Figure 7.27** Auxiliary oxygen outlet.

and legibly marked for their specific gases (air or oxygen) and their working pressure of 400 kPa approximately in the UK. They should also carry a warning symbol consisting of an exclamation mark within a triangle.

# 'Quantiflex' Machines

There is a range of continuous-flow machines for different purposes, all of which embody safety devices to prevent the administration of mixtures of gases containing less than a predetermined amount of oxygen. The Quantiflex MDM is described below, and the Quantiflex RA in Chapter 11. Note that the oxygen flowmeter is usually on the right and nitrous oxide flowmeter is on the left.

### The Quantiflex 'Monitored Dial Mixer' (MDM) surgical anaesthetic machine (Fig. 7.28)

The flow rates of nitrous oxide and oxygen are indicated by the two flowmeters, but the combined flow rate is controlled by a single knob. The relative percentages of nitrous oxide and oxygen are determined by the mixture control wheel, which is calibrated in steps of 10% from 30 to 100% oxygen. Thus never more than 70% nitrous oxide can be given. A carbon dioxide flowmeter and fine adjustment valve may be provided as an 'add-on' unit, but works independently of the flow rate and mixture controls.

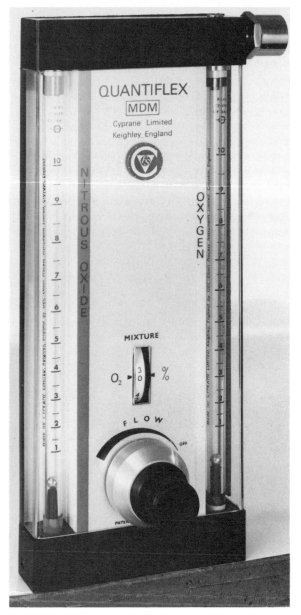

**Figure 7.28** The Quantiflex MDM anaesthetic machine. The lower knob controls the flow rate and the wheel above it adjusts the percentage of oxygen. Notice that 30% is the minimum amount of oxygen in the mixed gas flow. Note also that the nitrous oxide and oxygen flowmeters are in the reverse sequence to that which is customary in the UK.

# Maintenance of Anaesthetic Machines

In the UK it is recommended that all anaesthetic machines are serviced by competent engineers according to the manufacturers' advice. This has usually been four times a year, and that ventilators be serviced every six months. This service consists of cleaning all parts of the machine, including the flowmeter tubes; checking of flowmeters, regulators and all other parts such as corrugated tubing and breathing bags; and the cleaning and regreasing of the drums of vaporizers, circle absorbers, etc. as appropriate. It does not, however, usually include attention to the temperature-compensated vaporizers, which are serviced expertly by the appropriate manufacturer. Thymol, a normal constituent of halothane tends to collect in vaporizers, and most manufacturers advise that temperature-compensated vaporizers be returned to their factory once a year for an overhaul. It is usually possible to obtain a service exchange or other vaporizer on temporary loan while the original is away at the factory. As previously mentioned manufacturers recommend that the liquid agent be drained off, discarded and replenished at regular intervals, usually every two weeks.

Besides maintenance by service engineers it is wise for the anaesthetist to carry out his own checks (see Appendix IV).

# 8 Electronics in the Anaesthetic Machine

## Introduction

The modern anaesthetic machine has, not surprisingly, been invaded by electronics. This invasion has taken place, or will take place, in a number of ways, namely:

- integral physiological monitoring equipment;
- electronic monitoring of a conventional pneumatic anaesthetic machine;
- electronic control of gases and vapours in an entirely new form of pneumatic circuit;
- servo-control of gases and vapours;
- servo-control of depth-of-anaesthesia.

Monitoring of physiological variables is dealt with in Chapter 16 and the monitoring of gas composition and flow is dealt with in Chapter 15. This chapter will deal with the electronic control of gases and vapours and the principles of servo-control and will conclude with some remarks about including the patient in the servo-control loop.

## Ergonomics

*Ergonomics* is the study of the efficiency of persons in their working environment and *human factors engineering* is the design and development of equipment to improve the ergonomics of a task. This has the effect of making the working environment not only more pleasant but less tiring and less stressful, which should lead to increased safety (see Chapter 24). The conventional anaesthetic machine 'just grew' and there has been little attempt in the past to consider ergonomics. For example, when considering the fresh gas output of the anaesthetic machine, the anaesthetist has in mind a minute volume or fresh gas flow rate and an inspired oxygen percentage in either air or nitrous oxide. To acquire this output he has to select a flow rate for each of the component gases, add the flow rates mentally, and calculate the proportions of the constituents. It would be much more convenient to him or her if he could select:

- the *combination*: oxygen/nitrous oxide *or* air/oxygen;
- the *required total flow* in litres/minute;
- the *percentage of oxygen*.

Consideration also needs to be given to the display of any information, composition of gases, flow rates, airway pressure, etc. In order to make such changes to the ergonomics of the anaesthetic machine it is necessary to start from scratch, firstly asking what is required (as above) and then using new technologies to implement these goals.

## Control Engineering

*Control engineering* is a modern and complex subject concerned with automatic or semi-automatic control of variables and the correction of errors in their control. It also deals with the subject of *closed-loop systems* or *servo-control loops*.

The principle of a servo-control loop is shown in Fig. 8.1. A *system*, which may be part of an anaesthetic machine has its output varied by a controller device. In electronic servo-loops, the output is measured by the transducer which converts it to an electrical signal which may need amplification. This signal is then compared with the desired or *reference value* and the difference or error signal is then used to adjust the controlling element until the output of the system is at the required

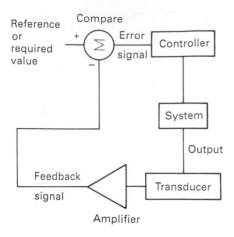

**Figure 8.1** The principle of servo-control loops.

value, at which point the error signal will be zero. The human analogy is of the anaesthetist continually adjusting the ventilator controls to maintain a particular end-tidal carbon dioxide level. The design of servo-control loops is complex as it is necessary to take into account delays, hysteresis, damping and stability.

# New Components

There are many ways by which the gases may be controlled, but to do so, different components are required in the interface between the gas circuit and the electronic circuitry, not only those to control the gas composition and flow, but also transducers for pressure, flow and composition.

## Control of gas flow

The electrical control of gas flow is usually by a motor-driven valve or by solenoid-operated valves. *Motor-driven valves* are in the form of conventional needle valves but a small geared-down electric motor replaces the knob that would normally be operated by hand. In a servo-loop system an infinite range of flows may be obtained from zero flow to the maximum flow permitted by the fully open valve. *Solenoid-operated valves* are usually valves that are either open or shut, with no intermediate positions, operated by an electromagnet (solenoid). They may be used in two ways to produce an apparently variable flow. (1) A bank of valves on a manifold, each having a pre-set flow rate, as shown in Fig. 8.2. Selection of combinations of the valves, by a microprocessor, produces the flow rates as

shown. (2) A single high-speed valve is operated at a high frequency with a variable *'mark–space ratio'* (Fig. 8.3); in other words, although the overall frequency is constant, the ratio between the periods of time during which the valve is open and when it is closed is varied. Thus the mean flow rate is infinitely variable between zero and the maximum, which is attained when the valve is constantly open. The disadvantage of this technique is that the flow is pulsatile. This is overcome by passing the gas into a damping chamber, which may be a simple

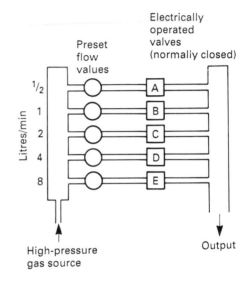

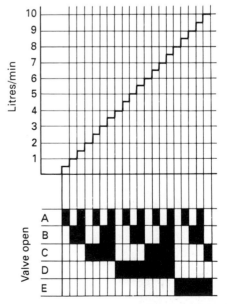

**Figure 8.2** Digital control of gas flow. The electrically operated or 'solenoid' valves are controlled by a microprocessor. Each valve may only be fully open or fully closed.

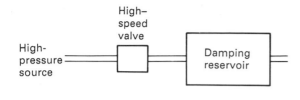

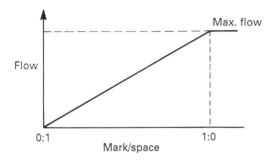

**Figure 8.3** Computer-controlled single high-speed solenoid valve providing continuously variable flow rate.

chamber or may also contain a spring-loaded piston, to smooth the flow.

## Transducers

A *transducer* is a device which converts one form of energy into another for the purposes of measurement. In general, this second form of energy is electrical. In the case of electronically controlled anaesthetic machines, pressure and flow transducers are needed to complete feedback loops for the control of these variables. Pressure transducers are described in Chapter 1 and flow transducers in Chapter 5.

# An Electronically Controlled Anaesthetic Machine

The Engström ELSA illustrates many of the principles of the anaesthetic machine of the future (Fig. 8.4). It has been developed with ergonomics and safety as prime considerations. A simplified description of the ELSA is given below.

The ELSA is divided into two sections, namely a lower anaesthetic delivery unit and an upper monitoring unit; although this layout is used for ergonomic reasons, the two units are fully integrated.

The supply pressures of oxygen, nitrous oxide and air are monitored electronically by semiconductor pressure transducers; the oxygen supply also has a conventional pneumatic alarm whistle. The pressure-regulated gases then pass to the gas mixer (Fig. 8.5).

Familiar controls are provided for oxygen, nitrous oxide and air, which operate conventional needle valves. These control knobs have pointers associated with them which give an approximate indication of the relevant flow rate so that a fresh gas flow can be maintained in the event of a power failure. The actual value of flow set is measured by an electronic thermistor mass-flow sensor and displayed electronically as a bar-graph. Flows down to 200 ml/min can be selected accurately by observing the bar-graph as the needle valve is adjusted. The mixer provides a minimum flow of 200 ml/min continuously, for safety, corresponding to the basic adult metabolic requirement. An oxygen-flush facility enables an emergency oxygen flow of about

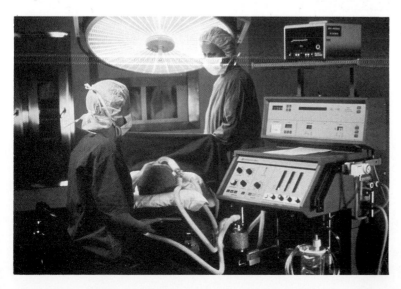

**Figure 8.4** Engström ELSA electronically controlled anaesthetic machine.

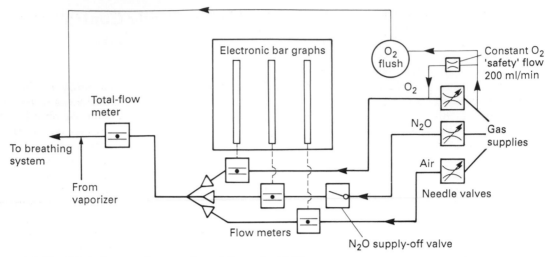

**Figure 8.5** Simplified diagram of a gas mixer of Engström ELSA.

50 litres/min to pass directly to the fresh gas outlet or the circle system. As an extra check on the function of the gas mixing valves, the total measured flow of the mixed gases is compared internally with the individual gas flows.

If a breathing gas mixture containing less than 21% oxygen is set and not corrected, the nitrous oxide flow is automatically shut off after 5 s. Simultaneous delivery of air and nitrous oxide is not possible.

### The vaporizer

The volatile anaesthetic agent is delivered directly into the fresh gas mixture as very small boluses of 100% vapour by a vaporizer which is unlike the conventional manually operated type (Fig. 8.6). There are three separate vaporizers, one for each of the agents: halothane, enflurane and isoflurane. The supply of volatile agent is stored on the machine in its original bottle, which is attached to the vaporizer assembly with a non-interchangeable adaptor. A pressure of 0.4 bar of oxygen is applied to the contents of the bottle to drive the liquid as required into the vaporizing chamber. A capacitive electronic sensor is used to measure the remaining contents of the supply bottle. This level is indicated on a bar-graph display on the front of the machine. The liquid then passes to the vaporizing chamber, which is electrically heated. The temperature at the

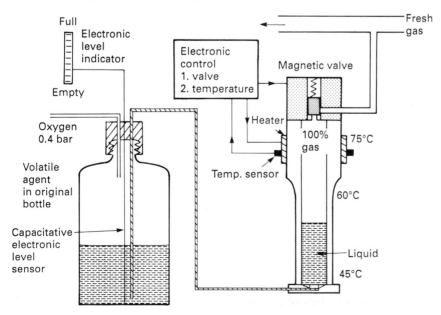

**Figure 8.6** Simplified diagram of a vaporizer — Engström ELSA.

top of the chamber is maintained at 75°C in the case of the halothane and isoflurane vaporizers, and 80°C in the case of enflurane. This falls to a temperature of about 45°C at the bottom of the chamber where the liquid enters. Thus the upper part of the chamber contains 100% anaesthetic vapour whilst the lower part contains the liquid form. One-millilitre boluses of this 100% vapour are then allowed to join the gases from the gas mixer by the opening, for short periods, of an electromagnetically controlled valve at the top of the chamber. The frequency with which these 1-ml boluses of vapour are allowed into the fresh gas flow is automatically varied so that the dialled vapour concentration is maintained irrespective of the fresh gas flow rate.

## The breathing systems

The fresh gas supply, with or without added volatile agent, is passed either to a fresh gas outlet for the addition of standard breathing systems, or to an integral circle absorber system with a built-in ventilator. The circle system is shown diagrammatically in Fig. 8.7. The gas flow is conventional but the parts shown within the boxed area may be removed as a single unit and autoclaved. Both the inspiratory and expiratory gas flows are measured using venturi flowmeters as described in Chapter 5. The airway pressure is monitored electronically and also displayed using a conventional mechanical aneroid pressure gauge. A safety inlet valve allows ingress of air if there is insufficient gas in the circle. The breathing bag is visible inside a transparent pressure chamber.

## The ventilator

The ventilator, shown schematically in Fig. 8.8, works on the bag-in-bottle principle. The reservoir (patient bag) inside the pressure chamber is filled with a continuous flow of respirable gases. By increasing the pressure inside the chamber, the bag is compressed and respirable gas is pushed into the circle system. During mechanical ventilation, the increased pressure is due to flow from the driving gas, and during manual ventilation by squeezing the manual bag. These two sources are connected to the pressure chamber via a bistable mechanical valve. This valve switches from one position to the other, depending upon the pressure difference between its two inputs. Whenever the manual bag is squeezed, the pressure increase automatically switches the bistable valve to connect the manual bag to the pressure chamber. To allow rapid adjustment of the gas volume in the manual bag, there is a filling valve that allows oxygen into the system. During the induction and spontaneous ventilation modes, the machine allows the patient to breath spontaneously from the patient bag. During spontaneous ventilation, the breaths are visible and may be 'felt' as the manual bag moves in sympathy with the patient bag.

During mechanical ventilation, the driving gas passes at a pre-set 'inspiratory flow rate', through a

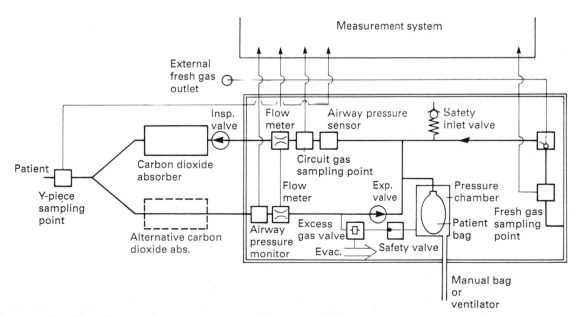

**Figure 8.7** Simplified diagram of a breathing system — Engström ELSA.

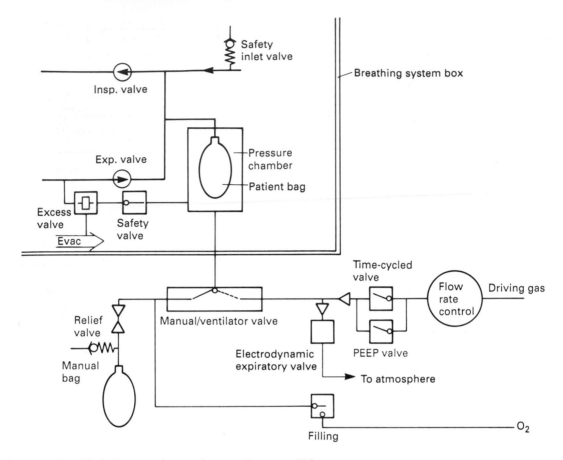

**Figure 8.8** Simplified diagram of a ventilator — Engström ELSA.

time-cycled solenoid valve into the pressure chamber, thus compressing the patient bag. During exhalation, inspiratory gas flow ceases and the driving gas is allowed to pass from the pressure chamber, via an electrodynamic expiratory valve, out to the atmosphere. This flow through an electrodynamic valve varies depending upon the electric current passing through it and may therefore be adjusted in conjunction with an extra amount of driving gas (via the PEEP valve) to provide a variable amount of positive end-expiratory pressure.

## Monitor functions

Transducers convert the following variables into electrical signals:
- gas supply pressures;
- airway pressure;
- inspired and expired breathing gas volumes;
- fresh gas flows, individually and total;
- fresh gas temperatures;
- vaporizer temperatures;

- volatile agent liquid levels;
- oxygen concentration (paramagnetic*);
- carbon dioxide (infrared*);
- volatile agents (infrared*).

The analogue signals from these transducers are all converted to digital format and two microprocessors, one for the ventilator and the other for all other functions, use the signals for control and safety monitoring of the machine function. Control messages and alarms are clearly displayed on the monitoring panel.

The control and safety functions of the microprocessors are fully integrated and will protect the patient from: gas supply failure; electrical supply failure; hypoxic mixtures; disconnections; soda-lime exhaustion; hypercapnoea; sum of fresh gas flows different from total fresh gas flow; vaporizer set too high; excessive airway pressure; exhaled minute volume outside pre-set limits; measured oxygen or volatile agents outside pre-set limits; measured end-

---

* The methods used to detect the concentration of gases/vapours are described in Chapter 15.

tidal carbon dioxide outside pre-set limit and technical failure.

Use of microprocessor technology in an anaesthetic machine in this way also means that automatic intervention can be made to occur under certain alarm conditions.

- Oxygen supply failure automatically shuts off the nitrous oxide supply.
- A delivered hypoxic fresh gas mixture instantly initiates an alarm, and if it is not corrected within 5 s the nitrous oxide is shut off.
- Nitrous oxide is automatically shut off if air flow is opened.
- If an excessive airway pressure occurs, it is automatically relieved.
- Vaporizer malfunction causes automatic shut-off and depressurization of the supply bottles.
- Anaesthetic agent concentration above a pre-set level *in the circle system* causes the vaporizer to shut off.

Most importantly, all of these conditions cause an alarm to sound and the nature of the fault condition to be displayed in words in the centre of the monitor panel.

## Servo-controlled Anaesthesia

There is currently much debate about the possibility of 'closing the loop' to servo-control the administration of anaesthesia. Figure 8.9 shows a commonly used servo-control loop for the control of blood pressure with vasoactive drug infusions. In essence this is once again the control loop of Fig. 8.1. Even with this simple system, complications are introduced, as there is a variable delay between the change in infusion rate and the change in blood pressure, and this delay is not constant in time or between patients. Also, as a closed-loop system is used to control more and more powerful drugs, safety becomes an even greater priority, with the necessity of one microprocessor system controlling a loop whilst an independent microprocessor monitors the loop for safety.

Ideally, some form of depth-of-anaesthesia moni-

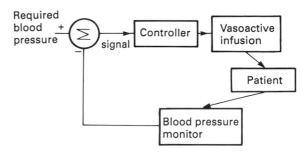

**Figure 8.9** Servo-control of arterial blood pressure.

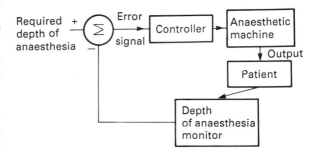

**Figure 8.10** Servo-control of depth of anaesthesia.

toring device is required as shown in Fig. 8.10. There is as yet no foolproof and easily applied monitor for depth of anaesthesia. The following techniques are under investigation but are at present outside the scope of this edition:

- electroencephalogram (EEG): zero crossing; spectral analysis; evoked response;
- monitoring of lower-oesophageal contractility;
- intravascular monitoring of arterial concentration of anaesthetic agents;
- monitoring of end-tidal exhaled concentration of anaesthetic agents.

None of these techniques has been proved to actually measure the depth of anaesthesia, and their reliability would have to be beyond reproach before their use could be contemplated in a closed servo-loop to control the administration of anaesthetic drugs.

# 9 Breathing Systems and their Components

## Introduction

The definition and classification of methods in which inhalation agents are delivered to a patient have undergone a number of changes since the beginnings of anaesthesia. Most current anaesthetic literature uses the following definitions and classifications.

## Definitions

*Breathing systems.* A breathing system (not a circuit) now describes both the mode of operation and the apparatus by which inhalation agents are delivered to the patient, i.e. a Mapleson A breathing system (generic terminology) would describe the mode of operation of a Magill breathing system (specific terminology). It was originally proposed that the actual apparatus be called an attachment (i.e. Magill attachment). Sadly however this is less commonly used.

*Rebreathing.* Rebreathing in anaesthetic systems now conventionally refers to the rebreathing of some or all of the previously exhaled gases, including carbon dioxide and water vapour. (Rebreathing apparatus in other spheres, e.g. fire fighting and underwater diving, has always referred to the recirculation of expired gas suitably purified and with the oxygen content restored or increased.) The previous edition of this book also used this definition to describe circle breathing systems, but this definition has now again disappeared from common useage in anaesthetic literature.

*Apparatus dead space.* This refers to that volume within the apparatus which may contain exhaled patient gas and which will be rebreathed at the beginning of a subsequent inspiratory breath (Fig. 9.1).

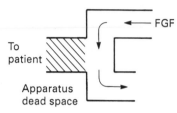

**Figure 9.1** Apparatus dead space in a breathing system. FGF = fresh gas flow.

*Functional dead space.* Some systems may well have a smaller 'functional' dead space owing to the flushing effect of a continuous fresh gas stream at the end of expiration replacing exhaled gas in the apparatus dead space (Fig. 9.2).

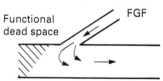

**Figure 9.2** Functional dead space in a breathing system with an angled FGF inlet. FGF = fresh gas flow.

### Classification of breathing systems

These are now usually classified according to function:

- non-rebreathing systems (with unidirectional flow of gas within the system);
- systems where rebreathing is possible, although not intended, (with bi-directional flow of gas within the system);
- non-rebreathing systems utilizing carbon dioxide absorption,
  (a) Unidirectional (circle) systems.
  (b) Bi-directional (to-and-fro) systems.

## Non-rebreathing Systems

The simplest way to develop an understanding of

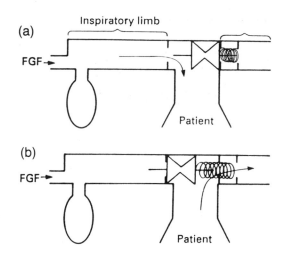

**Figure 9.3** Non-rebreathing valve: (a) inspiration; (b) exhalation. FGF = fresh gas flow.

gas delivery to a patient is to consider how a non-rebreathing system works using a non-rebreathing valve assembly (Fig. 9.3 a, b).

Fresh gas entering the system flows to the patient from the inspiratory limb (Fig 9.3a). It is either sucked in by the patient's inspiratory effort or blown in during controlled ventilation. The non-rebreathing valve is so constructed that when it opens to admit inspiratory gas, it occludes the expiratory limb of the system (see Fig. 9.3a). When the patient exhales, the reverse occurs, i.e. the valve mechanism moves to occlude the inspiratory limb and opens the expiratory limb to allow expired gases to escape (Fig. 9.3b). The mechanical principles by which the valve operates are discussed in Chapter 12 (page 190).

The inspiratory limb usually includes a distensible neoprene or rubber bag (2-litre capacity) which acts as a reservoir for fresh gas. This reservoir contains enough gas to cope with the intermittent high demand that occurs in inspiration. For example, a patient breathing normally (with a minute volume of 7 litres) may well have a tidal volume of 500 ml inhaled over approximately 1 s. This produces an average inspiratory flow rate (not peak flow rate) of 30 litres/min. Without this reservoir in the system, the fresh gas flow rate would have to at least match this figure (probably more, to match the patient's peak inspiratory flow rate) in order to avoid respiratory embarrassment.

The reservoir bag is refilled with fresh gas during the expiratory phase. It can also be compressed manually to provide assisted or controlled respiration since the non rebreathing valve works equally effectively in this mode as it does for spontaneous respiration (see Chapter 12).

In the non-rebreathing system described, the fresh gas flow rate needs to match the minute volume required by the patient.

## Systems Where Rebreathing is Possible (with Bi-directional Flow Within the System)

A miscellany of breathing systems was developed by early pioneers (largely intuitively) that allowed the to-and-fro movement of inspiratory and expiratory gases within the breathing system. Carbon dioxide elimination was achieved by the flushing action of fresh gas introduced into this breathing system, rather than by separation of the inspiratory and expiratory gas mixtures by a non-rebreathing valve described above. As it is mainly the flushing effect of fresh gas that eliminates carbon dioxide, these systems retain the potential for rebreathing of carbon dioxide when fresh gas flow rates are reduced.

Mapleson (1954) is credited with classifying these systems (A to E) according to their efficiency in eliminating carbon dioxide during spontaneous respiration. An F system, the Jackson Rees modification of system E (Ayre's T piece), was later added to the classification by Willis (1975), see below.

## Classification of Systems with Potential for Rebreathing

Figure 9.4 illustrates a modified Mapleson classification of breathing systems.

### Mapleson A breathing system (Fig 9.5)

The Mapleson A system illustrated is the Magill arrangement (or attachment) as popularized by Sir Ivan Magill in the 1920s. It consists of the following:

- at one end, an inlet for fresh gas linked to a 2-litre distensible rubber reservoir bag. (Not rebreathing bag, as the patient's exhaled gases should never be allowed to pass back into it.) This is attached to:
- a length of corrugated breathing hose (minimum length 110 cm with an internal volume of 550 ml). This represents slightly more than the average tidal volume in an anaesthetized adult breathing spontaneously. This volume is important as it minimizes the backtracking of exhaled alveolar gas back to the reservoir bag (see below). This is in turn connected to:

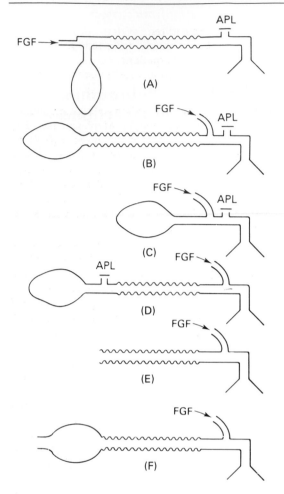

**Figure 9.4** A modified Mapleson classification of breathing systems in which there is potential for rebreathing. System (A) houses the gas reservoir in the afferent limb and is alternatively referred to as an afferent reservoir system. The fresh gas flow (FGF) need only be at or just below the patient's minute ventilation without functional rebreathing occurring. Systems (B) and (C) (junctional reservoir systems) require FGF of 1.5 times the minute ventilation to avoid rebreathing. Systems (D), (E) and (F) (efferent reservoir systems) require 2–3 times the minute ventilation to avoid rebreathing.

- variable tension, spring-loaded flap valve, for venting of exhaled gases. This valve should be attached at the opposite end of the system from the reservoir bag and as close to the patient as possible. It will be subsequently referred to as an APL (adjustable pressure limiting) valve.

The system makes efficient use of fresh gas during spontaneous breathing. This can be explained by examining its function during a respiratory cycle

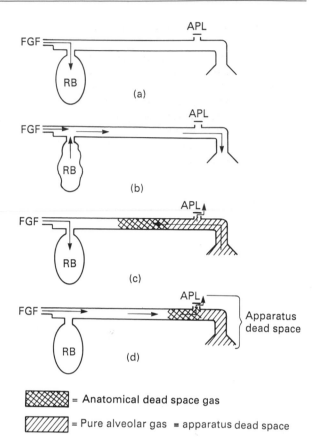

= Anatomical dead space gas

= Pure alveolar gas   = apparatus dead space

**Figure 9.5** The Mapleson A system used with spontaneous breathing (see text). FGF = fresh gas flow; APL = adjustable pressure-limiting (expiratory) valve. RB = reservoir bag.

consisting of three phases: inspiration, expiration, and an end-expiratory pause.

*Inspiration.* In Fig. 9.5a the reservoir bag and breathing hose have been filled by the fresh gas flow and the patient is about to take a breath. The whole system is therefore full of fresh gas. As the patient inspires, the gases are drawn into the lungs at a rate greater than the fresh gas flow and so the reservoir bag partially empties as shown in Fig. 9.5b.

*Expiration.* In Fig. 9.5c the patient has begun to exhale, and because the reservoir bag is not full, the exhaled gases are breathed back along the corrugated hose, pushing the fresh gases in the hose back towards the reservoir bag. However, before the exhaled gases can pass as far as the reservoir bag (hence the importance of the length of the inspiratory hose), the latter has been refilled by the fresh gases from the corrugated hose plus the continuing fresh gas flow from the anaesthetic machine.

A point is reached when the reservoir bag is again full and as the patient is still exhaling, the remaining exhaled gases have to pass out through the APL (expiratory) valve, which now opens.

The first portion of exhaled gases to pass up the corrugated hose from the patient was that occupying the patient's anatomical dead space and therefore apart from being warmed and slightly humidified (a satisfactory state of affairs) they are unaltered, having not taken part in respiratory exchange. This is followed by alveolar gas (with a reduced oxygen content, and containing carbon dioxide), some of which enters the corrugated hose, and some which is expelled through the APL valve when the reservoir bag is full.

*End-expiratory pause.* The next stage is the end-expiratory pause. The fresh gas flow entering the system now drives those exhaled gases, or some of them that had tracked back along the corrugated hose, out through the APL valve. It will be seen that the expiratory pause is important because it prevents the patient's rebreathing of exhaled alveolar gases contained in the hose at the end of expiration (Fig 9.5d).

During the end-expiratory pause, all the alveolar gases and some of the dead-space gases are expelled from the corrugated hose through the APL valve by the continuing fresh gas flow. Thus, during the next inspiratory phase, the gas inspired may well initially contain some of the remaining dead-space gases from the previous breath, along with fresh gas. As explained above, these dead-space gases may be re-inspired without detriment to the patient. The fresh gas flow rate may therefore be rather less than the patient's minute volume and rebreathing of alveolar gas is therefore prevented.

In theory, provided there is (a) no mixing of fresh gas, dead-space gas and alveolar gas, and (b) a sufficient end-expiratory pause, the fresh gas flow rate need only match alveolar ventilation (approximately 66% of the minute volume), as in this situation only alveolar gas will be vented through the APL valve. In practice, however, a number of factors dictate a higher fresh gas flow rate (70–90%).

- There is mixing of the various gaseous interfaces, which reduces the theoretical efficiency of the system.
- Occasionally, larger than expected tidal volumes may well be exhaled and therefore reach the reservoir bag, in which case carbon dioxide will contaminate the reservoir bag and the subse-

quent inspiratory gases.
- Rapid respiratory rates will reduce or even eliminate an end-expiratory pause and reduce the potential for carbon dioxide elimination that this pause allows.

Various other breathing systems containing similar components were evaluated by Mapleson (see Fig. 9.4). These systems are catalogued in order (B, C, D, E, F) of increased requirement of fresh gas flow to prevent rebreathing during spontaneous respiration. Systems B and C require 1.5–2 times the fresh gas flow and systems D, E and F (functionally similar) require 2–4 times the minute volume to prevent rebreathing (see below).

An alternative nomenclature has recently been proposed for the systems described above which relates to the position of the reservoir bag within the breathing system. The Mapleson A system in which the reservoir bag stores fresh gas is described as an afferent reservoir system. System D, in which the reservoir bag stores mixed expired gases, is described as an efferent reservoir system, and systems B and C, in which the reservoir bag stores mixed inspired and expired gases, are called junctional reservoir systems.

It was originally thought that the increased respiratory work produced by the expiratory resistance of APL valves in these breathing systems (Mapleson A–D) was detrimental to anaesthetized patients. This is without doubt true when the valve resistance is high (due to sticky valves, narrow valve apertures) or where the repiratory effort is severely compromised (e.g. in neonates). However, modern valve design (with wider valve apertures, more delicate springs, better screw threads) minimizes this resistance. Furthermore a small PEEP (positive end expiratory pressure) effect that these valves may produce is now thought to be positively beneficial, reducing the potential for the functional residual capacity of the lungs to fall below the closing volume in supine anaesthetized patients.

## Mapleson A system and controlled ventilation

The mechanical aspects of the Mapleson A (Fig. 9.6) (Magill attachment) system as described above relate to its use in spontaneous respiration. However, if controlled or assisted ventilation is used, with the patient's lungs inflated by means of squeezing the reservoir bag, a different state of affairs occurs.

*Inspiratory phase.* The APL valve has to be kept almost closed so that sufficient pressure can develop

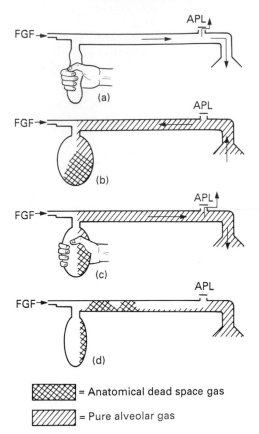

FGF→
APL↑
(a)

FGF→
APL
(b)

FGF→
APL↑
(c)

FGF→
APL
(d)

▨▨▨ = Anatomical dead space gas

▨▨▨ = Pure alveolar gas

**Figure 9.6** Mapleson A system with assisted or controlled ventilation: (a) at the end of inspiration; (b) at the end of expiration; (c) during subsequent inspiration; (d) at the end of the subsequent inspiration. Note that much rebreathing takes place (see text). FGF = fresh gas flow; APL = adjustable pressure-limiting (expiratory) valve.

in the system to inflate the lungs. During the first inspiratory phase with the anaesthetist squeezing the bag, it is fresh gases that are blown out of the valve.

*Expiratory phase.* At the end of inspiration, the reservoir bag may be almost empty, and as soon as the anaethetist relaxes his pressure on it, the patient exhales into the corrugated hose. The exhaled deadspace and alveolar gases may then pass right back into the reservoir bag. (The capacity of the standard 110-cm corrugated hose being about 550 ml.)

There is a natural tendency to allow little or no expiratory pause, so that when the anaesthetist squeezes the bag again, the first gases to enter the patient's lungs will be the previously exhaled alveolar gases. The volume of gases escaping via the APL valve during this second inspiratory phase is initially small (the valve being almost closed) but gradually increases as the pressure in the system

rises towards the maximum inspiration. Therefore, the greatest amount of gas will be dumped late in the cycle and will consist mainly of fresh gas. Under these circumstances there is considerable rebreathing (Fig. 9.6). Furthermore, as alveolar gas will have entered the reservoir bag, there will always be carbon dioxide contamination in any subsequent inspirate. In order to prevent this and thereby minimize the potential for rebreathing alveolar gas, a high fresh gas flow rate is required.

This is usually of the order of two times the patient's minute ventilation. This situation is highly wasteful of fresh gas and also increases the potential for pollution.

## Other Mapleson A breathing systems

### The Lack co-axial breathing system (Fig. 9.7a)

The traditional layout of a Magill system sites the APL valve as close to the patient as possible. This reduces the access to the valve in head and neck surgery and increases the drag on the mask or endotracheal tube when the valve is shrouded and connected to scavenging tubing.

The Lack system overcomes these two problems. The original version was constructed with a co-axial arrangement of breathing hoses. Exhaled gases passed through the orifice of the inner hose sited at the patient end of the system and then back towards the APL valve, which is now sited on the reservoir bag mount. The valve is thus conveniently sited for adjustment by the anaesthetist and its weight, and that of any additional scavenging attachment, is now supported by the anaesthetic machine (see Fig. 9.7). The system still functions as a Mapleson A system. The co-axial hosing on early models was criticized as being too narrow and having too high a flow resistance. In later models, the inner and outer breathing hose diameters were subsequently both increased, to 15 and 30 mm respectively to overcome this problem. Another problem was that the tubing was heavy and stiff, putting a stress on the connection to the facepiece or endotracheal connection.

### Lack parallel breathing system (Fig. 9.7b)

Co-axial breathing systems have not found universal favour. If the inner hose were to become disconnected or to split, as has been the case, the leak may pass unnoticed. It drastically alters the efficiency of the system in eliminating carbon dioxide and is therefore potentially very dangerous. A version of the Lack system with parallel hoses is now available (see Fig. 9.7b).

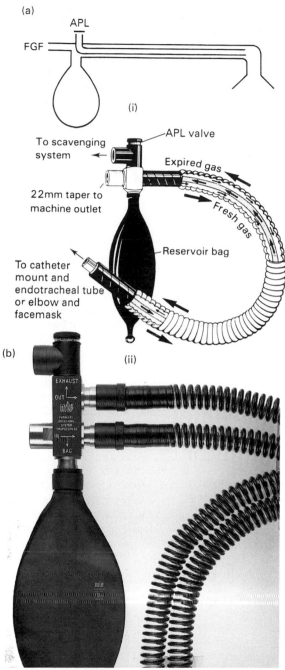

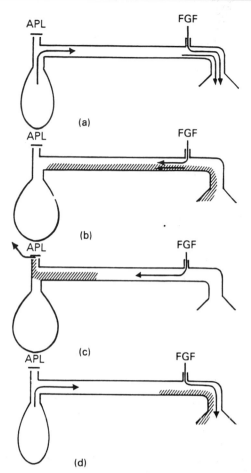

**Figure 9.8** The Mapleson D system with spontaneous ventilation (see text). FGF = fresh gas flow; APL = adjustable pressure-limiting (expiratory) valve.

## Mapleson D system

### The Mapleson D system with spontaneous respiration

The system is best explained if again, the three phases of the respiratory cycle are considered: inspiration, expiration and end-expiratory pause.

*Inspiration.* The system is initially assumed to be full of fresh gas so that during the first inspiration the patient breathes only fresh gas (Fig. 9.8a).

*Expiration.* During expiration, the exhaled gases, mixed with the fresh gas flow (FGF) pass down the corrugated hose to the reservoir bag (Fig. 9.8b) and when this has been refilled the remainder of the exhaled gases and the FGF are voided via the APL valve (expiratory valve). Of the expired gases it is those from the dead space that are voided first, followed by alveolar gases.

**Figure 9.7** (a) The Lack co-axial breathing system. (i) Working principles. (ii) The actual assembly. Note that the outer corrugated hose is partly transparent so that the inner tube may be seen to be intact. The adjustable pressure-limiting valve (APL) is fitted with a shroud having a 30-mm outlet so that it may be attached to a scavenging system. (b) The Lack parallel breathing attachment. The inner (expiratory) limb of the co-axial arrangement has been replaced by one that is parallel to the inspiratory limb. FGF = fresh gas flow; APL = adjustable pressure-limiting (expiratory) valve.

*End-expiratory pause.* During the end-expiratory pause the fresh gas flow passes down the outer hose, displacing some of the mixture of exhaled gas and FGF, which is now vented out through the APL valve (Fig. 9.8c). The amount of fresh gas occupying and thus stored in the patient end of the corrugated hose at the end of expiration, depends on the fresh gas flow rate, the duration of the end-expiratory pause, and the degree of mixing (due to turbulence) of the various gaseous interfaces within the corrugated hose.

At the next inspiration the inhaled gases consist initially of this stored fresh gas followed then by the mixture of exhaled gases and FGF that remain in the tube (Fig. 9.8d).

However, there are practical problems with this concept, since the expiratory pause may be short during spontaneous breathing (when volatile anaesthetics only are used *without opoid supplement*). In this case the fresh gas flow needs to be sufficiently high to flush the exhaled gases downstream prior to the next inspiration. In fact, rebreathing of exhaled alveolar gas occurs unless the fresh gas flow is at least 2 times and possibly up to 4 times the patient's minute ventilation.

It is worthy of note that the Mapleson D system is functionally similar to a 'T' piece (Mapleson E). However with a 'T' piece, the limb through which the ventilation occurs, if used without a reservoir bag, must be of such a length that the volume of gas in it when augmented by the volume of the fresh gas flow being delivered during inspiration is no less than that of the patient's tidal volume, otherwise dilution of anaesthetic by entrained air will occur.

## Mapleson D system with controlled or assisted ventilation

During the first inspiration, the fresh gas flow entering the system as well as fresh gases stored in the wide-bore breathing hose pass to the patient. At the same time some gases from the reservoir bag are lost through the partially open APL (expiratory) valve (Fig. 9.9a)

During the expiratory phase, a mixture of the fresh gas flow and exhaled gases passes along the hose, eventually entering the reservoir bag, which has been deflated during inspiration by the amount of both the patient's tidal volume and the volume of gases lost through the APL valve (Fig. 9.9b). Provided that there is an expiratory pause, the fresh

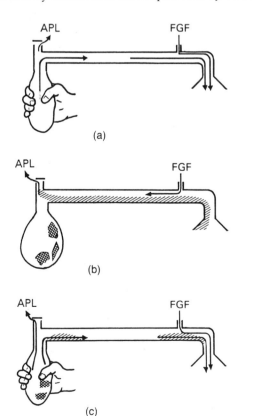

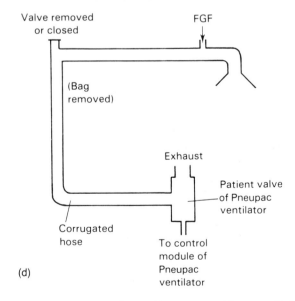

**Figure 9.9** The Mapleson D system with controlled ventilation. (a)–(c) With manual ventilation (see text). (d) With the employment of a ventilator such as the Pneupac. Note that in this case a standard length of corrugated hose (capacity approximately 500 ml) is required to prevent mixing of the driving gas from the ventilator with the anaesthetic gases in the breathing attachment. FGF = fresh gas flow; APL = adjustable pressure-limiting (expiratory) valve.

gas supply flows down the hose and continues to drive the mixture of fresh and exhaled gases out via the APL valve.

At the next squeeze of the reservoir bag (Fig. 9.9c), the continuing fresh gas flow plus the fresh gas now stored in the breathing hose plus any previously expired gases that may remain in the hose pass to the patient, while some of the mixed gases within the bag escape via the APL valve. The cycle then repeats itself. Thus to *prevent rebreathing* in the Mapleson D system during both spontaneous and controlled ventilation, the fresh gas flow must be sufficiently high enough to (a) purge the breathing hose of exhaled gases and (b) supplement the stored fresh gas in this breathing hose so that any mixed gas in the reservoir bag is prevented from entering the hose and reaching the patient. The amount of fresh gas required will always be greater than the patient's minute volume and will depend largely on the expiratory pause. The longer the pause, the more effective will be the ability of the fresh gas to purge the breathing hose of expired gas.

However, during controlled ventilation, deliberate use is often made of functional rebreathing. Theoretically, if slow ventilation rates (with long expiratory pauses) and large tidal volumes are chosen, then sufficient expiratory time will elapse to allow a modest fresh gas flow to fill the proximal part of the system with sufficient fresh gas to provide alveolar ventilation. This will enter the lungs first, followed by a mixture of previously expired gases (from the machine end of the system), which will then occupy anatomical dead space.

Hence, theoretically, it should be possible to reduce the fresh gas flow to the volume required for alveolar ventilation. In practice, there is turbulent mixing of the various gaseous interfaces. Even so, provided a sufficiently large controlled minute ventilation is delivered so that most of the fresh gas flow reaches the alveoli, adequate alveolar ventilation will occur with fresh gas flow rates of 70% of the anticipated minute ventilation since, as mentioned above, some rebreathing is acceptable.

Mapleson D systems are thus able to make efficient use of fresh anaesthetic gases during controlled ventilation and could have considerable cost saving benefits. Figure 9.9d shows how the Mapleson D system may be employed with an automatic ventilator. The reservoir bag is removed and replaced with a standard length of corrugated hose of sufficient capacity to accommodate the air or oxygen that is delivered by the ventilator, and which prevents it reaching the patient in place of the intended anaesthetic gases.

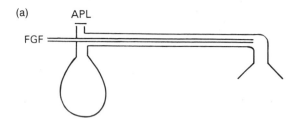

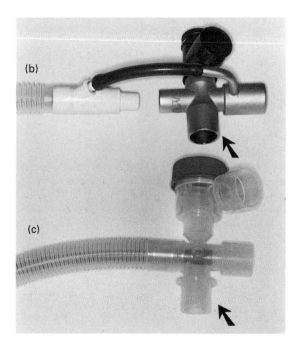

**Figure 9.10** The Bain breathing system. (a) Working principle. (b) and (c) show two different arrangements of the fresh gas flow (FGF) bypassing the bag mount (arrow). They are functionally identical. FGF = fresh gas flow; APL = adjustable pressure-limiting (expiratory) valve.

## The Bain system

The Bain breathing system (Fig. 9.10) is similar in function to the Mapleson D system. The only difference is that the fresh gas flow is carried by a tube within the corrugated hose (a co-axial arrangement). In the earlier models in particular, there was a risk that the inner tube could become disconnected at the machine end; if this happened a very big dead space was introduced. It could also become kinked, so cutting off the supply of fresh gases.

## Hybrid systems

A number of breathing systems have been described that, by means of a lever switch, can convert the

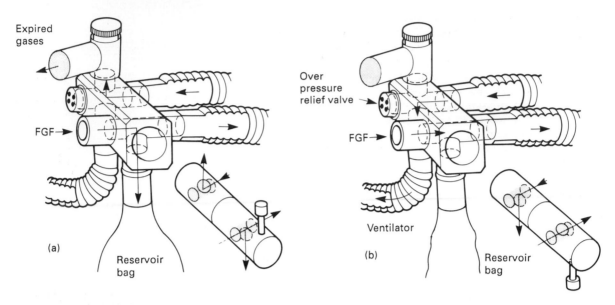

**Figure 9.11** Humphrey ADE system. With the lever set upright (a) the system functions in its Mapleson A mode as efficiently as the Lack for spontaneous respiration, with an average fresh gas flow (FGF) of approximately 3.6 litres/min. Without changing the setting or FGF, manual ventilation is easily instituted simply by partially closing the APL valve and squeezing the reservoir bag. For mechanical ventilation the lever is positioned downwards (b) in its E mode. The ventilator is now included while the reservoir bag and exhaust valve are excluded. The system now functions identically to the Bain. For children the lever settings are identical.

system from a Mapleson A to a Mapleson D or E, allowing a system to be chosen and used in its most efficient mode (i.e. System A, spontaneous respiration, System E, controlled respiration). The Humphrey ADE system (M&IE and Anaequip UK) seems to be the most popular version (see Fig. 9.11).

With the lever switch in the A mode, the reservoir bag is connected to the breathing system, just as it would be in a Magill system bag mount. The breathing hose connecting the bag to the patient is now designated as the inspiratory limb. However, expired gas is ducted down a separate limb back to an APL valve mounted on the 'Humphrey' block which is shrouded to facilitate scavenging. In practice it appears to function more efficiently than a traditional Magill attachment. The improved efficiency is thought to relate to the geometrical arrangement of the components at the patient end of the system. Towards the end of exhalation in the Magill attachment, the exhaled dead-space gas which has passed up the breathing hose is now returned towards the APL valve by the flushing action of the fresh gas flow entering the system. At the APL valve, it meets and mixes with alveolar gas in turbulent fashion, and a mixture of both is discharged from the valve. However, in the Humphrey (and Lack) systems alveolar gas is diverted in a more laminar fashion into a physically

separate expiratory limb, which minimizes any potential for mixing of the two gas phases in question. This arrangement, and the removal of the APL valve assembly away from the patient end of the system, also reduces apparatus dead space, so that with further modification (see below) it may be suitable for infants and neonates.

With the lever in the D/E mode, the reservoir bag and APL valve are isolated from the breathing system. What was the 'inspiratory' limb in 'A' mode now delivers gas to the patient end of the system as would a gas delivery system in a 'T' piece. The breathing hose returning gas to the 'Humphrey' block now functions as the reservoir limb of a 'T' piece. This hose is opened to atmosphere via a port adjacent to the bag mount. As this mode does not incorporate a reservoir bag, it is strictly a Mapleson E system. The port described above is usually connected to a ventilator of the bag-squeezer type, so that the system is used in its most efficient mode for controlled ventilation. If a reservoir bag and APL valve were to be attached to this port, it would function as a D system. However this is not recommended because it may encourage the system to be used uneconomically for spontaneous respiration, as a high FGF is required to prevent rebreathing.

The Anaequip version is supplied with 15-mm

smooth-bore non-kinking breathing hose. Interestingly, the use of this smooth bore hose reduces turbulence in the range of flows seen in quietly breathing adults, so that its performance is little different from that of 22-mm corrugated hose. The narrower bore hose also reduces the internal volume of the system to an extent that it is now also suitable for use with infants. A low internal volume is important in a paediatric breathing system in order that (a) during controlled ventilation, the small tidal volumes required are delivered more efficiently, and (b) during spontaneous respiration, the energy expended by the patient in overcoming the inertia of the gas present in the system is reduced, especially as with high respiratory rates the direction of gas flow is reversed very frequently.

## Mapleson E and F systems

### The T-piece system

However efficient an expiratory valve may be, it is bound to offer some resistance to exhalation, which may not be acceptable in certain anaesthetic techniques such as those used for neonatal and infant anaesthesia. To avoid this resistance, the T-piece system may be used. In Fig. 9.12 the fresh gases are supplied via a small-bore tube to the side arm of an Ayre's T-piece. The main body of the T-piece is within the breathing system and must, therefore, be of adequate diameter. One end of the body is connected by the shortest possible means to the patient. (The volume of this limb makes up apparatus dead space.) The other end is connected to a length of tubing that acts as a reservoir.

The FGF rate must be high in the case of spontaneous ventilation. During inspiration the peak inspiratory flow rate is higher than the FGF, so some gases are drawn from the reservoir limb. During expiration both the exhaled air and the fresh gases, which continue to flow, pass into the reservoir limb and are expelled to the atmosphere. During the end-expiratory pause the FGF flushes out and refills the reservoir limb. The dimensions of the reservoir limb and the FGF rate are governed by the following considerations.

- The diameter of the reservoir limb must be sufficient to present the lowest possible resistance (not more than 0.75 cmH$_2$O for a neonate and not more than than 2 cmH$_2$O for an adult at the appropriate flow rates).
- The volume of the expiratory limb should be

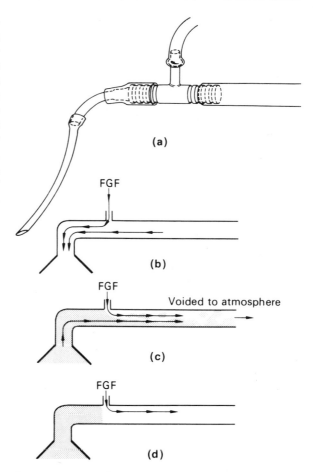

**Figure 9.12** (a) The Ayre's T-piece connected to an endotracheal tube. (b) During spontaneous inspiration. (c) During expiration. (d) During the expiratory pause. FGF = fresh gas flow.

approximately the same as the patient's tidal volume — too great a volume would matter only in that the greater length would lead to increased resistance. Too great a diameter would lead to mixing of the fresh gases with alveolar gas and to inefficiency of the system. For an adult a standard 110 cm length of corrugated hose is satisfactory.

- The optimum FGF rate depends not only on the patient's minute volume and respiratory rate but also on the capacity of the reservoir limb. If the latter is at least that of the patient's tidal volume, then a rate of 2.5 times the patient's minute volume is sufficient. This is the most satisfactory arrangement. However, if the capacity of the reservoir is reduced, the flow rate must be increased. If the capacity of the reservoir is reduced to zero, the flow rate must be in excess of the peak inspiratory flow rate so as to reduce the possibility of ingress of air.

The shape of the T-piece is also important. Normally the side arm is at right angles to the body. If it is at an angle pointing towards the patient, there is continuous positive pressure applied which would act as a resistance during expiration; similarly, if the gases were directed towards the reservoir, a sub-atmospheric pressure would be caused by a venturi effect. As mentioned previously this continuous positive airways pressure is thought to be beneficial in minimizing the fall in functional residual capacity (FRC), especially in neonates.

### Controlled ventilation with the T-piece

Controlled ventilation may be effected by intermittently occluding the end of the reservoir limb with the thumb. This should be done with care, since when the outlet is occluded the full pressure supplied by the anaesthetic machine is applied to the patient. It would seem prudent to include, in infant systems at least, a blow-off valve set to about 40 $cmH_2O$ pressure; but this is seldom done. A limitation in its use arises from the fact that the peak inspiratory flow rate is limited to that of the FGF. This is overcome in the Rees T-piece, described below.

The T-piece system is particularly suited to neonates and infants, where an expiratory valve presents a significant resistance. The scaling down of a system suitable for adults may be quite inappropriate for use with small children.

A disadvantage of the T-piece system is that it is not easy to observe the patient's respiration without the reassuring whistle of the expiratory valve. This can be overcome by attaching to the open end of the reservoir limb a small wisp of cotton wool, which can be seen to wave in the breeze, or by the use of an indicator devised by Marshall (Fig. 9.13).

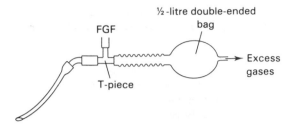

**Figure 9.14** The Rees T-piece. FGF = fresh gas flow.

### The Rees-T-piece (Mapleson F system)

A great improvement to the T-piece was made by Rees, who added a small double-ended bag to the end of the reservoir limb (Fig. 9.14). Note that the tubular portion of the limb should still approximate to the patient's tidal volume, or rebreathing could occur as a result of the mixing of expired and fresh gases. During spontaneous ventilation small movements of the semi-collapsed bag demonstrate the patient's breathing. During controlled ventilation the open end of the bag is partially or totally occluded by the anaesthetist's fifth finger during the inspiratory phase, while the bag is squeezed between his other fingers and thumb. The fifth finger is relaxed during expiration. This simple system is extremely efficient for infants and small children. Several mechanical devices are available which can be placed in the tail of the bag so as to provide a variable restrictor similar to that described above. These may all be accidently turned off, occluding the expiratory limb completely. As the system does not contain an over-pressure safety valve, a dangerously high pressure could build up which could damage the lungs of any infant connected to it. These devices cannot therefore be recommended.

Other paediatric breathing systems are described in Chapter 14.

## Non-rebreathing Systems with Facility for Carbon Dioxide Absorbtion

High flows of inhalation anaesthetic agents (i.e. at least approximately equal to the patient's minute ventilation) are regularly used with most breathing systems at the beginning of an anaesthetic for the following reasons:

- both to purge the system of air and to fill it with fresh anaesthetic agents;

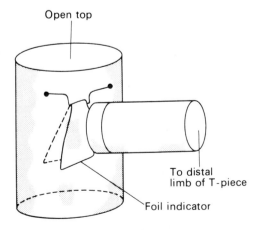

Open top

To distal limb of T-piece

Foil indicator

**Figure 9.13** Marshall's indicator.

- to provide a sufficient amount of inhalational agent for alveolar uptake (which is initially high at the onset of anaesthesia);
- to eliminate exhaled carbon dioxide. (As described previously the efficiency with which this is done depends on the characteristics of the breathing system chosen.)
- to eliminate body nitrogen.

However, when equilibrium between the patient's blood and inspired concentration of anaesthetic has been reached, this inspired concentration is exhaled relatively unchanged, and so the main function of high fresh gas flows in most breathing systems is the elimination of carbon dioxide (whilst at the same time providing oxygen!).

Thus to continue a high FGF after equilibrium has been achieved is both wasteful and expensive and may increase theatre pollution. This exhaled gas at near equilibrium can be re-used in suitable systems if it is purged of exhaled carbon dioxide, and has the oxygen concentration restored (oxygen is always removed from the inspiratory mixture by the lungs at a rate between 120–250 ml/min). The re-utilization of suitably modified exhaled gases can thus reduce the fresh gas flow to very low levels (see below).

### Carbon dioxide absorption

Carbon dioxide can be removed from exhaled gases by a chemical reaction with various metallic bases (hydroxides). This reaction requires the presence of water in order that these bases and carbon dioxide (as carbonic acid) can exist in ionic form. There are two types of commercial preparation of these metallic bases.

(1) SODA LIME. This is made up of approximately 80% calcium hydroxide, 4% sodium hydroxide and 14–20% added water content. The sodium hydroxide is included both to improve the reactivity of the mixture and for its hygroscopic properties (binding the necessary added water in the mixture). The addition of hardeners (silica and kieselguhr, a clay) to help form the required granule size in soda lime is no longer required in modern manufacturing processes. Similarly, potassium hydroxide, which was thought to improve the activity of soda lime when cold, is no longer added.

(2) BARIUM LIME. Barium lime is made up of 80% calcium hydroxide and 20% barium hydroxide (octahydrate). The barium hydroxide has its own naturally occurring 'water of crystallization' and in combination with calcium hydroxide has never required additional hardeners.

The main chemical reaction is

$$CO_2 \quad + \quad H_2O \quad = H^+ + HCO_3^-$$
Carbon dioxide        water          Carbonic acid

$$Ca(OH)_2 + H^+ + HCO_3^- = CaCO_3 + 2H_2O$$
Calcium      Carbonic acid    Calcium   water
hydroxide                      carbonate

The reaction is interesting in that (a) it produces heat energy (it is an exothermic reaction), (b) it changes the pH of the soda lime, which allows the use of indicator dyes to show when the soda lime is exhausted, and (c) it produces more water than that used up in the reaction.

The size of the granules is important. Too large a granule size produces large gaps in a canister of stacked granules, leading to poor contact with gases passing through, with a consequent inefficient absorption of carbon dioxide. Too small a granule may provide an unacceptably high resistance to gas flow along with the increased possibility of dust formation. The optimum size of granule is thought to be between 1.5 and 5 mm in diameter. The product is sieved through various meshes to retain sizes between these tolerances. Mesh standards differ between countries due to variations in thickness of the wire used to construct the mesh. In the USA soda lime granules are supplied at between 4 and 8 Mesh USP (2.36–4.75 mm). In the UK the granules are supplied to a BP (British Pharmacopoeia) standard of 1.4–4.75 mm (3–10 Mesh).

The dust is caustic and can produce burns in the respiratory tract if inhaled. This was a problem with the older type of system with 'to-and-fro' absorption (Waters canister, see below), where the absorber was placed in close proximity to the patient's airway. However, circle absorbers are usually separated from the patient by at least a metre of breathing hose, which normally hangs in a loop. This allows the dust, if present, to fall out before it can get to the patient.

### Absorptive capacity of soda lime

Soda lime is capable of absorbing 25 litres of carbon dioxide per 100 g, and barium lime 27 litres of carbon dioxide per 100 g. However, in continuous use, the soda lime appears exhausted (as indicated by the colour change) before these capacities are reached, because the outside of the granule is exhausted before the whole granule is used up. Furthermore, the contact time between the absorbent and carbon dioxide affects the efficiency of the absorbent. Smaller canisters containing 500 g of soda lime appear exhausted at a carbon dioxide load of 10–12 litres per 100 g of absorbent. 'Jumbo' absorbers containing 2 kg of soda lime, which allow a longer contact time between the carbon dioxide and absorbent, appear exhausted at a carbon dioxide load of 17 litres per 100 g.

When the system is allowed to stand for a few hours, the soda lime appears to 'regenerate' as the surface carbonate is diluted by hydroxide ions migrating from within the granule. The colour of fresh soda lime and barium lime depends on which indicator dye is added by the manufacturer. For example M&IE (UK) markets 'Durosorb' and 'Viosorb' soda lime. Durosorb has 'Clayton yellow' added, which turns from deep pink when fresh to off-white when exhausted, whereas Viosorb contains 'ethyl violet' as the indicator dye, which changes from white when fresh to purple when exhausted.

### The exothermic reaction

The heat and water produced by the reaction of soda lime on carbon dioxide are allegedly beneficial in that (at low flows) they warm and partially humidify the inspiratory gas. The temperature and humidity of the inspired gas is related to a number of factors. Firstly, for example, if the fresh gas flow rate is high, the dry gas entering the system reduces both the humidity and the temperature of the recirculating gas. Secondly, at low fresh gas flows, if the gas circulation time is high, the humidity and temperature rises. Thirdly, the longer the system is in use at low flows, the greater are the humidity and temperature of the circulating gas.

The heat produced, however, is not necessarily all beneficial. There is an increased chemical reaction with volatile anaesthetic agents in proportion to the temperature within the system. Trichloroethylene can be decomposed to dichloroacetylene (which is neurotoxic) and further to phosgene if the temperature within the soda lime exceeds 60°C. Older anaesthetic machines often incorporated a switching system on the back bar that could divert gas directly into a circle system rather than to the common gas outlet. The trichloroethylene vaporizer (where fitted) was always positioned downstream of this switch so that it could never be used with the circle absorber system (see page 106). Modern anaesthetic agents are known to be mildly degraded even by dry soda lime, but this is not known to be harmful.

### Anaesthetic non-rebreathing systems which include carbon dioxide absorption

Carbon dioxide absorption can be used in two types of system:

- a 'to-and-fro' absorption system;
- a circle absorption system.

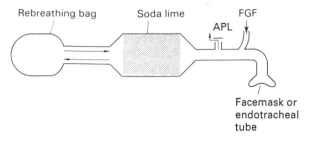

**Figure 9.15** A 'to-and-fro' system incorporating a Waters' canister. FGF = fresh gas flow.

## 'To-and-fro' absorption systems

### The Waters' canister (Fig. 9.15)

Here the patient breathes in and out of a closed bag, which is connected to the facemask or endotracheal tube via a canister containing soda lime. The part of the system between the patient and the soda lime is dead space and therefore its volume must be kept to a minimum. This means that the soda lime canister must be close to the patient's head, and this leads to mechanical difficulties. A length of wide-bore tubing may, however, be interposed between the canister and rebreathing bag without detriment. The fresh gases are introduced at the patient end of the system, and the expiratory valve is usually mounted close by, though it may equally well be put at the bag end. The canister is usually placed in the horizontal position for convenience, and it is most important that it is well packed, since if there were a space above the soda lime, 'channelling' would occur and absorption would be incomplete (Fig. 9.16). Furthermore, the soda lime at the patient end of the system becomes exhausted first and so increases the functional dead space of the system. The soda lime may conveniently be compressed to prevent gaps by the insertion of a nylon pot scourer at one end. When the canister is closed, the sealing washer should be checked to ensure that it is in the correct position. Any soda lime on the threads of the canister or the sealing washer should be carefully removed. The whole system should be tested for leaks before use.

Apart from being cumbersome, the 'to-and-fro' system has the disadvantage that the patient could inhale soda lime dust. The anaesthetist may prove this by taking a few breaths through a canister himself. Cotton wool filters may be inserted in the patient end of the canister to prevent this.

The main advantages of the Waters' canister over circle systems is the ease in which it may be cleaned

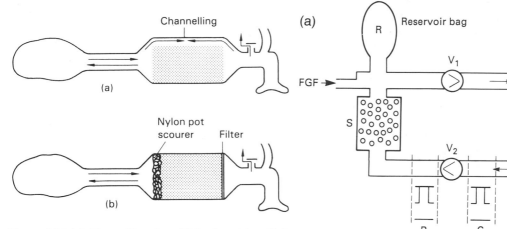

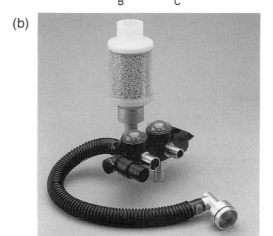

**Figure 9.16** (a) Channelling in a Waters' canister. If the canister is not completely filled with soda lime and is placed in a horizontal position, the gases can pass through the void at the top and therefore fail to come into adequate contact with the soda lime. (b) The prevention of channelling by the insertion of a nylon pot scourer to compress the soda lime. Note also the filter at the patient end that prevents particles of soda lime reaching the patient.

and sterilized. It is therefore very useful for use with infected patients.

## Circle absorption systems

Here the disadvantages of the soda lime canister being so close to the patient are avoided. The patient is connected to the absorber by two corrugated hoses, one inspiratory and the other expiratory, as shown in Fig. 9.17a. The one way or 'circle' flow of gases through the system is determined by two unidirectional valves $V_1$ and $V_2$, which are accommodated in transparent domes so that their correct action may be observed.

The fresh gas port and the reservoir bag are usually sited in the inspiratory pathway close to the inspiratory valve $V_1$. This reduces the resistance to inspiratory effort. (Some older circle systems positioned the reservoir bag in the expiratory limb of the system downstream of the valve $V_2$ which required some added inspiratory effort to draw the gas through the absorber.) The APL valve is usually mounted downstream of the valve $V_2$ in the expiratory limb, but before gas entry into the absorber. Here, it can dump excess exhaled gas prior to entry of gas into the absorber. At one time it was considered that an APL valve could be added to the breathing system at position A for use with spontaneous respiration. This would preferentially dump exhaled *alveolar* gas during the expiratory cycle, increasing carbon dioxide elimination prior to

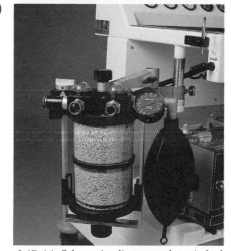

**Figure 9.17** (a) Schematic diagram of a circle breathing system with absorber. The diagram highlights the alternative siting of the APL valve (points A, B or C) (see text). (b) Conventional circle type carbon dioxide absorption system. It uses disposable and stackable soda lime canisters. (c) A 2-kg circle type carbon dioxide absorber that uses fully autoclavable polyethersulphone canisters and valve domes.

(a)

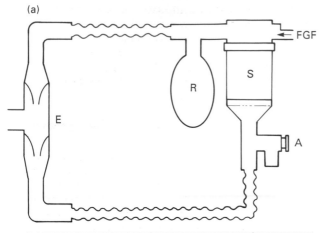

(b)

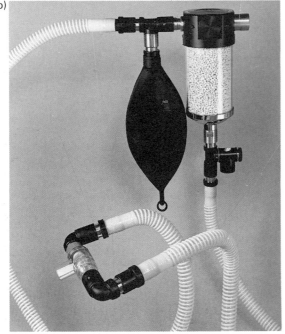

**Figure 9.18** M&IE 'Exeter' circle breathing system. (a) Working principles, showing the replacement of the conventional unidirectional valves in a circle breathing system by an Ambu E valve. E = Ambu E valve; R = reservoir bag; S = soda lime; A = APL valve; FGF = fresh gas flow. (b) The system.

the entry of expired gas into the absorber, thus conserving soda lime. However, as scavenging has assumed a greater importance, the inconvenience of connecting scavenging hoses to a valve in this position has limited its usefulness. Figures 9.17b, c show two commercial versions of the system described. In the simple system shown in Fig. 9.18, valves $V_1$ and $V_2$ can be replaced by an Ambu E valve which performs the same function.

## Apparatus dead space

The apparatus dead space is low in this system. It consists only of that volume inside the male taper at the end of the Y piece which joins the inspiratory and expiratory breathing hoses to the patient. The functional dead space of this system should be identical. However, if the unidirectional valves malfunction and do not fully close, rebreathing will occur. Furthermore, some circle systems position the APL valve just upstream of the expiratory unidirectional valve (position C, Fig 19.17). If this APL valve is mounted horizontally, and the valve screw is opened fully, the valve disc may not seat correctly (although it is supposed to do so) and will cause rebreathing due to ingress of air or exhaust gases through this valve during spontaneous respiration.

## Flow resistance

Circle systems impose a greater resistance to breathing than other commonly used breathing systems (Mapleson A–F systems), although less than co-axial arrangements of D systems (Bain system). This is largely due to the fact that there are two extra valves and a soda lime canister in the system. A number of factors further influence this resistance. A high fresh gas flow rate will assist flow in the inspiratory side of the system, thus decreasing any inspiratory resistance, but will increase expiratory resistance through the unidirectional and APL (expiratory) valves. The reverse occurs with low gas flows. Low fresh gas flow rates will also increase the relative humidity and thus increase the 'stickiness' of the unidirectional valves owing to water vapour condensation, therefore further increasing flow resistance. Lastly, the flow rates developed by respiratory excursion (tidal volume and rate) produce the greatest swings in flow resistance (see Table 9.1). These factors may not matter in healthy adults, but

**Table 9.1** Flow resistance in circle breathing systems*

| Frequency (min) | Tidal volume (ml) | Pressure swing (cmH$_2$O) |
|---|---|---|
| 12 | 500 | $-1 +\frac{1}{2}$ |
| 12 | 1000 | $-1 +1$ |
| 12 | 1600 | $-2 +1\frac{1}{2}$ |
| 24 | 500 | $-1 +1$ |
| 24 | 1000 | $-3 +1\frac{1}{2}$ |
| 44 | 500 | $-4 +3$ |

*Reproduced from Young, T. M. Carbon dioxide absorber. *Anaesthesia* vol. 26 (1971), p. 78, with permission.

they can be unacceptable in young children. Several devices have been described (Revell's circulator, etc.) which reduce this problem (see page 138).

### Efficiency of soda lime absorbers

The efficiency of carbon dioxide absorption in a canister depends on the freshness of the soda lime, the available surface area of the granules, and the length of time the gas to be treated is in contact with the granules. Early canister designs contained approximately 480 g of soda lime. These required frequent changes (after approximately 2–2.5 h of continuous use at low fresh gas flows). Most current absorbers are of the 'Jumbo' type which contain 2 kg of soda lime and, since this has a large volume and surface area of granules, the expired gas is in contact with them for a relatively long period of time, so increasing the efficiency of absorption. It has been shown that a 2-kg canister lasts five times longer than a 0.5-kg canister. When a 2-kg canister is employed it usually has two chambers, one above the other. When one half appears exhausted it is refilled and then the canister is inverted so that the previously unused half now bears the brunt of absorption. Not only is the absorption thought to be more efficient in the larger absorbers, but also less frequent recharging is necessary.

With the recent introduction of routine expired carbon dioxide monitoring these last two considerations appear to be less of a problem in clinical practice, and the reintroduction of smaller absorbers (Fig. 9.17b) may well have advantages. These are easier to maintain, to use, to keep clean and have fewer leaks. The soda lime can also be supplied in disposable cartridges.

### Absorber switch

Traditionally, a switch is included in a circle system which channels expiratory gas either through the absorption chamber or across a bypass directly into the inspiratory limb. When the switch is of the flow-splitting type, it can also proportion the flow of expiratory gas through the two channels.

Some newer European and American models omit this switch completely or make the switch to be either on or off with no intermediate flow-splitting facility (Ohmeda Mark 5a UK). The rationale for excluding this switch involves safety reasons. Rebreathing of carbon dioxide is rendered impossible under normal operating conditions.

However, partial rebreathing during controlled respiration is an acceptable technique (see Mapleson D systems above) and this facility with a circle

system is still useful with many currently used 'bag-in-bottle' ventilators whose minimum respiratory rate setting cannot be reduced below 10 breaths per minute. With these ventilators, normocarbia may sometimes be achieved only by the use of inappropriately small tidal volumes if the facility for partial rebreathing is eliminated.

## Daily maintenance of circle absorber systems

During prolonged administration at low fresh gas flow rates, water vapour condenses in the expiratory hose and this needs to be emptied from time to time. Condensation also occurs in the expiratory unidirectional valve. Not only may this obscure the glass dome so that the correct operation of the valve cannot be observed, but also a drop of water on the cage retaining the valve disc may cause the latter to adhere to it by surface tension. This holds the valve permanently open, causing the patient to rebreathe repeatedly substantial amounts of exhaled gas from the expiratory pathway in the system. This gas would eventually have a very low oxygen content which would be catastrophic for the patient. The tendency of the valve discs to stick is a result of their being made of increasingly lightweight materials in order to reduce the resistance to gas flow.

Ideally, to avoid this complication, a low resistance bacterial/hydrophobic filter should be fitted upstream of the expiratory valve $V_2$. This will protect this valve and absorber system from both bacterial and water contamination. Alternatively, the breathing hoses should be disposed of between cases.

In locations where the cost of the above exercise would be prohibitive, the tubing should be washed and hung out to dry between cases. Secondly, the expiratory valve should be dismantled and wiped clean with isopropyl alcohol; and thirdly, the system should be flushed with dry gases between cases. When, after dismantling, the glass dome of the expiratory valve is screwed back on again, it is important to ensure that the sealing washer is correctly in place, otherwise a serious leak may occur. If a low-resistance bacterial filter is not used, then the circle absorber housing should be autoclaved (where possible) on a regular basis. Some circle absorbers cannot be autoclaved but may be cleaned by chemical means.

The soda lime should be changed at regular intervals either when the dye indicates that the majority of the granules are exhausted or, when using an analyser, when carbon dioxide appears in the inspiratory mixture.

The soda lime container usually has a mark above

which it should not be filled. Overfilling may result in granules of soda lime clogging the threads of canisters that screw into position, or may prevent the correct seating of the sealing washer, thus causing a leak or bypassing of the soda lime. Furthermore, leaving this space at the top reduces the preferential 'channelling' effect of the gas stream along the sides, and ensures a more even flow through the container. Since the canister is held in the vertical position, channelling is less of a problem than in the Waters' canister, although some channelling does occur between the granules and sides of the canister as the air spaces are bigger here than those between granules within the canister.

### Gas and vapour concentration in a circle system

Circle systems are unique in that they function effectively (when a steady state of anaesthesia has been reached) using a wide variety of fresh gas flow rates. However, the fate of the various gases within the system needs to be understood in order that it may be used safely and effectively. For example, the internal volume of the apparatus, which consists of the intergranular air space in the absorber (1 litre), the breathing hoses (1 litre) and pathways within the absorber (1 litre), totalling 3 litres, along with the functional residual capacity of a patient of 1.25 litres, provides a large reservoir into which the anaesthetic gas is diluted at the beginning of anaesthesia.

In order to minimize this dilution and provide adequate concentrations of anaesthetic agent, high flows of fresh gas and vapour are initially required in order to flush the residual gas out the circle system; the higher the flow the faster this 'wash out' occurs. Lung 'wash out' will of course depend on the patient's minute ventilation. The greater this is, the less time the process takes.

Secondly, the alveolar uptake of anaesthetic agent is greatest at the beginning of anaesthesia. Therefore, the higher the initial fresh gas flow rate (up to a value equal to the patient's minute ventilation) the greater is the delivery of anaesthetic agent into the system. This in turn minimizes any reduction in concentration of agent caused by uptake by the patient. When near equilibrium of anaesthetic agents has occurred between the alveoli and blood, exhaled agent concentration almost equals that in the inspiratory mixture, and therefore the high initial fresh gas flows may safely be greatly reduced.

In practice the fresh gas flow is usually reduced in stages. *First stage*: the initial flow for patient and breathing system washout, as well as supply of

adequate anaesthetic agent to match alveolar uptake, usually takes approximately 5–10 minutes. If this flow rate is at or greater than the patient's minute ventilation, then most or all of the exhaled gas will leave the system via the APL (expiratory) valve without passing through the absorber. *Second stage*: an intermediate flow rate of 70% of the minute ventilation for a further 5 minutes will allow purging of the soda lime canister without major changes in anaesthetic concentrations. *Third stage*: finally, a low flow may be selected, the value of which will depend on (a) the availability of gas and vapour monitoring within the system, (b) the efficiency of the vaporizer (in or out of circle) and (c) personal preference.

### Oxygen concentrations in circle systems at low fresh gas flows

As the fresh gas flow in a circle is decreased, exhaled gas that is allowed to recirculate exerts an increasing influence on the final subsequent inspired gas mixture. The oxygen concentration of this exhaled gas depends on (a) its original inspired concentration and (b) the alveolar oxygen extraction,

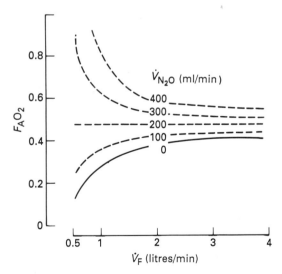

**Figure 9.19** Predicted variations in alveolar oxygen concentrations ($F_{A}O_2$) produced by decreasing fresh gas flow ($V_F$) and assuming different levels of nitrous oxide uptake in a 50 : 50 mixture of oxygen in nitrous oxide. A constant oxygen consumption of 200 ml/min and a constant ventilation required to produce an alveolar $CO_2$ concentration of 5% have been assumed. The heavy line shows the fall in alveolar oxygen concentration with decreasing fresh gas flow when the inspired and body levels of nitrous oxide have reached equilibrium (zero uptake). (Reproduced with kind permission from *Scientific Foundations of Anaesthesia*, Butterworth/Heinemann.)

which may be unpredictable. Figure 9.19 shows the decrease in alveolar oxygen concentrations of a 50% nitrous oxide and 50% oxygen mixture under controlled conditions. It can be seen that at a fresh gas flow of 1 litre/min the oxygen concentration has dropped to 27% and drops even further at a FGF of 0.5 litre/min. Therefore, in clinical practice the oxygen concentration in a circle at low flows is most unpredictable and monitoring of inspired oxygen with an analyser is essential. In fact, moniting of all gases and anaesthetic vapours should be considered mandatory for circle systems at low flows.

### The use of volatile agents in the circle system

Volatile inhalational agents can be introduced into the system either by being added to the fresh gas flow (vaporizer outside circle/VOC) or by incorporating the vaporizer within the circle (vaporizer in circle/VIC)

#### Vaporizer outside circle

This is probably the most common method of introducing inhalational agents into the breathing system. At high fresh gas flows, the vapour concentration in the circle is reliably represented by the dial setting of the vaporizer. However, as the fresh gas flow is reduced two phenomena occur.

- Expired gas, which is recycled (and which has a reduced concentration of inhalational agent due to uptake), dilutes the fresh gas flow within the system. This reduces the delivered concentration of inhalational agent to below that anticipated by the dial setting on the vaporizer.
- At low fresh gas flow, vaporizer efficiency may well be altered, providing a lower or higher than expected output concentration of inhalational agent (e.g. TEC 2 vaporizer, see Chapter 6, vaporizers and flow charts of vaporizers).

At low fresh gas flows, therefore, the anaesthetist needs to know: (a) the performance of the vaporizer in use at that given fresh gas flow; (b) the expired concentration of inhalational agent; and (c) the degree of dilution of the fresh gas flow with expired gas (which in turn depends on the patient's minute ventilation). The lower the fresh gas flow, the more difficult it is to predict the inspired concentration of agent. At flows below 2 litres/min it is highly advisable to incorporate a vapour analyser into the system, especially during controlled ventilation when signs of light anaesthesia may be more difficult to determine, to ensure that adequate amounts of agent reach the patient.

#### Vaporizer in circle

If the vaporizer is incorporated into the circle system, it must have a low resistance to gas flow so as to minimize the respiratory work required of a spontaneously breathing patient. High-resistance Plenum vaporizers are unsuitable.

With a vaporizer incorporated in the circle, recirculating gas picks up vapour to add to the vapour already being carried, and therefore the vapour concentration may well be greater than intended. Calibration of vaporizers in this system is therefore impossible. The vapour concentration in this type of system depends on a number of factors when equilibrium has been reached:

- the fresh gas flow. The lower the fresh gas flow, the greater will be the recirculation of gas already carrying vapour and the higher will be the concentration of inspired agent;
- the efficiency of the vaporizer. The more efficient the vaporizer the higher will be the inspired concentration of agent. This has important implications with potent inhalational agents. At a low fresh gas flow and a large assisted or controlled minute ventilation, the anaesthetic gas may well become saturated with agent at that temperature. For halothane, this will represent a concentration of 33% at 21°C (the saturated vapour pressure for halothane).

Therefore, for potent agents, an *inefficient* vaporizer is preferable. The presence of a wick in a vaporizer in the circle is also unsuitable, since water vapour will condense on the wick, reducing its efficiency and possibly increasing the resistance to gas flow.

Ether, for which much higher concentrations are appropriate, has, however, been widely and safely used with a VIC. Adequate vaporization may be assisted by the use of baffles within the vaporizer that cause the gases to impinge repeatedly on the surface of the ether, or even by bubbling the fresh gas flow through the liquid ether. It may also be increased to some extent by the heat from the recirculating expired gases.

## Modifications of Breathing Systems and their Components

It has long been appreciated that part of the energy required to propel the gases along the passages of a breathing system must be derived from the patient's respiratory effort. The latter, being prejudiced by the depressant effects of narcosis, becomes inefficient, and any form of resistance would further impair respiratory function. On the other hand, any form of assistance to flow or of reduction of resistance would be beneficial. To this end various 'circulators' have been devised and expiratory valves that are not spring-loaded have been advocated. Some of these are described below.

## Breathing systems with assisted circulation

These attempt to reduce the problems of resistance to flow, the inertia of gases, and dead space discussed on page 134.

### Revell's circulator

A small fan helps to assist the circulation of gases in a closed system. It will be noted that this is used in conjunction with a 'chimney' which is part of the facemask mount or catheter mount. As is shown in Fig. 9.20, this causes a continual flow of fresh gases into the facemask, thereby reducing the effects of dead space. The Revell's circulator may be incorporated in a circle system and thereby help to overcome the resistance of the valves and other parts of the system. The design features are of particular benefit in paediatric anaesthesia, and enable a circle system designed for adults to be used for small children.

### Neff's circulator

In 1968 a venturi circulator was described by Neff, Simpson, Burke and Thompson. This makes use of the power that is latent in the fresh gas flow at regulated pressure entering the breathing attachment from the back bar (Fig. 9.21).

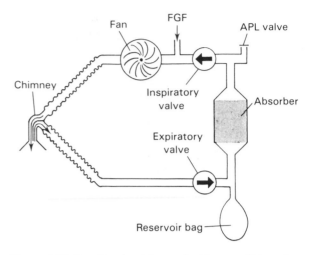

**Figure 9.20** Revell's circulator and chimney. Driven by compressed air or other gas, a fan induces the circulation of anaesthetic gases within a circle breathing system. The 'chimney' directs a flow of fresh gases into the facepiece, thus minimizing the effective dead space. FGF = fresh gas flow; APL = adjustable pressure-limiting (expiratory) valve.

These circulators enabled the exploitation of the advantages of the circle system, such as the economy in fresh gas flow and the retention of water vapour and heat, but without the disadvantages of resistance, dead space and the inertia of gases in a large apparatus volume.

## Further developments

When scavenging systems were devised, this led to the development of the various Hafnia breathing systems (Fig. 9.22) The common feature of these is

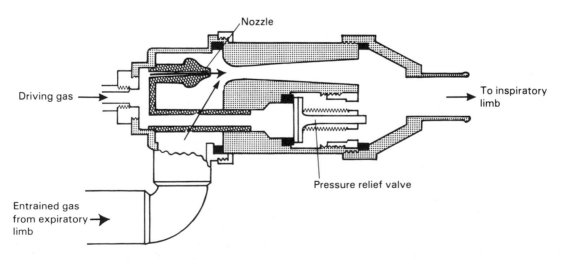

**Figure 9.21** Neff's circulator, which is a venturi powered by the fresh gas inflow.

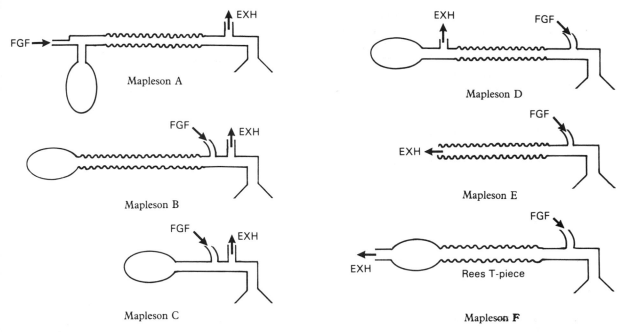

**Figure 9.22** The Hafnia modifications of the breathing systems described by Mapleson. Note that in each case the expiratory valve is replaced by a connection to the scavenging system. FGF = fresh gas flow; EXH = exhaust to scavenging system.

that there are no valves but simply one port delivering the fresh gas flow, and another through which excess gases are removed by the scavenging system, the flow rate of the latter being adjusted so that the reservoir bag is never fully distended, nor completely emptied. One method of controlling the rate at which excess gases are extracted is the use of the ejector flowmeter. In this device a jet of oxygen or compressed air, or any other gas, utilizes the venturi effect to draw the gases through a flow-meter. The rate of extraction may be controlled by a flow control valve so that it balances the combined inflow of the fresh gases (Fig. 9.23, see also page 285).

A more recent embodiment of all these features is to be seen in the system described by Jorgensen (Fig. 9.24), in which the circulation of gases is assisted by a venturi, and the excess gases are removed by an ejector flowmeter. It will be seen that this is a circle closed system with spill which enables the fresh gas inflow to be reduced to well below the minute volume of the patient. This affords economy of gases and also a reduction of the total volume of gases to be scavenged. During the first few minutes of anaesthesia, with a high fresh gas flow, the control may be turned to 'D', whereupon the system will behave as a Mapleson D system.

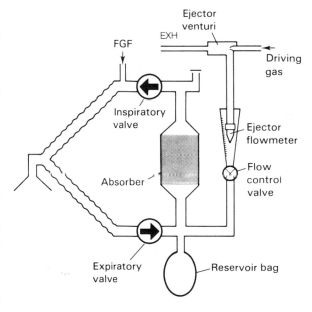

**Figure 9.23** The principle of the ejector flowmeter. By means of a flow control valve, the total volume of gases drawn from the breathing system and delivered to the scavenging system is adjusted so as to be equal to the fresh gas flow (FGF) rate. EXH = exhaust to scavenging system.

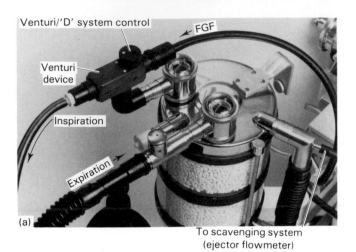

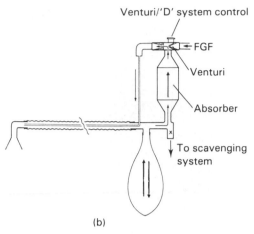

**Figure 9.24** (a) Jorgensen's venturi circulator. (b) Diagrammatic representation of its use with a Mapleson D coaxial breathing system. Note that the control knob may be turned to 'D' during induction and the first few minutes of maintenance of anaesthesia, while a high fresh gas flow (FGF) rate is used.

# The Components of a Breathing System

### Rebreathing and reservoir bags

Rebreathing and reservoir bags (Fig. 9.25) are identical, the distinction being solely in the use to which they are put, as explained previously. The commonly used size in adult breathing systems is 2 litres (i.e. that which when fully but not forcibly distended has a capacity of 2 litres; in clinical practice it is seldom filled beyond this capacity). Larger bags are used as reservoir bags in ventilators, and smaller ones in paediatric anaesthesia.

In adult breathing systems, the capacity to which the bag may easily be distended must exceed the patient's tidal volume. A larger capacity, bag (2 litres), however, is safer as it more easily absorbs pressure increases. Bags are frequently provided with a loop at the bottom end that makes it possible to double the bag back on itself by hanging the loop from a knob on the top of the bag mount. This manoeuvre, or tying the bag around with string, is used when anaesthetizing small children. It does not alter the mechanics of the breathing system, and is justified only in that it makes movements of the bag easier to observe. Certainly it should not be used if it makes the bag 'stiffer'.

'Double-ended' bags may be used in two ways. The narrow end may be connected to the fresh gas flow, provided that rebreathing is prevented as in the Digby–Leigh paediatric attachment (see Fig. 14.5). In the Rees T-piece paediatric attachment, a double-ended bag is added to the expiratory limb

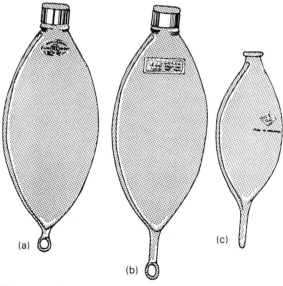

**Figure 9.25** Reservoir (and rebreathing) bags. (a) A single-ended 2-litre bag. (b) A 2-litre bag in which the extended tail loop may be removed to convert it into a double-ended bag. (c) A 0.5-litre bag with a small neck, which may be converted into a double-ended one, for paediatric use.

(see Fig. 9.14) and the smaller end acts as an expiratory port which can be controlled by the anaesthetist's fifth finger.

The 'pressure-limiting' bag (Fig. 9.26), seldom used now, was intended for use as a reservoir for ventilators. When it is distended, a string within it pulls open the flap of a valve in its wall, allowing the escape of excess gases. It should be noted that it would be dangerous to use such a bag in a Magill attachment, since if the opening pressure of the valve on the bag were less than that of the

(a)

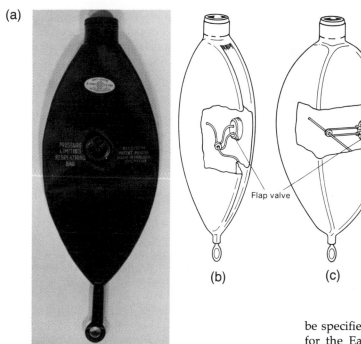

(b)    (c)

Flap valve

**Figure 9.26** (a) The 'pressure-limiting' bag. (b) The bag before it is distended. (c) The bag when it is full and the flap valve has been opened.

expiratory valve, the latter would fail to open and so expired gases would not escape through it. Fresh gases would escape from the bag, and the patient would rebreathe the gases in the corrugated hose, the capacity of which would present a dead space of about 500 ml.

The material of which the bag is constructed is important. Where ventilation is spontaneous, the opening pressure of the expiratory valve must exceed that required to prevent the bag from emptying spontaneously owing to its weight or resistance to distension. Therefore, to maintain a low expiratory pressure, the bag must be 'soft'.

A stiffer bag with stronger walls is required for use with minute volume divider ventilators such as the East–Freeman Automatic Vent (page 203), where the back pressure on the bag may rise to 4kPa (40 cmH$_2$O) or more, and the elasticity of the bag plays a part in the operation of the valve.

The black antistatic rubber of which it is constructed may make movements of the bag difficult to observe under some conditions. In this case a couple of strips of white adhesive plaster stuck diagonally on the bag may help. The observed movement of the bag depends on several factors, such as its shape, size, degree of filling, the tension of the expiratory valve and the fresh gas flow rate, as well as on the patient's tidal volume. An accurate estimate of the patient's tidal volume cannot be made simply by watching the bag.

When ordering bags, the size of the neck should be specified. Whereas in some bags, including those for the East–Freeman Automatic Vent, the neck is integral with the bag itself and relatively easily stretched, in others the neck includes a stiff moulded rubber fitting that is suitable only for the appropriate size of bag mount.

The bag mount may incorporate a valve that can exclude the bag from the breathing attachment. This is no longer widely employed, but where an intermittent flow machine is used 'on demand', either the valve should be closed or the bag and its mount should be removed from the machine. The bag also needs to be disconnected when minute volume divider ventilators such as the Manley are used.

## Expiratory ('pop-off' or adjustable pressure limiting) valves

In the latest British and International Standards this valve is called the *adjustable pressure limiting valve*, or APL valve, but it is likely that for a long time the older terms *expiratory valve* (EXP) or 'pop-off' valve will be used.

The purpose of this valve is to allow the escape of exhaled (expired) and surplus gases from a breathing attachment, but without permitting entry of the outside air, even during a negative phase. Usually it is desirable that the pressure required to open the valve should be as low as possible, in order to minimize resistance to expiration. It must, however, present sufficient resistance to prevent the reservoir bag from emptying spontaneously, particularly when a scavenging system is employed that exerts a subatmospheric pressure upon it.

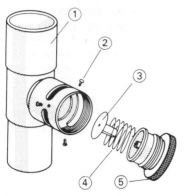

Figure 9.27 The Heidbrink valve: 1, female taper; 2, retaining screws; 3, disc; 4, spring; 5, valve top.

A commonly used type of expiratory valve is the Heidbrink (Fig. 9.27). The valve disc is as light as possible, and rests on a 'knife-edge' seating that presents a small area of contact. This lessens the tendency to adhesion between the disc and seating due to the surface tension of condensed water from the expired air, or after washing or sterilizing. The disc has a stem that is located in a guide, in order to ensure that it is correctly positioned on the seating, and a coiled spring, of light weight, which promotes closure of the valve.

Some people prefer to remove the spring in order to reduce resistance to the opening of the valve. When this is done, if the valve is orientated so that the disc is in a horizontal plane over the seating (i.e. upright), it would seem that gravity would be sufficient to close it, obviating the necessity for the spring. However, as the disc is very light, dampness might lead to surface tension holding it open. Also, if the valve is placed obliquely or sideways, friction between the stem and the guide might prevent it from closing, and if it is upside-down, gravity could keep it open. Another problem arising from the absence of the spring is that there may be some delay in the closing of the valve at the start of inspiration, in which case air could be drawn in.

The spring is a delicate coil and is of such dimensions that when the valve top is screwed fully 'open' there is minimal pressure on the disc when seated. However, during the 'blow-off' phase the disc rises and shortens the spring so that the pressure it exerts on the disc is greater and will close it at the appropriate time. Screwing down the valve top produces progressively increasing tension in the spring. When the top is screwed fully down the valve is completely closed. If, owing to damage or fatigue, the spring is shortened, the top may have to be screwed down a little in order to ensure closure at the start of inspiration. If it has been

elongated, the pressure at which it opens may be excessive. Small screws in the body of the valve, and a groove in the skirt of the top, prevent it from being unscrewed so far that it falls apart.

## Breathing hoses

The hoses connecting the components of a breathing system must be of such a diameter as to present a low resistance to gas flow. Its cross-section must be uniform to promote laminar flow where possible, and although it should be flexible, kinking should not occur. It should drape easily so that a deep loop may hang between the patient, and, say, a circle absorber since this tends to trap droplets of moisture that could carry infective organisms back to the apparatus.

The most commonly used type of hosing has for a long time been a corrugated hose of rubber or neoprene (Fig. 9.28). The corrugations allow acute angulations of the hose without kinking. The disadvantages of these materials are that the irregular wall must cause turbulence and may har-

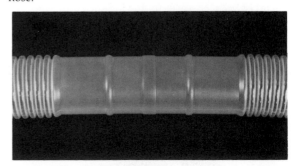

Figure 9.28 A standard length of wide-bore corrugated hose.

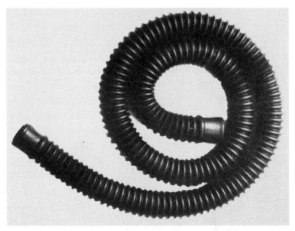

Figure 9.29 Lightweight plastic corrugated hose. At frequent intervals the corrugations give way to a shaped connector, where a long roll of this hose may be cut.

bour dirt and infection. They are also heavy and if unsupported, may drag on a facemask or endotracheal tube. The advantage is that the ends are more easily stretched, and will make a good union with other components of different diameters.

Various other materials such as silicone rubber and plastics, both in corrugated and smooth form, are in use. Plastic hosing (Fig. 9.29) has become very popular because it is lightweight, cheap to manufacture, and therefore disposable. Some of these plastic hoses are supplied in long coils, the appropriate length of which may be cut off at one of the frequent intervals where the corrugations give way to a shaped connector. Silicone rubber hosing

is autoclavable, unlike many plastics which would melt if so treated. Plastic apparatus is normally sterilized by gamma irradiation if it is intended for single use only, or by chemical sterilization, boiling or pasteurization if it is reuseable. Most manufacturers supply guidelines with their products as to the suitability of the various sterilizing methods.

There are several standard sizes of corrugated hose (sometimes known as 'elephant tubing'), both ends of which have smooth walls for about 2–3 cm. These ends are designed to fit either tapered connectors (see Fig. 9.30a, b), or tapered components of a breathing system (see Fig. 9.30e, f, k). Breathing hose for adult use is normally 22-mm

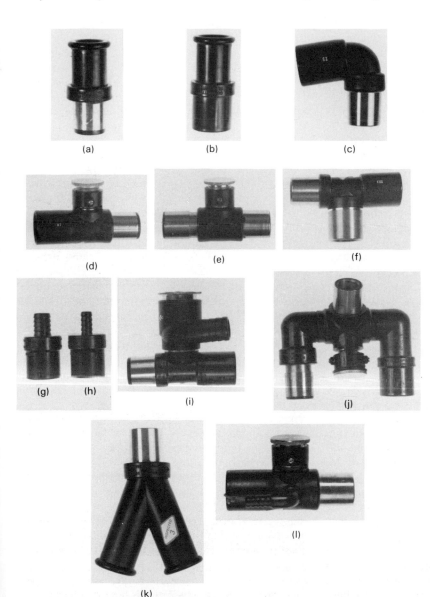

Figure 9.30 Various Superlite connections for breathing attachments. (a) Hose adaptor (male). (b) Hose adaptor (female). (c) Facemask angle mount (elbow). (d) APL (expiratory) valve. (e) APL valve with double male tapers. (f) Bag mount. (g) Catheter mount. (h) Feed mount. (i) Exhaust valve. (j) Swivel Y-piece. (k) Fixed Y-piece. (l) APL (expiratory) valve with side feed. Note that (d), (f), (i), (j) and (l) no longer meet ISO and BS requirements as they include a female taper (see text). Note also that (h) should not, mistakenly be used for a catheter mount since the resistance is high.

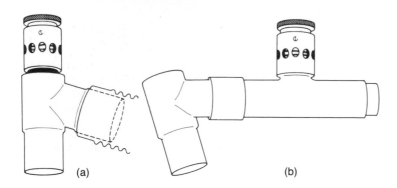

**Figure 9.31** (a) A Heidbrink valve attached to an elbow in order to lessen both dead space and the weight of ironmongery hanging on the facemask, as shown in (b).

wide so as to reduce the resistance to breathing to a minimum. Paediatric breathing hose has a narrower bore (15 mm) to reduce its internal volume (see Chapter 14) and to make it less cumbersome.

Smooth bore breathing hose produces less turbulence than the corrugated variety at similar gas flows. It can also be produced so that it resists kinking (by the attachment of a reinforcing spiral of a similar material to its external surface). With smooth bore hosing, a smaller diameter (e.g. 15 mm) may well be acceptable for use with adult breathing systems (see Humphrey ADE breathing system, Fig. 9.11).

As described above, breathing hoses may be fitted with either a rigid metal, a hard rubber or a plastic tapered connector which fits other components in a breathing system. These tapered connectors and other parts of the breathing system sometimes present as a large mass of 'ironmongery' that can drag on the face mask or endotracheal tube, particularly if the patient is a child. The dead space may also be greater than necessary. By using the end of the corrugated hose as a simple push fit much of this trouble can be prevented (as seen in Fig. 9.31).

## Tapered connections

Tapered connections (conical fittings) provide a useful way of joining rigid tubes or other components together in such a manner that the joint will not leak. The joint is described as having a male half and a female half which are pushed together and twisted to form a gas-tight fit. The joint may be easily dismantled and reassembled, a feature which makes it useful for the interconnection of breathing systems, catheter mounts and endotracheal connectors. A leakproof joint relies on its components being completely circular and having the same angle of taper so that the maximum contact between the components of the joint will occur. Prior to the introduction of any standards, manufacturers were free to decide the size and angle of tapers used with

their equipment (see Table 9.2). However there is now an internationally agreed size for tapered connections for use with anaesthetic breathing systems and endotracheal tubes so that there is compatibility between equipment from different manufacturers. The International Standards Organization (ISO.5356, 1987) and the British Standard (BS 3849) specifies the use of 30-mm tapered connections for the attachment of scavenging hose to breathing systems, 22-mm tapers for connections within a breathing system, and 15-mm connections for the attachment of a breathing system to an endotracheal tube. Some 22-mm male breathing hose connections are so manufactured that they incorporate a 15-mm female taper for direct connection to an endotracheal tube.

In the UK, the original standard prior to 1988 stated that the tapers should be directed in the same way, i.e. a male taper upstream and a female one downstream, in order to minimize the chance of a component of the breathing system being omitted. Unfortunately, it is not successful in this respect. Furthermore, it increased the number of tapered components in a breathing system. For example breathing hose is always manufactured with similar sized ends (female) so that with the original British Standard, one end would require the fitment of an extra (male) taper (Fig. 9.32a). The current ISO and revised BS recommendations on the sequence of tapers are set out in Fig. 32b. The standard also requires male tapers to be fitted with a recess behind the taper so that when rubber and plastic hosing is pushed on to a male connector, its leading edge can contract into this recess to provide a more secure fitting (see Fig. 9.33). It is worthy of note that the current British Standard requires that a reservoir bag now should have a female inlet, whereas previously it had a male one. This could have disastrous consequences should one bag fail and the replacement be fitted with a different standard. Departments have been advised to make a planned change over to the new system.

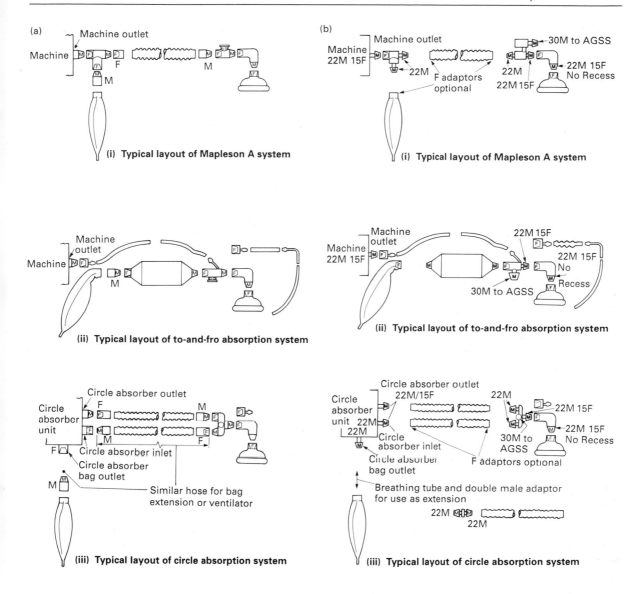

**Figure. 9.32** (a) Sequence of tapers in anaesthetic breathing systems in the UK from 1965 to 1988 (BS 3849). (b) Current sequence of tapers in anaesthetic breathing systems as recommended by the International Standards Organization and British Standards (BS 3849) as from 1988. M = male conical fitting, F = female conical fitting.

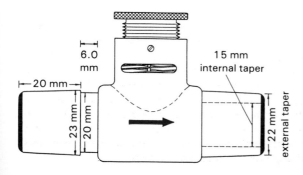

**Figure 9.33** An expiratory valve with the British and International Standard 22-mm taper. Note that the proximal taper may be pushed directly into the end of a corrugated hose and the square shoulder will help to secure this joint. The distal 22-mm taper will also accept a 15-mm endotracheal connector.

**Table 9.2**  Details of various types of tapered connections

| Name or nominal diameter | M → F = male upstream<br>F → M = female upstream | Maximum diameter of spigot or socket (mm) | Purpose | Angle of taper |
|---|---|---|---|---|
| 15-mm | F → M | 15.47 | Endotracheal connectors<br>Paediatric breathing systems | 1 in 40 |
| 22-mm<br>British and ISO Standard | M → F | 22.37 | Adult breathing systems<br>Paediatric facepieces<br>Vaporizers in breathing system | 1 in 40 |
| Cagemount<br>23-mm | F → M | 23.75 | Back bar fittings including high-resistance vaporizers | 1 in 36 |
| 30-mm | M → F | 30.9 | Scavenging | 1 in 20 |
| McKesson<br>M & IE | M → F<br>M → F | 19.75 | McKesson fittings<br>M & IE back bar | —<br>— |
| Nosworthy connectors | M → F | 15.4 | Endotracheal connectors | — |
| Knight's connectors | M → F | 9.7 | Paediatric endotracheal connectors | — |

## Problems with tapered connections

Many accidents have occurred as a result of the accidental and unobserved disconnection of tapered joints. The material used in the construction may either wear with frequent use (most plastics and rubber), or become distorted by damage (metal connectors). Disconnection can be minimized by giving the components of the joint a slight twist following their insertion.

Devices designed to prevent accidental disconnection are described on pages 165–166.

Conversely some metal connectors made from aluminium alloys may stick together by the phenomenon of cold welding produced by the recommended twist above, and may be very difficult to separate.

## Facemasks

Facemasks are also referred to as facepieces. They are designed to fit the patient's face perfectly, without any leaks, and yet to exert the minimum of pressure, which might either depress the jaw and cause respiratory obstruction or cause pressure sores. A snug fit is achieved by anatomical shaping and by the use of an air-filled cuff that has a soft cushioning effect or a flap that takes up the contour of the face. The facemask (Fig. 9.34) consists of three

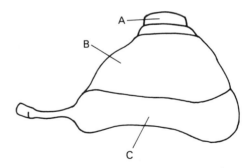

**Figure 9.34** The parts of an anaesthetic facemask: A, the mount; B, the body; C, the edge.

parts; A, the mount; B, the body; and C, the edge.

The mount is normally a 22-mm female taper if made to ISO or BS standards, although other sizes do exist. When ordering facemasks, it is therefore important to specify the size. It is usually constructed of hard rubber but may be plastic or metal.

The body may be of rubber, neoprene, plastic or polycarbonate. In some cases a wire stiffener or a wire gauze is incorporated so as to make it malleable in order that its shape may be altered to fit the patient's face. The transparent body of the Ambu and other facemasks is particularly useful in resuscitation as it permits the early detection of vomit.

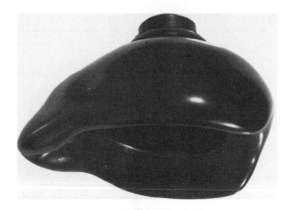

**Figure 9.35** The Everseal facemask (M&IE).

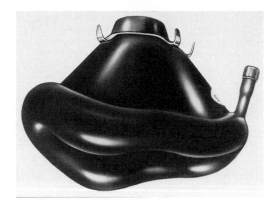

**Figure 9.36** The anatomical facemask (Ohmeda).

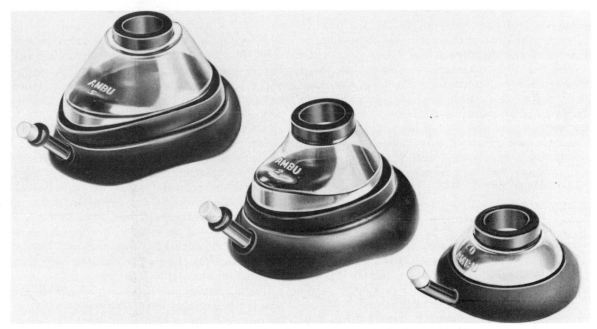

**Figure 9.37** Three examples of the Ambu facemask, which has a transparent body that enables the presence of vomitus to be seen.

The edge may be anatomically shaped and fitted with a cuff or a flap. Where there is a possibility of explosive anaesthetic agents being used, the cuff, like the rest of the equipment, must be of antistatic material, but otherwise a soft latex one is very satisfactory. There is a small filling tube fitted with a plug to enable the degree of inflation of the cuff to be regulated. Inflation is normally carried out using a hypodermic syringe. The plug must also be removed and the cuff deflated if the mask is to be autoclaved.

It is advisable to stock a variety of types of facemask, since none will fit every type of face well.

Facemasks are made in various sizes and examples of some types are shown in Figs 9.35–9.38.

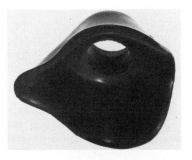

**Figure 9.38** The Rendell–Baker paediatric facemask.

(a)  (b)

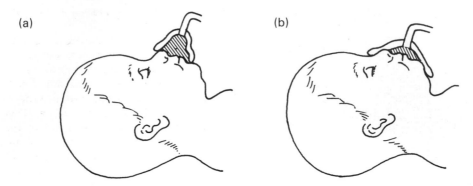

**Figure 9.39** The use of the smallest facemask (a) does not necessarily result in the minimum dead space. The patient's face may fit into a larger facemask (b), resulting in less dead space.

Note that the smallest facemask does not necessarily give the lowest dead space (Fig. 9.39).

Whereas some facemasks withstand the high temperatures of autoclaving, others do not. Since these are not easily distinguished, it is advisable to adopt a uniform policy of disinfection. This may be by boiling, pasteurizing or by chemical means, although some chemicals, e.g. chloroxylenol (Dettol) are known to have been absorbed by the material of the facemask and have resulted in injury to the patient's skin.

### Endotracheal tubes

There are various situations in which it is not feasible to administer anaesthetic gases via a facemask, laryngeal mask or nasal mask. In these cases an endotracheal tube (Fig. 9.40), or occasionally a tracheostomy tube is used. Where positive pressure ventilation is contemplated, it is also necessary to make an airtight connection with the trachea. Traditionally, endotracheal tubes have been made of red rubber or latex. However plastics, and to a lesser degree, silicone rubber are rapidly replacing them as primary materials for the following reasons.

Although red rubber and latex can be cleaned and sterilized, these materials are opaque and inadequate cleaning is not always apparent from a superficial examination. Occlusion of the lumen occurs occasionally with foreign objects and dried mucus. Perishing may cause cuff failure, sometimes at awkward moments, and also causes the wall of the tube to weaken, increasing the possibility of kinking. The material itself (red rubber) is potentially irritant when used for long periods and has been blamed for producing laryngeal granulomata. The cuffs made from these materials are usually thick

and require high pneumatic pressures to inflate them. If a small degree of inadvertent overdistension of the cuff occurs, these pressures are transmitted to the tracheal mucosa, resulting in mucosal ischaemia when the tubes are used for prolonged periods.

Plastic tubes possess several advantages over red rubber ones in that they are non-irritant and are now cheaper to produce. They can be sterilized more reliably during manufacture (as they are not meant to be reuseable) and, as the material is usually clear, blockages may be visible. Plastic used for the manufacture of cuffs can be made so that it is both thin as well as inelastic. Large volume cuffs may then be constructed requiring only low inflation pressures to effect a tracheal seal, with a lower potential for mucosal damage.

The manufacturing tolerances are much closer with plastics, so that there is much less variation in the size of the lumen (important in neonatal endotracheal tubes).

Plastic tubes do not have the 'springiness' of rubber and may be more difficult to insert in difficult situations. Also, the relative rigidity of plastic tubes at room temperature appears to cause more trauma when they are inserted via the nasal route compared to rubber ones. However prewarming, by immersing them in warm water, does make the plastic softer.

The type of plastic used in the construction of endotracheal tubes is tested on a 'once only' basis to make sure that it is non-irritant. Each endotracheal tube is marked with a test number, which can be seen on the body of the tube labelled 'I.T.' (implant tested) Z.79. This refers to the Z79 Toxicity Subcommittee of ANSI (American National Standards Institute) set up in 1968 in the US, which established the current method of test. The test

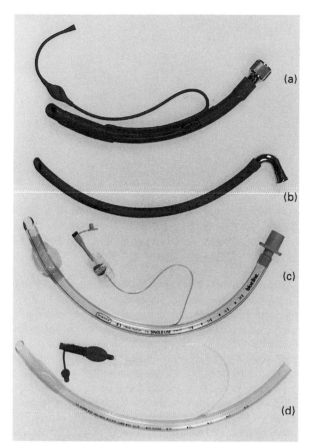

**Figure 9.40** Endotracheal tubes. (a) Red rubber orotracheal tube with high-pressure low-volume cuff. (b) Red rubber plain nasotracheal tube. (c) Plastic oro-/nasotracheal tube with high-volume low-pressure cuff. (d) Silicone rubber oro-/nasotracheal tube with streamlined medium-volume, medium-pressure cuff.

consists of implanting four samples of the plastic, under sterile conditions, into the paravertebral muscle of anaesthetized rabbits along with two samples of Reference Standard Negative Control plastic, for 70–144 h. The rabbits are then killed by giving them an overdose of an anaesthetic and the implant sites examined both micro- and macroscopically for signs of inflammation.

Silicone rubber is increasingly used in the manufacture of endotracheal tubes. These have a high production cost per unit but may be resterilized. They are softer than red rubber and plastic and are non-irritant and can be used very many times.

Modern methods of production allow cuffs to be made of silicone rubber which are relatively thin (medium-volume, medium-pressure) but without the bulkiness of the plastic high-volume, low-pressure variety. These properties make tubes with

these 'slimline' cuffs ideal for use via the nasal route.

Tubes for orotracheal use are usually cuffed (sizes 6.0–11.0-mm internal diameter). Below 6.0-mm internal diameter, the cuff, added to the size of the tube wall, increases the relative bulkiness of the tube so that a smaller size is required in order to pass as easily into the larynx and trachea. This causes a reduction in the internal diameter of the resultant air passage and produces a sharp rise in resistance to gas flow (see Chapter 1, Poiseuille's law), so that below this value (6 mm) the use of a plain tube is preferable. Also, the larynx of a child or infant is almost circular and a more snug fit is possible, therefore reducing the need for a cuff on a tube. There are a few exceptions to this rule however (see the section on Special Tubes). (See also page 249.)

## Endotracheal cuffs (Fig. 9.40a, c, d)

Cuffs are inflated via a small bore inflation tube either welded onto the outside of the endotracheal tube or built into its wall. The inflation tube is connected to a small pilot balloon which is designed to give an indication of the distension of the cuff. The cuff and pilot balloon are inflated, usually with air, via a syringe. The inflation tube is often fitted with a self-sealing valve which prevents air escaping when the syringe is removed. Earlier designs of these tubes required the application of forceps to the pilot tube between the syringe and pilot balloon to maintain cuff inflation. Cuffs on tubes should be inflated with just sufficient air or gas to prevent leaks. This limits the pressure on the ciliated columinar epithelium of the trachea, so as to prevent damage or even necrosis. Also, if there were overpressure in the breathing system it would permit leakage around the cuff thereby (a) allowing excess gas under pressure to escape and (b) giving a warning by the gurgling noise produced.

Nitrous oxide diffuses into a cuff filled with air. A 50% mixture of nitrous oxide will eventually increase the number of molecules of gas present in the cuff by a factor of 2 and 75% nitrous oxide will increase it by a factor of 3. The rate at which this occurs depends on the permeability of the material from which the cuff is constructed (rubber being more permeable than plastic) and upon the surface area of cuff exposed to the nitrous oxide. The rise in pressure caused by this diffusion into the cuff depends on the compliance of the cuff. Low-volume, high-pressure cuffs suffer the greatest pressure rise and may well transmit this rise in pressure to the tracheal mucosa. High-volume, low-pressure cuffs, constructed of plastic, expand with only a slight

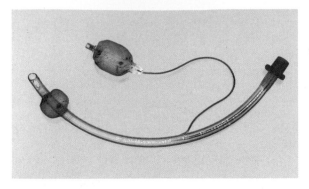

**Figure 9.41** The Mallinckrodt Brandt device.

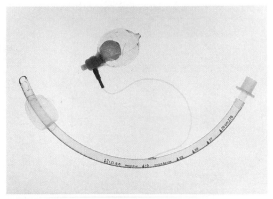

**Figure 9.42** The Mallinckrodt Lanz device.

increase in pressure until all the slack in the cuff is taken up. At this point, owing to the inelasticity of plastic, the pressure rise increases rapidly (up to 12 kPa/90 mmHg) so that the tracheal mucosa may become damaged. This phenomenon can be avoided if the cuff is filled with either sterile water or a gas mixture identical to that of the inspired gas. Alternatively, there are several devices which limit the pressure rise. For example the Mallinckrodt Brandt device allows the nitrous oxide, which has diffused into the cuff, to diffuse out through the pilot balloon into the atmosphere (Fig. 9.41). The Mallinckrodt Lanz device uses a secondary balloon made of thin latex which is placed inside the plastic pilot balloon on the tube. When air is introduced into the system, the tube cuff and this latex balloon are both inflated. As the cuff pressure starts to rise due to the diffusion of nitrous oxide, the latex balloon absorbs this pressure by expanding (Fig. 9.42).

## Nasotracheal intubation

The size of the tube that can be passed via the nasal route is limited by the size of the nares and the potential obstruction caused by the nasal turbinates. Tubes made from harder materials (certain plastics) as well as those with cuffs may well be more difficult to insert and may increase the likelihood for epistaxis. Unless spontaneous respiration is contraindicated, plain (uncuffed) red rubber tubes still seem to be the least traumatic. If a cuffed tube has to be used, then one with the softest and smoothest exterior surface is best. This will include one that incorporates the inflation tube within its walls, and one that has a close fitting streamline cuff of fine latex or plastic material. Plastic tubes may be preheated to body temperature by immersion in warm water to soften them prior to insertion.

## Maintenance of reuseable endotracheal tubes

Endotracheal tubes may be sterilized by immersion in a cold solution of chemical sterilizing agent or by being pasteurized or autoclaved. In either case, connectors should be removed and cuffs deflated before treatment. The self-sealing valves fitted to endotracheal tubes should be kept open with an autoclavable syringe (with the plunger removed) so as to release any residual gas which might expand during the autoclaving process. Tubes may be wrapped separately, in which case a transparent packet should be used so that they may be inspected before opening. The cuff should be tested before reuse and if it shows any weakness or herniation, it should be rendered unuseable and discarded. Tubes should be also tested for resistance to kinking, and any that show signs of ageing or perishing should also be discarded.

## Endotracheal tube lengths

Endotracheal tubes are supplied from the manufacturer longer than normally required. Many anaesthetists cut these tubes to shorten them so that when inserted they are less likely to enter a main bronchus (see Table 9.3).

## Common faults with the use of endotracheal tubes

These are as follows.

- A tube may be passed too far down the trachea and enter the right main bronchus. This occurs because the tube selected is too long and it needs shortening.

**Table 9.3**    Lengths of endotracheal tubes

| Internal diameter (mm) | | Age (years) | Length (cm) | |
|---|---|---|---|---|
| Oral | Nasal | | Oral | Nasal |
| 2.5 | 2.5 | PREMATURE | 10.5 | 13.0 |
| 3.0 | 3.0 | | 10.5 | 13.0 |
| 3.5 | 3.5 | 0–1 | 11.0 | 14.0 |
| 4.0 | 4.0 | | 12.0 | 14.5 |
| 4.5 | 4.5 | 1–2 | 13.5 | 15.0 |
| 5.0 | 5.0 | | 14.0 | 16.6 |
| 5.5 | 5.5 | 2–4 | 14.5 | 17.0 |
| 6.0 | 6.0 | | 15.0 | 17.5 |
| 6.5 | 6.5 | 5–12 | 16.0 | 18.5 |
| 7.0 | 7.0 | 13–16 | 17.5 | 19.0 |
| 8.0 | 8.0 | | 18.5 | 19.5 |
| — | 6.0 | | — | 24.0 |
| — | 6.5 | | — | 24.0 |
| 7.0 | 7.0 | ADULTS — Small women | — | 24.0 |
| 7.5 | 7.5 | | — | 25.0 |
| 8.0 | 8.0 | | 23.0 | 26.0 |
| 8.5 | — | | 24.0 | — |
| 9.0 | — | | 25.0 | — |
| 9.5 | — | Large men | 25.0 | — |
| 10.0 | — | | 26.0 | — |
| 11.0 | — | | 26.0 | — |

A widely used formula for selecting the diameter of an endotracheal tube suitable for children over the age of one year is:

$$\frac{\text{Age in years}}{4} + 4.5\ \text{mm}$$

The exact length to which a new tube should be shortened cannot be categorically specified. In some operations it is necessary to pass the tube further down the trachea than in others. Cuffed tubes are generally trimmed to a centimetre or so longer than plain ones.

- There may be a leak between the cuff and the trachea. This may be either because the cuff has not been sufficiently inflated in the first place, or because it has leaked. The latter may be due to a fault in manufacture, or to over-inflation. The presence of a leak may be demonstrated by immersing the whole tube, pilot and all, in water, inflating the cuff and watching for bubbles. It is possible to kink the pilot tube accidentally and prevent inflation of the cuff even though the pilot balloon is blown up.

The cuff may become stretched and baggy after repeated use and autoclaving, and it is possible for it to form a 'diverticulum' that can protrude over the open end of the tube and obstruct it (Fig. 9.43). This is more likely to occur if the tube is withdrawn or allowed to slip out a little after the cuff has been inflated. For this reason it is a better practice to fix the tube into position before

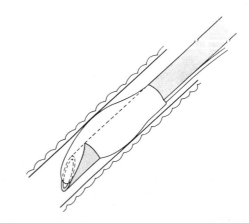

**Figure 9.43** A herniation of the cuff that may occlude the distal end of the tube.

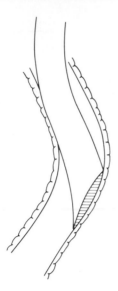

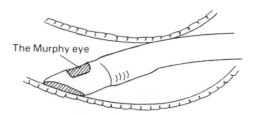

Figure 9.45 The distal end of an endotracheal tube with a 'Murphy eye'.

Figure 9.44 If there is marked deviation of the trachea, the end of the tube may be obstructed.

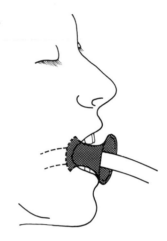

Figure 9.46 The London Hospital airway prop.

inflating the cuff. With age, the cuff may become wrinkled and prune-like, and this can make extubation difficult.

- The tube may be obstructed in one or more of several ways. The opening may be occluded if the larynx or trachea is deviated to one side as seen in Fig. 9.44. This may happen particularly during thyroidectomy, when the gland is being pulled to one side by the surgeon. The 'Murphy eye' (Fig. 9.45) will prevent this hazard. During nasal intubation the tube may be blocked as it harvests a polyp or adenoidal tissue. It may also kink when bent to too small a radius, particularly if soft from frequent use. If it must be acutely bent, an armoured tube or one that is specially shaped should be used (see below). A tube may be compressed by a throat pack that has been inserted too firmly, and it may also be ostructed if the patient is lightly anaesthetized and bites it. This may be prevented either by inserting an airway alongside the tube or by using a 'London Hospital airway prop' (Fig. 9.46).

All sorts of foreign bodies have been found within endotracheal tubes, blocking them, including the tops of ampoules. This emphasizes the fact that tubes, airways, etc. that are to be reused should not be placed in the same 'dirty dish' as discarded syringes, needles, ampoules, etc. A diaphragm of dried mucus or K-Y Jelly has been found blocking a tube, and even if the tube is straightened so that one can look through it to confirm patency, it is almost invisible.

For neurosurgical anaesthesia it may be considered wiser to use an anatomically shaped tube such as the Oxford non-kinking tube (Fig. 9.47) which may be either cuffed or plain. There is a special stylet or 'director' available to assist the insertion of these tubes. Alternatively, armoured tubes may be used. These are made of latex, plastic or red rubber and contain in their wall a spiral of metal wire or tough nylon. The latest models are constructed of silicone rubber and are of considerably superior quality. If they are to withstand repeated use they must be sterilized with care. On autoclaving, the cuff must not be over-distended by steam, and to this end the self-closing valve or the pilot tube should be kept open, if necessary by a dummy syringe (Fig. 9.48). In the resting state they may be either straight or curved. A stylet or 'director' may be needed to introduce them, but care must be taken to avoid injuring the larynx or trachea (see below). Typical armoured tubes are shown in Figs 9.49 and 9.50. They must be handled with care since if the armouring is distorted by handling roughly with forceps, especially while hot after autoclaving or boiling, there will be a con-

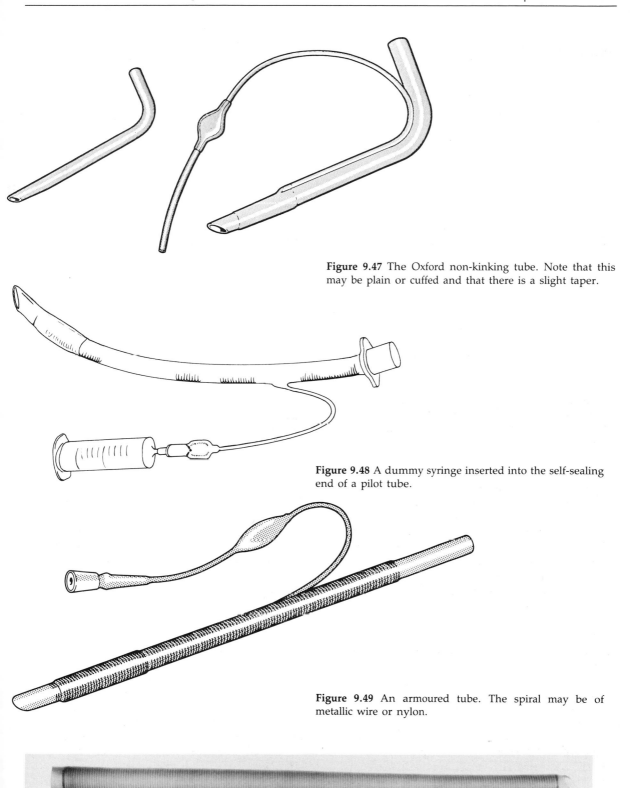

**Figure 9.47** The Oxford non-kinking tube. Note that this may be plain or cuffed and that there is a slight taper.

**Figure 9.48** A dummy syringe inserted into the self-sealing end of a pilot tube.

**Figure 9.49** An armoured tube. The spiral may be of metallic wire or nylon.

**Figure 9.50** The Enderby paediatric armoured tube.

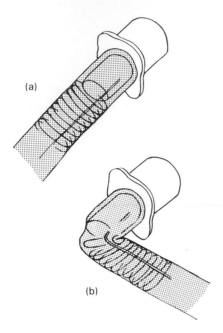

(a)

(b)

**Figure 9.51** Obstruction at the 'soft spot' between the connector and the spiral of an armoured tube. (a) With the connector placed correctly. (b) With incorrect placement leaving an unarmoured segment of tube.

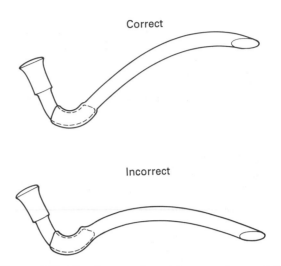

Correct

Incorrect

**Figure 9.52** The lumen of a tube may be partially obstructed if a Magill nasal connector has been wrongly fitted.

siderable narrowing of the lumen. When an endotracheal connector is being inserted into an armoured tube it is important to ensure that there is no 'soft spot' between the end of the connector and the start of the spiral reinforcement, since kinking could occur at this point (Fig. 9.51). A little of the unreinforced end of the tube may need trimming off. However, if the unreinforced end is removed altogether it is difficult to insert a connector of the appropriate size, since the reinforcement will not

stretch to admit it. The use of an unsuitable connector may obstruct the lumen of the tube (Fig. 9.52).

With any endotracheal tube it is important that it is cut to the correct length so that the connector is as close as possible to the patient's mouth. If there is an excess of tube sticking out of the mouth, kinking may easily occur at that point. A tube may also be obstructed by being twisted in its long axis if the position of the catheter mount is altered.

Endotracheal tubes may be kinked in the mouth (Fig. 9.53) or nasopharynx when the patient's neck is flexed, and this is particularly likely when procedures such as oesophagoscopy are being performed, or during operations when extreme flexion of the head on the neck is required, as in

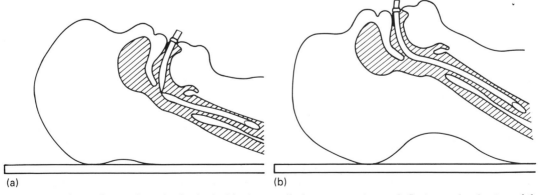

(a)

(b)

**Figure 9.53** (a) Kinking of an endotracheal tube inside the mouth due to excessive neck flexion and softening of the tube owing to its becoming warmer during anaesthesia, all having seemed to be well at induction. (b) Head in correct position.

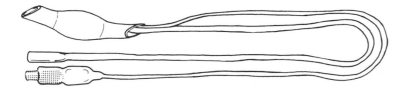

**Figure 9.54** A Carden tube.

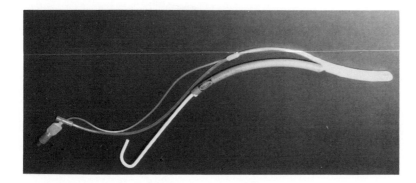

**Figure 9.55** A method of inserting the Carden tube.

some neurosurgical procedures.

Tubes for children, infants and neonates require special consideration. The thickness of the wall is important. Since it must be adequate to prevent kinking, it represents a considerable proportion of the cross-sectional area of a small tube. (It will be seen below that there may also be a similar problem in the case of connectors.) The resistance of such a narrow tube may be decreased by tapering it (see Fig. 9.50), the narrow end being just small enough to enter the larynx, but the larger end leading to a less resistive connector. It is true that a tapered tube has a slightly larger dead space, but the disadvantage of this is more than offset by the decrease in resistance.

### Endotracheal tubes for special purposes

Many 'special' tubes have been devised — they are too numerous to all be described here. A few examples are shown in Figs 9.54–9.57.

THE CARDEN TUBE. This was developed to facilitate microsurgery of the larynx. As will be seen in Fig. 9.54 the part occupying the larynx during surgery is very slender, and can be kept out of the way of the surgeon's manipulations. The tracheal portion has a cuff which, when inflated, prevents aspiration of blood or debris and may also make artificial ventilation feasible. The tube may be inserted either by grasping it with the Magill's endotracheal forceps, or as follows. A Carden tube and a plain nasal tube are threaded in series onto a stylet (Fig. 9.55). This assembly is then introduced through the

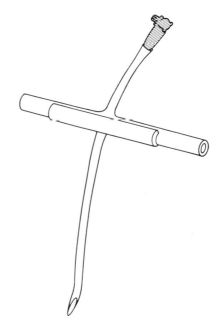

**Figure 9.56** The Jackson Rees paediatric T-tube. Note the provision for suction.

larynx so that the Carden tube and a centimetre or so of the nasal tube pass into the trachea. The stylet is then withdrawn, and until all is ready for the laryngoscopy, the anaesthetic is maintained through the plain tube. When the laryngoscopy is to be performed, the cuff on the Carden tube is inflated and the plain nasal tube is removed. The breathing system is then discarded and the anaesthetic

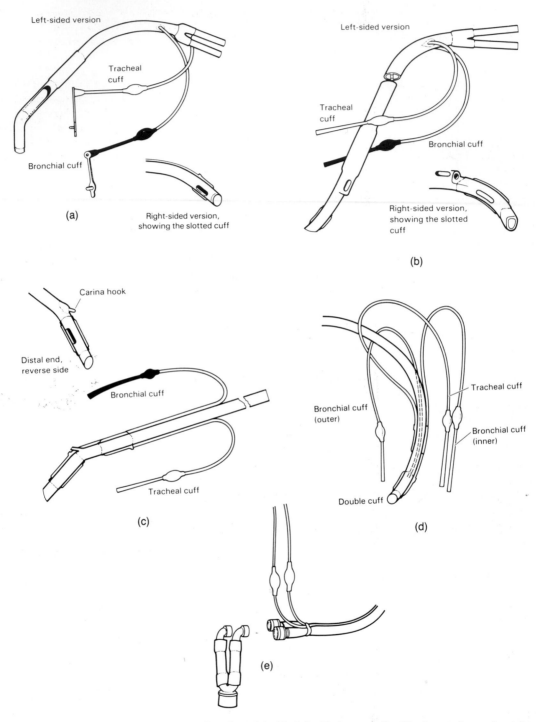

**Figure 9.57** Various endobronchial tubes. (a) Robertshaw left-sided double-lumen tube. The insert shows the right-sided version, which has a slotted cuff to connect with the right upper lobe bronchus. Note that in each case there are two cuffs, one for the trachea and the other for the bronchus. (b) Bryce-Smith double-lumen tube. Note the slot for the right upper lobe bronchus on the right-sided version, shown in the insert. (c) Gordon-Green tube. Note the slot for the right upper lobe bronchus and the hook which engages the carina. (d) Brompton left-sided triple-cuffed tube. If the outer bronchial cuff is damaged during surgery, the inner one may be inflated. (e) Catheter mount for a double-lumen tube. Note that either side may be blocked by a robust pair of artery forceps, if required.

gases are delivered directly to the Carden tube through a feed mount. The expired gases escape via the lumen of the Carden tube.

*THE JACKSON REES PAEDIATRIC TUBE* (Fig. 7.56). This is especially useful for cases of prolonged intubation and incorporates its own T-piece and suction facility.

*ENDOBRONCHIAL ANAESTHESIA.* There are several special tubes for endobronchial anaesthesia during lung surgery. Examples of these are shown in Fig. 9.57. These enable the anaesthetist to administer the anaesthetic via one lung, the other being 'blocked'. In some cases, suction tubes are also incorporated. Detailed description of these specialized tubes can be obtained from the manufacturers.

*TRACHEOSTOMY TUBES.* There are also many varieties of these; most have a 15-mm female taper which connects to a catheter mount. Various swivelling adaptors, some with facilities for suction, are available. Two examples of tubes are shown in Fig. 9.58.

*MICROLARYNGEAL TUBE* (Fig. 9.59). This is designed to be a narrow tube with a very small internal diameter (5–6 mm) but with a high-volume, low-pressure cuff. It is supplied uncut for insertion either nasally or orally. Its small external diameter takes up little space in the laryngeal inlet so that endoscopy and surgical procedures on the larynx may be performed relatively unhindered. The high-volume cuff provides a tracheal seal to enable controlled ventilation to be performed during anaesthesia. (The high resistance to gas flow in these tubes is probably too great for spontaneous respiration for anything but the shortest of periods.)

*LARYNGECTOMY TUBE* (Fig. 9.60). The pre-formed cur-

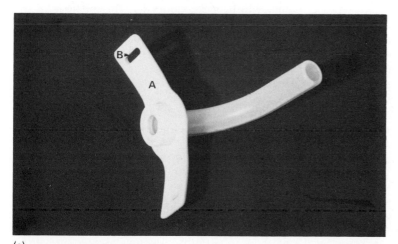

(a)

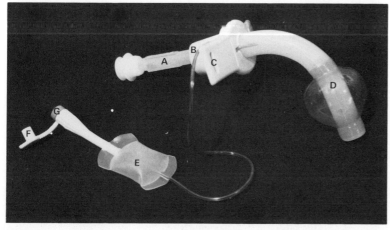

(b)

**Figure 9.58** (a) A plain tracheostomy tube (which is supplied by Portex in a variety of sizes). Note that there is a flange A with slots B, to which the securing tape may be tied. Another version has a 15-mm male taper for connection to a condenser/humidifier filter. (b) The Portex siliconized PVC cuffed tracheostomy tube with a replaceable internal cannula, A, which may be changed with minimal disturbance to the patient. The cuff inflating tube has a self-sealing inlet, but there is also a bung to ensure that the cuff does not accidentally deflate before it is required. This tracheostomy tube has a 15-mm male taper that fits the International 15 catheter mount, even when the internal catherer is in place, provided that it is correctly installed. B, 15-mm OD connector; C, flange with slot for tape; D, cuff; E, pilot balloon; F, bung; G, one-way valve.

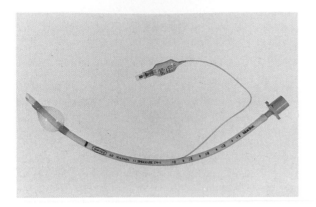

Figure 9.59 A tube for microlaryngeal surgery.

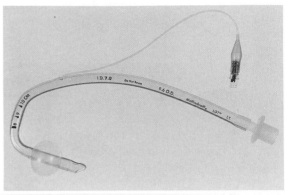

Figure 9.60 A laryngectomy tube.

vature of this tube makes it ideal for placement through tracheostomies. The relatively large, straight, portion conveniently allows direct connection to a breathing system away from the operation site without producing an excessive apparatus dead space.

TUBES FOR USE IN THE PRESENCE OF LASERS (Fig. 9.61). Conventional endotracheal tubes of either rubber, silicone rubber or plastic, may be damaged by the carbon dioxide laser. These materials burn more fiercely in the presence of oxygen (as well as nitrous oxide) than in air, at temperatures generated by a 'direct hit', with a laser beam. The resultant fire can produce serious upper airways burns. Figure 9.61 shows samples of tubes that can be used in the presence of a carbon dioxide laser beam. These include flexible metal tubes (Oswald/Norton tubes, Fig. 9.61a b,) which deflect laser beams. These tubes are made up of circular links of metal (similar to a shower hose) to make them flexible. However, they are not supplied with cuffs. They are intended to be reuseable. The Bivona 'Fome-Cuff' laser endotracheal tube (Fig. 9.61c) is constructed in a similar fashion. However the metal links are incorporated into the wall of the tube which is made of silicone rubber. The cuff is packed with a sponge which can be filled with either air or water, so that if the cuff were to burst, the sponge would prevent the cuff from deflation. The cuff can be forcibly deflated by extracting the air or water from within so that atraumatic insertion and removal of the tube from the larynx is possible. The tube however is intended for single use only.

An alternative approach used by many anaesthetists, is to wrap a suitably small tube (microlaryngeal tube) spirally with a narrow strip of good quality aluminium foil, ensuring that the ends are well secured and the edges are smoothed down. A commercial version of this is available (Fig. 9.61e). The Laser-Shield II is coated in such a fashion. The aluminium foil is then overwrapped with Teflon to provide an outer, smooth coat. The pilot balloon contains methylene blue crystals which dissolve in saline which is recommended for inflation of the endotracheal cuff. Should this cuff puncture, the leak of dye would then cause this hazard to be detected easily at operation.

## Airways

The maintenance of a clear airway under anaesthesia need not routinely require endotracheal intubation. In fact, for shorter procedures where controlled ventilation is not essential, or where regurgitation of gastric contents is extremely unlikely, endotracheal intubation may be unnecessary. Intubation may increase morbidity by the increased use of drugs, with the attendant risks of anaphylaxis, suxamethonium myalgia and apnoea, as well as the risk of pharyngeal and dental trauma and problems with the tube itself. The airway may just as easily be secured by the use of a Guedal artificial airway or a nasopharyngeal airway (Fig. 9.62). There have been many patterns of artificial airway, but these seem to be the most popular.

### The laryngeal mask airway (LMA/Brain airway)

The LMA (Fig. 9.63) may well be the most exciting innovation in anaesthesia since the endotracheal tube was introduced. It is usually inserted blindly into the pharynx of an anaesthetized patient without the use of muscle relaxants. When the mask seal is inflated, it reliably secures the airway in most patients. In fact, the seal is usually so effective that controlled ventilation may well be possible without an obvious perilaryngeal leak. Persistent minor leaks can be minimized by a soft pharyngeal pack

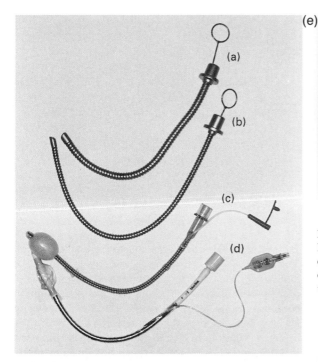

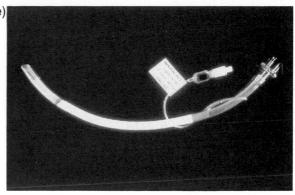

**Figure 9.61** (a) Oswald/Norton adult endotracheal tube. (b) Endobronchial version of (a). (c) Bivona 'fome cuff' laser endotracheal tube. (d) Foil-wrapped plastic microlaryngeal endotracheal tube. (e) Xomed Laser-Shield II endotracheal tube.

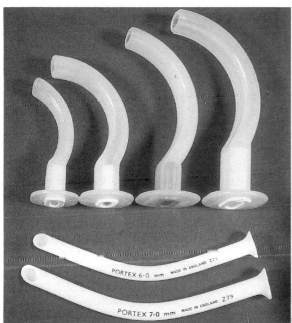

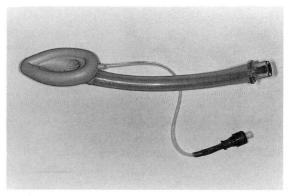

**Figure 9.63** The laryngeal mask airway.

The LMA has also been used to secure the airway first so that blind introduction of a soft gum-elastic bougie through the LMA into the larynx can be performed. The LMA is then removed so that an endotracheal tube can be 'railroaded' down over the bougie and through the larynx.

### Aids to difficult intubation

There are occasions when intubation by the nasal or oral route may be difficult, owing to anatomical abnormalities in the patient, or other factors.

In some of these situations intubation may be assisted by prior insertion of a stylet of gum-elastic, plastic or wire, into the tube so as to maintain it in a

**Figure 9.62** A selection of Guedel oropharyngeal (upper) and nasopharyngeal (lower) airways.

placed behind the 'mask'. Its use in different anaesthetic situations is being extended as familiarity with the device is gained. It is extremely useful in securing airways in patients who are difficult to intubate but who have adequate mouth opening.

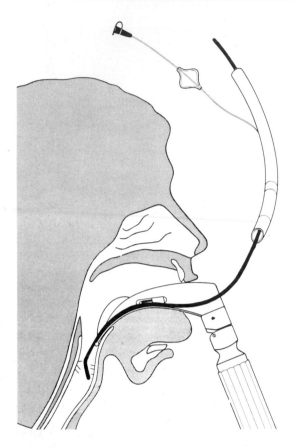

**Figure 9.64** The Eschmann endotracheal introducer.

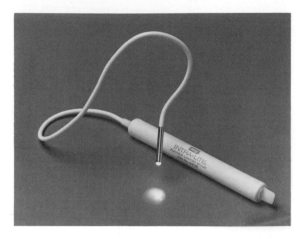

**Figure 9.65** A torch on which endotracheal tubes may be 'railroaded'.

particular shape. This is especially useful for tubes of silicone rubber, etc. which may be very floppy. When the tube has been inserted into the larynx, the stylet is withdrawn.

This procedure is not without dangers, especially with wire stylets, which may protrude from the end of the tube and injure, or even perforate, the trachea.

There are gum elastic stylets available of extra length, such as the so-called 'endotracheal introducer' manufactured by Eschmann (Fig. 9.64). This is of such a length that it may first be passed on its own and then, when the tip has passed through the larynx, there remains outside the mouth a sufficient length on which the tube may be threaded and railroaded through the larynx into the trachea. It is the safest and most useful stylet currently available.

In recent years a fibreoptic endoscope (see Chapter 21) has been used in place of a stylet, and in skilled hands this may be very useful. However this skill must be acquired by using the instrument on a regular basis before depending on it in times of difficulty.

A more recently used aid to intubation consists of

a disposable electric torch, which has a small bulb at the end of a long, narrow, flexible limb. The endotracheal tube is threaded upon this and then inserted. The light from the bulb may be seen through the skin of the neck and serve as a guide when passing it into the larynx (Fig. 9.65).

There is a variety of other stylets, hooks, etc. designed to facilitate intubation. In the authors' view, however, it is prudent to avoid dependence on these potentially dangerous devices, and if assistance is required it is safer to grasp the tube with Magill's endotracheal forceps.

## Endotracheal connectors

Endotracheal connectors join the endotracheal tube to the catheter mount. Various types are shown in Figs 9.66–9.75. Their particular features are:

- the two-part design of the connectors, which permits rapid disconnection and reconnection;
- the provision for suction;
- the incorporation of a special angle, as, for example, for nasal tubes.

When delivered from the suppliers, connectors frequently have a length of wire threaded through them, as seen in Fig. 9.67. This is to demonstrate that the lumen is patent and was introduced following an accident in which one was found to be blocked by a metal diaphragm as a result of faulty manufacture. Obstruction may also result from the improper fitting of a nasal connector, as may be seen in Fig. 9.52. Another cause of obstruction is the use of an unsuitable bung in a Magill suction connector (Fig. 9.76).

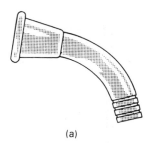

(a)

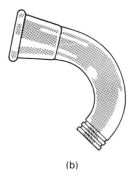

(b)

Figure 9.66 Magill connectors: (a) oral; (b) nasal.

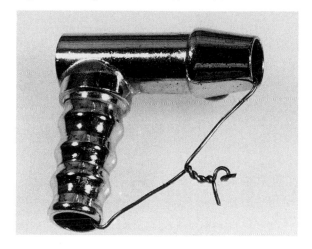

Figure 9.67 Rowbotham connector. Note that there is a piece of wire threaded through this connector when supplied, to demonstrate that the lumen is patent.

In selecting a connector, thought should be given to using one with an adequate internal diameter, which should be no less than that of the endotracheal tube. Any abrupt reduction of bore will result in resistance and this is rendered even greater by turbulence.

Turbulence may also be caused by an acute bend,

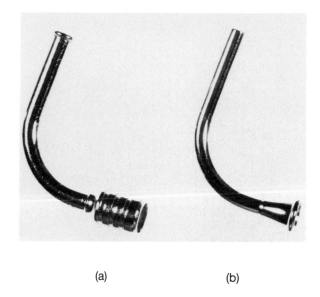

(a)                              (b)

Figure 9.68 (a) The Worcester and (b) the Doughty connector.

as in the Rowbotham connector (Fig. 9.67), but is considerably reduced in the Rink connector (Fig. 9.72). The disadvantage of the latter is either that it protrudes a long way from the patient's mouth and the pressure of towels, etc. covering it may cause kinking of the tube, or that the point of attachment of the tube is well within the mouth, and accidental disconnection here would be unobserved. It is also difficult to fix the tube and connector securely with adhesive plaster. These dangers are minimized with the Rowbotham connector and it is difficult to recall any harm resulting from turbulence due to the acute bend.

In paediatric anaesthesia, connectors of small size are used. When choosing these, one should be careful to avoid those with very thick walls, since their lumen is likely to be smaller that the tubes into which they can be inserted (Fig. 9.77).

If the need for bronchial suction is envisaged, the most convenient type of connector is either one such as the Cobb or Magill suction connector, or a two-piece connector such as the Nosworthy or the Knight's paediatric connector, which may easily be disconnected and reconnected (Figs 9.69 and 9.70).

Metal endotracheal connectors may be autoclaved or cold sterilized. When fitting them to a tube they will be found to slip in very much more easily if they are lubricated by dipping them in ethanol (surgical spirit).

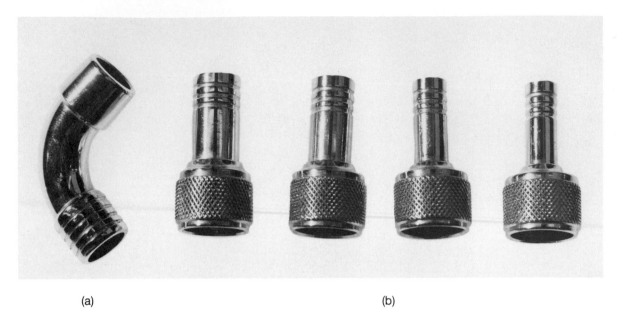

(a)                                        (b)

**Figure 9.69** Nosworthy adult connectors (14 mm taper). (a) To attach to the catheter mount. (b) To be inserted in the endotracheal tube.

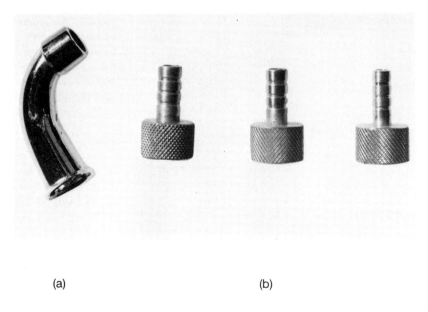

(a)                                        (b)

**Figure 9.70** Knight's paediatric connectors (9.7-mm taper) (a) To attach to the catheter mount. (b) To be inserted in the endotracheal tube.

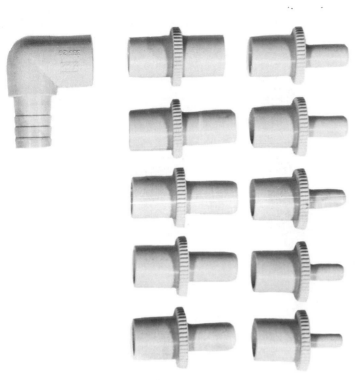

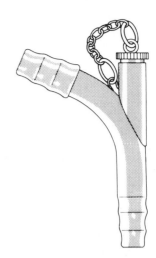

Figure 9.72 Rink connector.

Figure 9.71 'International 15' connectors.

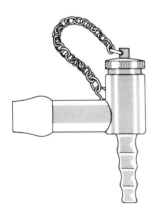

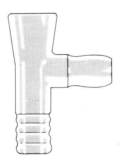

Figure 9.74 The Magill suction connector. Note that a cork is required to occlude the suction limb.

Figure 9.73 The Cobb suction connector.

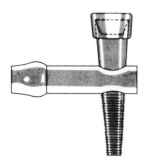

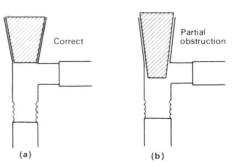

Figure 9.76 The lumen of a Magill suction connector may be obstructed by the use of an inappropriate bung. (a) Correct. (b) Too long a cork has been used.

Figure 9.75 The Cardiff paediatric suction connector.

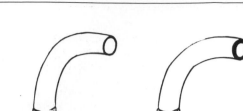

**Figure 9.77** Two Magill oral connectors of the same size but supplied by different manufacturers. Note that owing to the thickness of the wall in one of them the lumen is considerably smaller that that of the other.

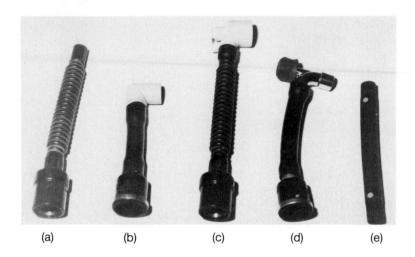
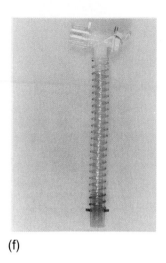

(a)  (b)  (c)  (d)  (e)  (f)

**Figure 9.78** Catheter mounts (endotracheal adaptors). (a) For use with Magill, Rowbotham or similar connectors. (b) For use with International 15 connectors. (c) For use with International 15 connectors, with a facility for suction. (d) For use with Nosworthy connectors. This fitting has a side branch for suction, which is closed by a rubber bung. (e and f) With spiral reinforcement to prevent kinking. Note that this mount should not be shortened by cutting, since the part that is reinforced cannot be distended to accommodate the nozzle of a 22-mm tapered fitting catheter mount or an endotracheal connector. NB. The corrugated tubes also resist kinking when flexed.

## The catheter mount (Fig. 9.78)

The term 'catheter mount' does not appear in BS 6015 (ISO 4135), which is the official glossary of terms used in anaesthesiology. Its modern equivalent 'tracheal tube adaptor' will probably be slow to replace the older and more familiar term, as will the term 'tracheal tube' rather than the older 'endotracheal tube'. Some explanation of these terms would perhaps be apt.

Before the introduction of the Boyle's machine with the Magill breathing attachment, the mixed gases, with added vapour of volatile agents, were fed via a narrow-bore tube to the patient, with no reservoir bag or expiratory valve in the positions in which we now know them. The end of the tube could be attached to a Boyle–Davis gag, a modified open-drop mask such as the Tyrrell, a bag on a Hewitt's stopcock, or to a catheter that was passed

through the larynx into the trachea. In the latter case, the gases and/or vapours were blown constantly down the catheter and were exhausted to the atmosphere by passing out through the trachea but outside the catheter. Spontaneous ventilation became very shallow, respiratory exchange being mainly by diffusion. A thoracotomy was possible under these conditions. This technique was known as intratracheal insufflation. Thus, when the catheter was replaced by a wider bore tube through which the patient could breathe (or be ventilated) in both directions, this was called endotracheal intubation.

Modern techniques with high-frequency jetting seem to hark back to the older technique and the authors would therefore have preferred to retain the older terms, 'catheter mount' and 'endotracheal'.

The catheter mount acts not only as an adaptor between the breathing attachment and the tracheal tube (or tracheostomy tube), but also to minimize the transmission of accidental movements of the

(a)

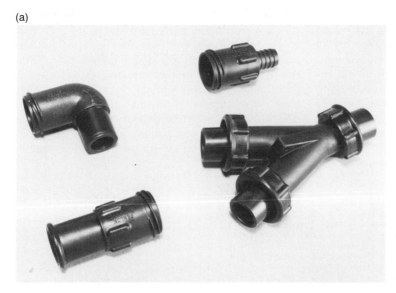

**Figure 9.79** (a) Penlon 'Safelock' tapered connections showing the nut on the male component and the screw thread on the female connection. (b) Dräger 'Isoclic' safety connection. (i) End on view showing the distortion required on the female component to retract the claws to enable separation of the connection. (ii) Side view showing the components being engaged.

(b)

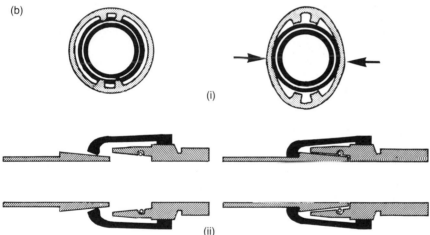

breathing attachment to the endotracheal tube. Repeated movements of the tube within the trachea are undesirable since they can cause injury to the tracheal mucosa. Various types of catheter mount are shown in Fig. 9.78.

## Anti-disconnect devices

Perhaps one of the saddest, and most common of accidents associated with anaesthetic equipment is the unobserved disconnection of some part of the breathing system. Although antidisconnect devices have been available for several years, they are seldom used. Two such systems are described below.

### The Penlon 'Safelock'

In this system (Fig. 9.79a), which is made of plastic,

the male taper has a threaded 'cap' which can be screwed onto a matching male thread on the female taper, thus securing the union. The cap is kept on the fitting by an 'O' ring, but the latter does not contribute to the gas-tight seal. The advantage of this kind of system is that items fitted with it can still be joined in the conventional manner with other standard tapers, although the 'safelock' will be ineffectual. The disadvantages are that it is rather bulky, and that its efficacy depends on the anaesthetist taking the trouble to secure the connection. This may be neglected by the same person who fails to give an ordinary tapered connection that important twist as he engages it.

### The Dräger 'Isoclic'

This system (Fig. 9.79b) consists of a female taper which is shrouded by a cone that ends in four claws. These engage in the 'groove' ('notch' or 'undercut'), on the latest version of the male taper of the ISO connector. A simple push-fit is all that is needed to ensure a secure engagement. Release is achieved by gentle squeezing of the appropriate two sides of the shroud, thus disengaging the claws. The taper is the ISO 22-mm. The gas-tight nature of this joint is completed by an 'O' ring set within the female taper. The correct seating of this system is therefore assured, *provided that the male taper onto which it engages has the appropriate groove* (see Fig. 9.33). In the absence of the latter, which is the case with many parts currently in use, not only is the lock impossible, but the union is far less secure than that with two simple metal tapers. Thus, this system would promote safety only in a department where all appropriate items of equipment have male tapers with the groove. Otherwise disconnections might become even more common.

Certainly, all hard rubber tapered connectors, which are renowned for jumping apart, should be discarded.

# 10 'Intermittent Flow' and 'On Demand' Apparatus

## Introduction

The Boyle's machine, the components of which have been described in previous chapters, is known as a *continuous* flow machine. This means that when the fine-adjustment valves have been set, the various gases flow at a regular, continuous rate to the breathing attachment. The inspiratory effort to the patient, as he inhales, may vary the amount of

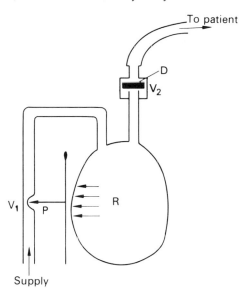

**Figure 10.1** Basic principles of demand flow apparatus. The supply gases pass through the valve $V_1$ and enter the reservoir bag R. The outlet of R is closed by the gravity valve $V_2$. As R distends it pushes the plate P sideways and by this lever action closes $V_1$. No more gases enter R and it remains in the filled (ready) position. The weight of the disc D in $V_2$ is just sufficient to prevent gases flowing to the patient until he makes an inspiratory effort, which produces a subatmospheric pressure above D just sufficient to raise it and the gases flow to the patient on demand.

mixed gases drawn from the reservoir bag, but the fresh gas flow rate remains constant until readjusted by the anaesthetist.

In a *demand* flow apparatus the gases flow only in response to the patient's respiratory effort. Figure 10.1 shows the basic principles upon which such a system operates. In order to fill the reservoir bag R, the gases pass through the valve $V_1$. As R becomes progressively distended, the plate P is deflected; this operates $V_1$, which is eventually closed, whereupon the supply of gases ceases. Under static conditions the weight of the disc D in the valve $V_2$ (assisted by a spring, the tension of which is set in the factory) is just sufficient to prevent gases escaping from R. However, when the patient inhales, $V_2$ is drawn open and the gases flow from R to the patient. When this happens R partially empties, P returns towards its former position and $V_1$ reopens to admit more gases, refilling R.

If we add to the demand flow apparatus a means of applying variable counter-pressure to P, e.g. a screw T and spring S (Fig. 10.2), a greater pressure has to be built up in R in order to close $V_1$. This pressure is too great to be contained by the weight of D, which is therefore lifted and gases flow from R even when they are not demanded by the patient. When the patient inhales there is an even greater flow of gases. The 'intermittent' flow machine has now been converted into one which gives an uninterrupted but *varying* flow of gases. The flow rate is not indicated, and the only calibration that is possible is that of the pressure against which the gases are able to flow, this being dependent on the force with which S acts on P. Even when this 'pressure setting' is constant, the flow rate varies with the demand from the patient. This principle is used in the McKesson anaesthetic machine.

Some readers will question the need to retain descriptions of intermittent flow machines in this edition. They will be surprised to know that they

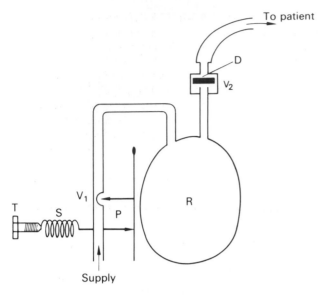

**Figure 10.2** A similar arrangement to that shown in Fig. 10.1 except that a spring S and screw T are added. The pressure exerted on the plate P by S prevents the reservoir bag R from pushing P sufficiently to close valve $V_1$. The pressure in R therefore rises enough to overcome the weight of the disc D and gases flow without demand.

are still used widely in dental chair anaesthesia, for which they are particularly suited. At the time of going to press, McKesson UK service over 770 of them on a regular basis, and about the same number are repaired or serviced as the need arises. The AE and Walton Five are also still both in common use. They tend to be omitted from the standard textbooks of anaesthesia and are afforded scant mention in training courses.

# The McKesson Simplor Machine

As shown in Fig. 10.3, nitrous oxide and oxygen are delivered to their respective reservoirs at a pressure of 60 psi (420 kPa) either from the pipeline or from cylinders via 60 psi regulators. For each gas there is a gauge for regulated pressure. On some models this is not calibrated in units of pressure, but shows a segment of the scale marked 'operating range' to indicate that the pressure is sufficiently close to 60 psi to assure accuracy of the mixing mechanism. Each gas passes to the appropriate reservoir via a cut-off valve V. This valve is closed by the pivoted lever L, when the latter is pushed by the fully distended reservoir. This cuts off the gas flow. When gas is drawn from the reservoir, L returns

towards its former position allowing V to reopen.

The outlets of the two reservoirs lead through variable ports to the mixing chamber M. The gravity valve is just heavy enough to prevent the flow of gases during stand-by conditions ('0' on the dial). When the patient inhales, the gravity valve is lifted and the mixed gases pass to the breathing system.

The mixing chamber consists of a drum that rotates within a cylinder, both being drilled with corresponding ports. By rotating the drum, the relative degree of opening of the ports may be varied, so determining the proportions of the two gases delivered to the outlet. The dial on the mixing chamber is calibrated in percentage of oxygen in the mixture, and there is a fine-adjustment knob calibrated from 0 to 50, which makes two complete revolutions between the positions for pure oxygen and pure nitrous oxide. So, for example, if the latter reads 15, the mixture may contain either 15 or 65% oxygen and reference to the main mixing valve dial will determine which is the case.

Under the conditions so far described, the McKesson delivers gases only when demanded, and it is therefore called a *demand flow* or *intermittent flow* machine. However, it can be made to deliver a continuous flow as follows. The pressure dial, when rotated, actuates a balanced mechanism that presses equally on the oxygen and nitrous oxide levers, pushing them against the reservoirs. This prevents the valves from closing until a higher pressure is reached in the reservoirs. This increase in pressure is sufficient to open the gravity valve, producing a flow of mixed gases even when not demanded by the patient. The pressure control, which is calibrated in mmHg, indicates the pressure at which the gases flow (or more precisely, the back pressure required to stop gas flow). With the dial set at '0', flow is on demand only, and when at 'OFF', there is no flow under any circumstances.

There is an oxygen flush control which delivers oxygen directly to the mixing chamber above the gravity valve, so that the latter is closed and the flow of nitrous oxide is stopped when it is operated.

Originally the McKesson was fitted with a rebreathing bellows, the volume and compliance of which could be varied (Fig. 10.3c). Later this was replaced by a simple bag with an on-off tap but in present-day models this too has been omitted for reasons that will be explained below, and the connection to it blanked off by a plate and gasket. In the UK, at least, there are many of these old Nargraf heads still in existence, though kept with the bellows closed and out of use. Since the latter are made of rubber and prone to perish, the risk of a leak occurring at this point should be prevented by the removal of the Nargraf head, which should be replaced by the blanking plate referred to above.

A vaporizer may be fitted to the outlet of the McKesson. This may be one that is appropriate for halothane, but the older model had, as a fixture, a vaporizer that was intended for diethyl ether, and if this were used for halothane, it would give a lethally high concentration.

## The practical use of the McKesson breathing systems

With *demand flow*, as seen in Fig. 10.4a there is no rebreathing bag (if one is fitted it is turned off or the bellows are closed). A vaporizer may be included but there is no reservoir bag. There is an expiratory valve at the patient end of the corrugated hose.

The disadvantage of this system is that it depends on a slight subatmospheric pressure in the breathing attachment to produce a supply of gases. If the facepiece is not a perfect fit, air is drawn in and dilutes the gases. Thus it is quite inappropriate for dental anaesthesia, which is the sole scene where the McKesson is now used.

With *varying flow and intentional rebreathing*, as seen in Fig. 10.4b and c, the pressure control is turned sufficiently to produce a low fresh gas flow

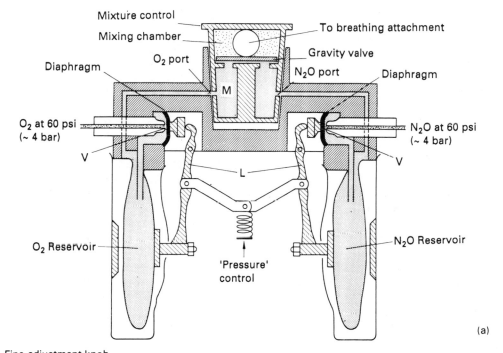

(a)

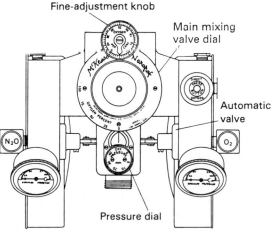

(b)

**Figure 10.3** McKesson intermittent flow gas and oxygen apparatus. This consists of two demand flow arrangements, one for oxygen and the other for nitrous oxide. The gases are mixed in the mixing chamber and passed through the gravity-operated check valve to the patient. (a) A diagrammatic representation showing the principle of operation (see text). (b) The top view, showing the dials, pressure gauges and oxygen bypass.

*(Continued overleaf.)*

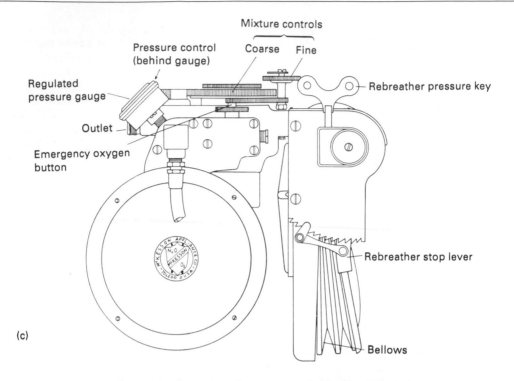

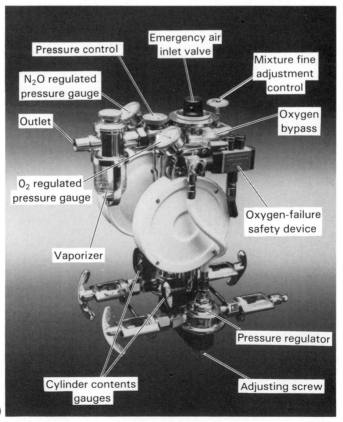

**Figure 10.3** (*Continued*). (c) The side view, including the Nargraf rebreathing bellows. (d) A recent model incorporating an oxygen-failure safety device, an emergency air inlet valve and facility for minimum oxygen concentrations.

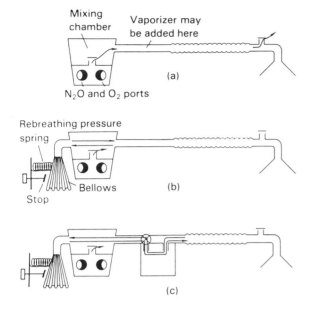

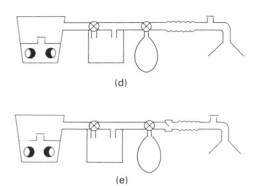

**Figure 10.4** Breathing systems used with the McKesson intermittent flow machine (see text). (a) Demand flow. (b) No vaporizer — continuous flow with intentional rebreathing (not now acceptable). (c) With vaporizer. (d) With continuous flow and no *intended* rebreathing. (e) Rebreathing prevented by the interposition of a check valve.

rate — less than the patient's minute volume. As rebreathing into the bellows occurs, the gases pass backwards and forwards through the vaporizer. This might have been deemed satisfactory when ether was employed, but now that halothane is used it is inadvisable, since a dangerously high vapour concentration would result, owing to the gases passing repeatedly through the vaporizer. Also there would be an undesirable accumulation of carbon dioxide.

With *continuous flow and no rebreathing*, as seen in Fig. 10.4d, a vaporizer and a Magill's attachment (Mapleson A) have been added. The McKesson is now being used in much the same way as the Boyle's machine — except that there is no precise indication of the mixed gas flow rate, the percentages only of the gases being known. If the flow rate

is too low, rebreathing occurs.

It is not easy to determine in practice the exact setting of the pressure control to guarantee an adequate flow rate, and very often an excessive rate is used not only to prevent rebreathing but also to make sure that the patient does not inhale air. However, it is possible to prevent rebreathing by interposing a check valve between the reservoir bag and the corrugated hose (Fig. 10.4e).

It is most important that, if there is no check valve, the reservoir bag should be fitted on the downstream side of the vaporizer to prevent the gases being exposed more than once to the halothane, which would then produce too high a concentration (Fig. 10.5).

From time to time the regulated pressure should be checked and, if necessary, corrected so that the

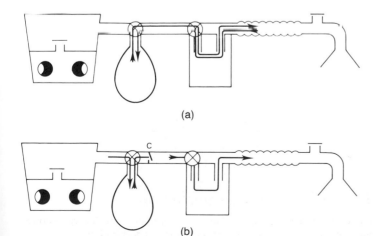

**Figure 10.5** (a) The effect of mounting a vaporizer between the reservoir bag and the patient on a varying flow machine. If there is a low fresh gas flow rate, gases pass more than once through the vaporizer, generating an excessive vapour concentration. (b) A check valve C prevents rebreathing and the gases pass only once through the vaporizer.

gauges read 60 psi or indicate the middle of the segment marked 'operating range'.

In the author's experience the McKesson Simplor is the most reliable of all anaesthetic machines. Some of those used are over 40 years old and still working satisfactorily, in spite of the fact that the dentists who own them have had them serviced and recalibrated far less often than should have been the case. The accuracy of the percentage of oxygen tends to vary with flow rate, but it is rare for it to be less than that indicated (see Further Reading, Naimby-Luxmore).

## The Walton Five Machine

The Walton Five machine (Fig. 10.6) works on a different principle from that of the McKesson. There are two low-pressure regulators to which gas is supplied at about 11 psi (80 kPa). The chambers above the diaphragm of each of these are interconnected by a pressure loading tube, thereby making the oxygen regulator a slave of the nitrous oxide regulator. The latter contains a sensing diaphragm which, when deflected by the inspiratory effort of the patient, causes the valve to open and nitrous oxide to flow to the mixing chamber and the outlet. This nitrous oxide is mixed with oxygen which flows from its regulator at the same time. There is a pressure control knob analogous to that of the McKesson machine. This causes deflection of the diaphragm of the nitrous oxide regulator and a rise of pressure therein. This change is transmitted by the loading tube to the oxygen regulator. The nitrous oxide and oxygen flow to the mixing drum, the percentages being determined by the relative degree of opening of ports $X_1$ and $X_2$, which are varied by means of the mixture control lever.

The machine also includes high-pressure regulators for nitrous oxide and oxygen, an emergency oxygen control valve, a pressure relief valve and a cut-out unit which will prevent the flow of nitrous oxide should there be a failure of the oxygen supply. There is also an air inspiratory valve, complete with a whistle, which will act if the supply fails and the patient makes a respiratory effort. Note that this might not operate if the breathing attachment includes a reservoir bag.

As with the McKesson and the AE (see below), if large wall-mounted cylinders or a piped gas supply are used, the high-pressure regulators are mounted on the cylinders so that the tubing carries the gases at the regulated pressure.

The Walton Five is accurate, economical and very convenient to operate. Many anaesthetists regret that it has been declared obsolete by the manufacturer.

Although in Fig. 10.6 it is depicted with neither reservoir bag nor vaporizer, it is most commonly used in the manner described above for the McKesson intermittent flow machine, and a non-return valve downstream from the reservoir bag is recommended.

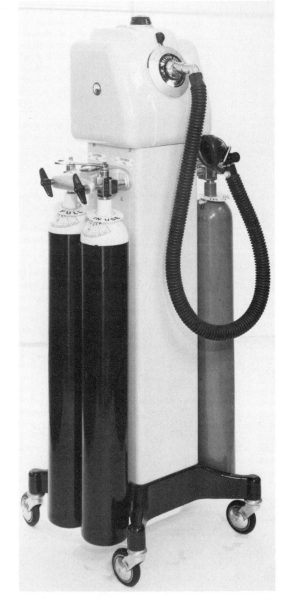

**Figure 10.6** (a) The Walton Five machine.

(b)

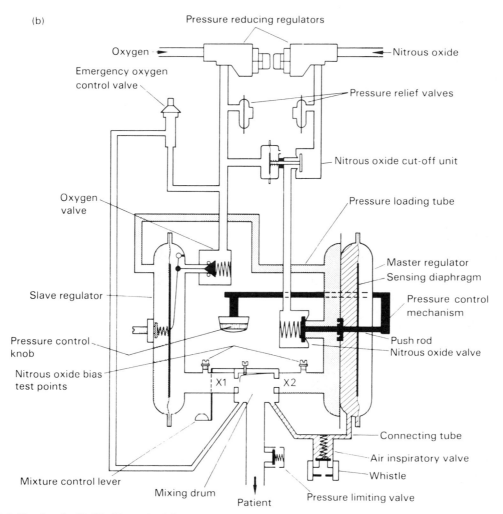

Figure 10.6 (*Continued*). (b) Working principles.

# The AE Gas–Oxygen Machine

The working principles of this machine (Fig. 10.7) depend on three stages of pressure regulation. In the first stage there are two high-pressure regulators $R_1$, one each for nitrous oxide and oxygen. The cylinders or pipelines are attached at HP, and there is a pressure gauge P for each gas. The output pressure from these regulators is 60 psi, and from them the nitrous oxide and oxygen pass to their appropriate second-stage regulators $R_2$. These two regulators have a spring S, which is common to both and ensures that their output pressures are maintained equal — at about 70 cmH$_2$O (52 mmHg). The gases then pass to the mixing chamber MC, where they are mixed in any proportion required,

depending on the position of the mixture control lever and the consequent degree of opening and closing of the ports in the mixing chamber. They then pass to the third stage, which is a simple regulator $R_3$, the output pressure of which can be varied by a spring which is controlled by the pressure control knob PC. The gases then pass via a unidirectional valve UDV to the outlet and the breathing attachment. The unidirectional valve has a glass dome so that the anaesthetist can see the disc move as an indication of the fact that the patient is breathing, if he is unable to hear the 'hiss' of the expiratory valve.

Also incorporated in the AE machine is a device that cuts off the nitrous oxide supply if the oxygen fails, an oxygen flush, and gauges showing the pressure at the output of the first stage (60 psi).

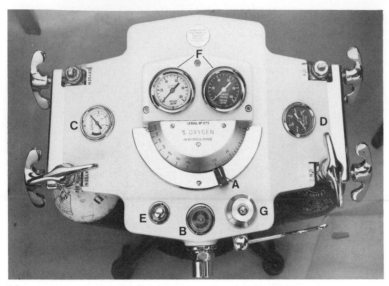

(a)

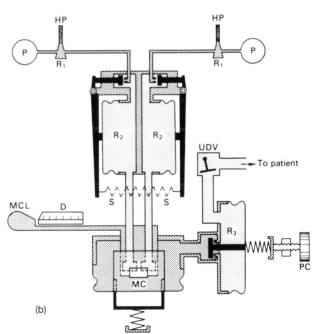

(b)

**Figure 10.7** (a) The AE intermittent flow anaesthetic machine. A, mixture control lever; B, unidirectional valve; C, oxygen cylinder contents gauge; D, nitrous oxide cylinder contents gauge; E, oxygen flush button; F, first-stage regulated pressure gauges; G, pressure control knob. (b) Working principles. $R_1$, $R_2$ and $R_3$, first-, second- and third-stage regulators; P, first-stage regulated pressure gauges; S, balancing spring; MC, mixing chamber; MCL, mixing control lever; D, mixture indicating dial; PC, pressure control knob; UDV, unidirectional valve.

None of these machines incorporates devices to assure the delivery of a set minimum percentage of oxygen. In each case, a simple adaptation could be made to achieve this. It is the opinion of one of us (C.S.W.) that the ideal might be an arrangement resembling the 'dead man's handle', where the percentage of oxygen could be reduced below the intended minimum only as long as the anaesthetist was actually holding the control knob.

See also the McKesson 882 RA/GA machine (Chapter 11).

## 'Demand' Valves

Demand valves may be used by the patient for self-administration. Suitable instruction and only general supervision, which may be by a nurse or ambulance man, is required. Two valves for the delivery of Entonox — a 50/50 mixture of nitrous oxide and oxygen, supplied in cylinders by BOC — will be described.

**Figure 10.8** (a) The Entonox valve. (b) Working principles (see text).

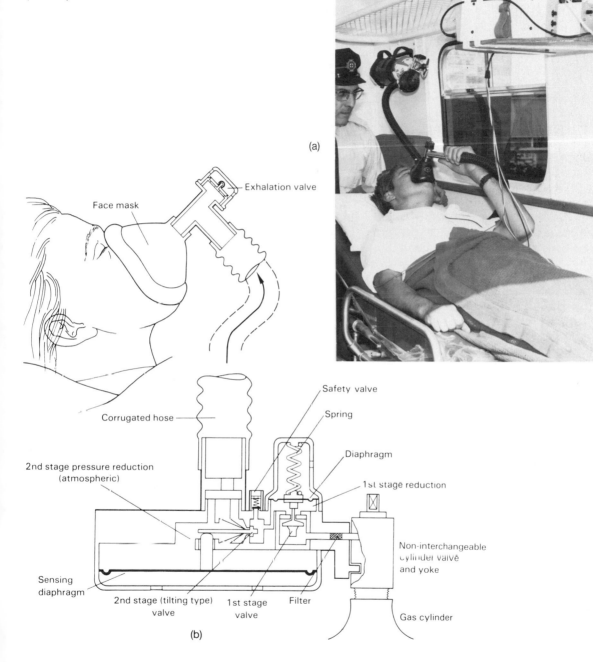

(a)

(b)

## The BOC Entonox valve

The Entonox apparatus is used to administer 'pre-mixed' nitrous oxide and oxygen (50% of each) to produce analgesia.

The valve (shown in Fig. 10.8) clamps directly onto a pin-index cylinder. It contains a first-stage regulator and a second-stage demand valve. A sensitive diaphragm, which is deflected by the patient's inspiratory effort, operates a push rod which tilts the valve lever, opening the valve and letting the gases flow. Very little inspiratory effort is required to achieve a high gas flow rate, making this a most efficient demand valve.

Since the nitrous oxide is in the gaseous state in the cylinder of premixed gases, the pressure gauge gives a direct indication of the cylinder contents. When small cylinders are used they may be placed in any position, but large ones should be maintained upright.

As mentioned on page 44, Entonox cylinders should not be allowed to cool below 0°C, since if it gets very much colder the nitrous oxide and oxygen may separate out, with serious consequences.

### The Pneupac analgesia valve

Although the valve shown in Fig. 10.9 also uses Entonox and may be used on demand by the patient, it embraces some additional features to those mentioned above.

A pressure regulator is attached to the cylinder yoke and clamps directly onto the cylinder. A narrow-bore delivery tube connects this to the demand valve which is mounted directly onto the facepiece. Two versions of the demand valve are available, one having a push-button manual override by which the attendant can inflate the lungs of a patient in respiratory failure.

The delivery tube between the regulator and demand valve may be several metres long and this may facilitate its use in the roadside treatment of accident cases and also allows the cylinder to be

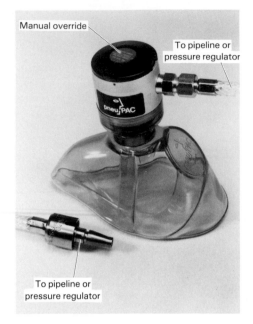

Figure 10.9 The Pneupac analgesia valve.

kept inside the ambulance so that during cold weather it will not become too cold. The joints at either end of the tube are secure, and this makes disconnection less likely.

# 11 Equipment for Dental Chair Anaesthesia

## Introduction

For the purposes of this chapter, dental anaesthesia is defined as general anaesthesia for the removal or conservation of teeth, in the dental operatory (surgery) and exclusively for outpatients. Whereas it is possible to intubate inpatients undergoing oral surgery in hospital, to pack the pharynx completely and afterwards to let the patient remain in a recovery ward for a prolonged period, this is often impracticable in dental anaesthesia.

In the dental operatory rather different circumstances appertain, namely:

- the patient is required to be fit to leave for home within a short period of time;
- the induction of anaesthesia is often by inhalation;
- during the operation the anaesthetist must allow the dentist access to the open mouth, thereby sharing the air passages with him, usually without the advantage of endotracheal intubation.

These seemingly impossible requirements are met by the use of a nasal inhaler. For inhalational induction the patient is instructed to keep his mouth closed so that he breathes through the nose. When anaesthesia is established the mouth is opened and a pack is inserted to prevent mouth-breathing and the inhalation of blood or dental debris during the operation.

The patient may be sitting upright, semirecumbent or lying prone, each position having its advocates. It is not always possible to obtain a good fit between the inhaler and the face at the start of induction, so a high flow rate of gases must be available to prevent the inhalation of air rather than the anaesthetic mixture. It is desirable to be able to make changes to flow rate and to the percentage of

nitrous oxide and oxygen independently of each other, on a 'breath to breath basis' and with minimal manual manipulation.

Therefore a so-called intermittent flow machine with an $N_2O/O_2$ percentage control is preferable to a continuous flow machine. It is, however, usually used with the pressure control turned somewhat 'up' so that there is always some flow of mixed gases. This resembles 'continuous flow', but since the rate is dependent on the patient's demand, which is continually altering, it may conveniently be called 'varying flow'.

## Continuous Flow Machines for Dental Anaesthesia

An ordinary Boyle's machine can be used, but it may present difficulties. The maximum flow rate of nitrous oxide may be lower than is convenient and the manipulation of the flow control valves may require more movements of the hand than are desirable.

The Quantiflex RA dental machine (Fig. 11.1) does have flowmeters — but they are capable of a greater flow rate than those on the average Boyle's machine (see page 101). Note that the Quantiflex RA always gives at least a minimum flow rate of oxygen, usually pre-set at 3 litres/min.

The McKesson 883 RA and 882 RA/GA machines (Fig. 11.2) both have flow control valves for oxygen and nitrous oxide and an on/off switch. The regulated pressure is 60 psi ($\sim$ 420 kPa) and they both have not only an emergency oxygen flush button but also an arrangement whereby a fall in the oxygen regulated pressure is automatically accompanied by a fall in nitrous oxide pressure so that the percentages of the gases remain the same. If the oxygen pressure falls below 10 psi ($\sim$ 70 kPa),

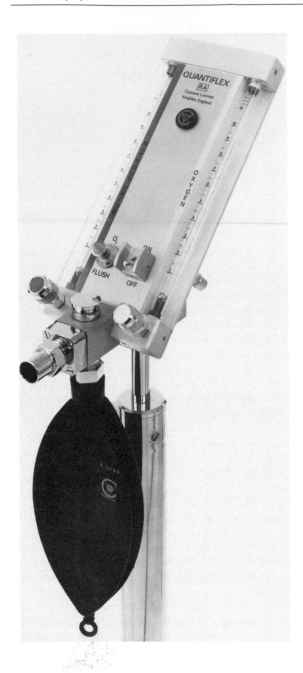

**Figure 11.1** The Quantiflex RA machine. Note that in this range of machines there are many models in which the control and flowmeter for oxygen is on the right-hand side. This is contrary to the custom in the UK and many other countries where it is traditionally on the left-hand side.

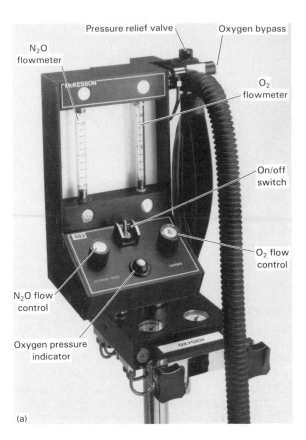

(a)

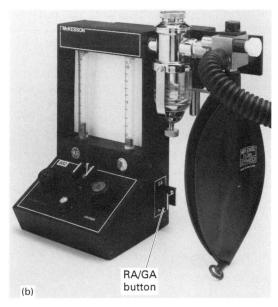

(b)

**Figure 11.2** (a) The McKesson 883 RA machine. (b) The 882 RA/GA machine.

the nitrous oxide is cut off altogether. In the 883 RA there is a minimum flow rate of oxygen of 3 litres/min. The 882 RA/GA machine has a special refinement. When it is initially turned on, it is in the 'RA mode' and will give a minimum oxygen flow of 3 litres/min. When the GA button mounted on the side of the control block is depressed, setting it in the 'GA mode', the oxygen flow can be reduced to zero. Whenever the switch is turned off and on again, the machine is automatically returned to the RA mode. It is understood that the GA button will be omitted in some future models. The 882 also carries a halothane vaporizer. Both machines have a valve that admits air if the oxygen and nitrous oxide supply fails, and the reservoir bag is mounted on the machine itself with a one-way valve in the mount for the corrugated tube.

# Intermittent (Varying) Flow Machines

Intermittent flow machines were described in Chapter 10. They may be used for demand flow, or a modified Magill attachment (Mapleson A) may be employed with the 'pressure' control turned up. The modified Magill attachment differs from the traditional one in that a non-return (check) valve downstream from the reservoir bag prevents rebreathing. This modification is made because there is no indication of flow *rate*, and therefore there would be no indication of an inadequate fresh gas flow rate, resulting in rebreathing. Where true demand flow is required, the reservoir bag may be omitted, but theoretically this is not necessary if there is a non-return valve.

# Vaporizers for Dental Anaesthesia

The halothane vaporizer is often detachable. It must be mounted upstream of the reservoir bag — otherwise gases might flow repeatedly backwards and forwards through the vaporizer as the patient breathes and would contain a higher concentration of halothane than intended. The check valve mentioned above would also prevent this (see Fig. 10.5).

## Choice of vaporizers for dental anaesthesia

Although other volatile agents are used, halothane is at present the most popular, and will be considered here. When selecting a vaporizer, distinction should be made between static apparatus, as kept in a hospital or group dental practice, where bulky or heavy apparatus may be used, and the type of vaporizer that may be conveniently carried by the itinerant dental anaesthetist in his case.

With a continuous flow machine, such as the Boyle's, the usual temperature- and level-compensated vaporizer, such as the Fluotec, may be used, but with the so-called 'intermittent flow' machines, such as the McKesson, Walton Five or AE, vaporizers of low resistance are required, since they are within the low-pressure breathing system and would better be described as VIBS (vaporizer in breathing system). The patient draws gases through them on demand. Vaporizers containing wicks may be used, since the moist exhaled gases do not pass through them. A most satisfactory type is the AE halothane vaporizer by Ohmeda (Fig. 11.3). This is suitable more for static apparatus, since it is rather bulky and older models need to be drained before transportation. It is a calibrated, compensated vaporizer of satisfactory accuracy.

The three small portable vaporizers that can best be recommended, in spite of their limitations, are the Goldman, McKesson and Rowbotham which are mentioned in Chapter 6 (see Figs 6.25, 6.26, 6.27 and Tables 6.3, 6.4 and 6.5). The limitations of, and care needed in the use of these vaporizers, described below, should be noted.

Most of the suitable portable vaporizers are neither calibrated nor compensated for temperature or level, but tables giving typical performance characteristics are available. Provided that the vaporizers are used correctly, they do not give a dangerously high concentration of halothane.

It must be emphasized that only a vaporizer designed for halothane should be used for this agent, since those designed for other volatile anaesthetics might give a dangerously high concentration of halothane.

Agitation or tilting of such vaporizers increases the vapour concentration. If the vaporizer is accidentally overturned and then used soon afterwards, liquid halothane in the bypass or tubing could give rise to a lethally high concentration of vapour.

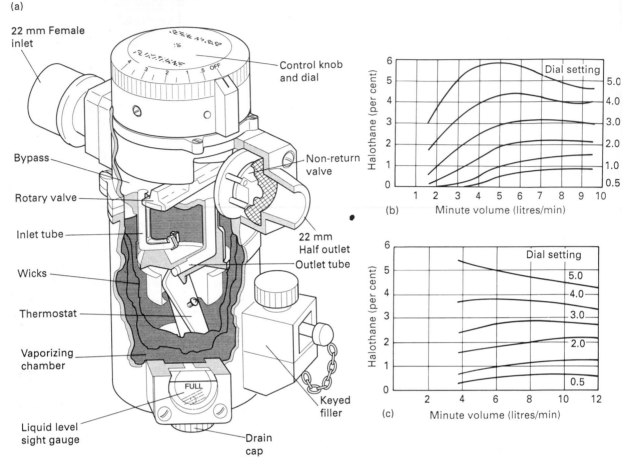

(a)

22 mm Female inlet

Control knob and dial

Bypass

Non-return valve

Rotary valve

Inlet tube

22 mm Half outlet

Outlet tube

Wicks

Thermostat

Vaporizing chamber

FULL

Liquid level sight gauge

Keyed filler

Drain cap

(b) Minute volume (litres/min) — Halothane (per cent) — Dial setting 5.0, 4.0, 3.0, 2.0, 1.0, 0.5

(c) Minute volume (litres/min) — Halothane (per cent) — Dial setting 5.0, 4.0, 3.0, 2.0, 0.5

**Figure 11.3** (a) The Ohmeda Draw-Over TEC Vaporizer. This strongly resembles the AE Draw-Over vaporizer, of which there are very many still in use. Note that it is available with either a screw cap or a keyed filler. There are alternative inlet and outlet tapers available, some of which have a screw coupling to prevent it falling off the front of the anaesthetic machine and causing expensive damage, as well as allowing liquid agent to spill into the bypass and give a dangerously high fault concentration. *Working principles:* All the gas passages are wide, so as to reduce flow resistance. The Control knob is linked to the Rotary valve. When set to 'off', the inlet and outlet tubes are closed to prevent leakage of liquid during transportation. Note that there is a non-return valve in the outlet. Different models have maximum calibrations for halothane of 3, 4 or 5%, and this should be noted before use. (b) Performance characteristics with Halothane in the older AE models. (c) Performance characteristics with halothane in later models. Characteristics for vaporizers for other agents are available from the manufacturer.

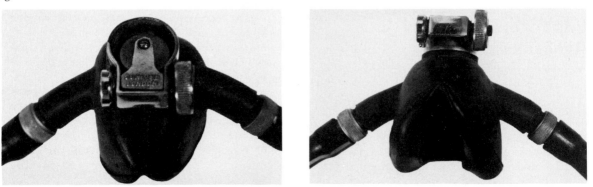

**Figure 11.4** The McKesson nasal inhaler. Note that the lever-action valve manufactured by Coxeter was used at one time.

# Nasal Inhalers

There are two traditional types of nasal inhaler (or hood) — the McKesson and the Goldman, and from these numerous modifications have been made.

The *McKesson inhaler* (Fig. 11.4) is constructed of rubber and fits over the nose. It is quite flexible and can be widened or narrowed. The gas enters through two narrow tubes, one on each side of the inhaler. These tubes pass round each side of the patient's head and are held together by means of a sliding clamp behind the head. Thus, when properly applied, the inhaler stays in place on its own, thereby freeing the anaesthetist's hands for other manipulations. It may be fitted with either a Heidbrink expiratory valve (Fig. 11.5) or a Coxeter lever-action valve (Fig. 11.4) the former being the more satisfactory. The latter has the disadvantage that it may be closed by accidental pressure from the dentist's hand as he works.

The McKesson inhaler may be augmented by a mouth cover, as shown in Fig. 11.6. This is used if the patient persists in mouth breathing, particularly before the pack is inserted. When the mouth cover is out of use it falls downwards, automatically turning off the supply of gas to it. Mouth covers are rather objectionable to the patient, and most experienced dental anaesthetists manage without them.

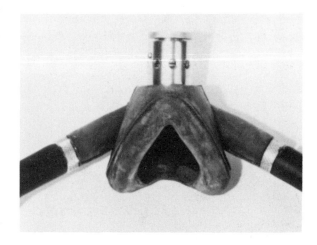

**Figure 11.5** The Heidbrink valve used in a nasal inhaler.

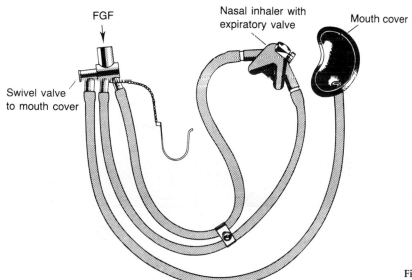

**Figure 11.6** The McKesson nasal inhaler complete with a mouth cover.

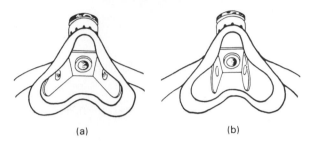

**Figure 11.7** (a) The Braun nasal inhaler. Note the metal stiffener. (b) An inhaler with a stiffener made of too flimsy a material that has become bent.

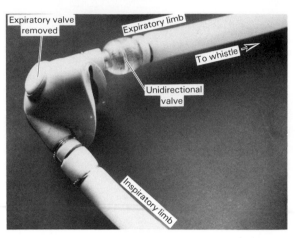

**Figure 11.9** A prototype nasal inhaler manufactured by Cyprane.

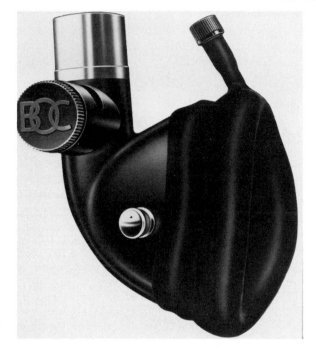

**Figure 11.8** The Goldman nasal inhaler. Note the studs for the attachment of a head harness.

The *Braun modification* of the McKesson inhaler (Fig. 11.7) has a metal stiffener inside to spread it open and prevent it from pinching the nose. This makes it much more acceptable to the patient. It may also be used to cover both the mouth and nose of an infant during induction. The stiffener should be made of strong metal, since otherwise the two sides may be pressed together and become impaled on the patient's nose, so defeating the object of the exercise.

The *Goldman inhaler* (Fig. 11.8) is rigid and has a rather larger capacity than that of the McKesson. The pad, which is moulded to fit the face, can be replaced when damaged or perished. Gases enter

via a wide-bore hose, which passes over the top of the patient's head, and escape through a Heidbrink expiratory valve. The inhaler can be held in place by a harness of the Connell type (see Fig. 21.27b).

The advent of the vogue for scavenging exhaled anaesthetic vapours and the partial relaxation of regulations concerning the employment of electrically conductive materials (containing black carbon) have led to the diminution of the use of the 'black mask over the face', the insensitive and unsympathetic use of which has, in the past, kindled such fear in the patients on whom it was imposed.

Figure 11.9 shows a prototype nasal inhaler produced by Cyprane several years ago. It has been in use for many thousands of cases with great success. The hood is of pale grey plastic, and much more acceptable to the patient. The fresh gases pass along the inspiratory limb, and expired gases via a unidirectional flap valve, down the expiratory limb, which incorporates a whistle. The intermittent sound of the latter is most useful in reassuring both anaesthetist and dentist that there is no respiratory obstruction. It can be attached to a scavenging system, but even if it not, it discharges the expired gases at floor level rather than into the faces of the operator, nurse and anaesthetist.

Another dental nasal inhaler is the Brown scavenging mask, manufactured by Narco-McKesson (Fig. 11.10), in which the fresh gases are delivered through an internal nasal hood and the expired gases pass via an external hood to the disposal system. The author has no experience in the practical use of this inhaler, but found on examining it that the various components were easily disconnected, which may prove unsatisfactory during a 'lively' induction!

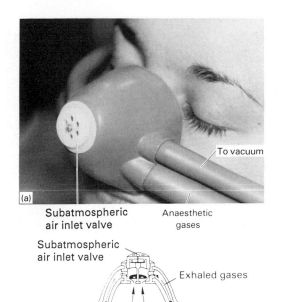

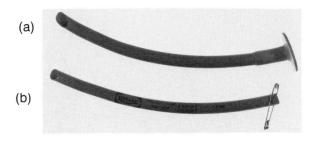

Figure 11.12 Nasopharyngeal airways. (a) Purpose-made with a flange. (b) The improvised version (to be used only in an emergency situation).

Figure 11.10 (a) The Brown scavenging nasal inhaler (manufactured by Narco-McKesson). The anaesthetic gases are delivered through the wider bore tubes and the vacuum for scavenging is connected to the narrower pair. The subatmospheric air inlet valve admits air only if the reservoir bag has been emptied. The inhaler has a double skin, as shown in (b), the anaesthetic gases being delivered to the interior and the vacuum to the gap between the two layers.

Figure 11.11 shows the scavenging mask by McKesson of the UK. It is intended for both anaesthesia and relative analgesia. A head strap is available for securing it during longer cases.

Further information on scavenging will be found in Chapter 17.

Nasal inhalers may be sterilized by cold methods such as immersion in chlorhexidine solution, but not all can be autoclaved. Usually, however, they are simply washed in hot running water after use on each patient and may then be dipped into a sterilizing solution. In busy dental practices it is rather expensive to provide a fresh inhaler for each patient.

An anaesthetist who has to resort to the use of the 'full facepiece' for a difficult patient more than *very* infrequently must admit that he is deficient in technique.

Endotracheal tubes used in dental anaesthesia are described in Chapter 9. Nasopharyngeal tubes (or airways) may be purpose-made, with a flange to prevent their slipping out of reach from the nostril, or may be improvised (but only where an emergency situation justifies this) by inserting a safety pin through an old nasotracheal tube cut short (Fig. 11.12). A No. 7 tube, 17-cm long, or a No. 6 tube, 15-cm long should suit most adults.

Since this chapter was written, clinicians have started to use laryngeal masks (see page 158) in dental anaesthesia. To date, reports have been encouraging, especially when these masks have been used in cases for multiple extractions and conservation.

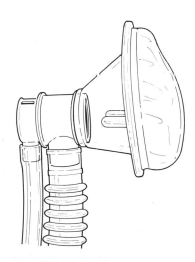

Figure 11.11 The scavenging mask of McKesson for both RA and GA.

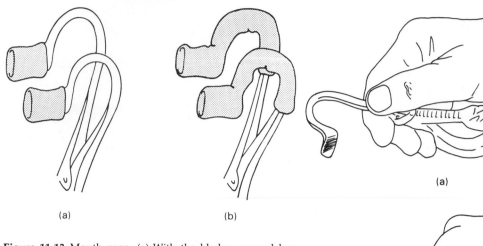

(a)                              (b)

**Figure 11.13** Mouth gags. (a) With the blades covered by inadequate lengths of tubing that might easily become dislodged and be inhaled by the patient. (b) With the blades covered by longer lengths of tubing.

# Gags and Props

Mason's and Ferguson's gags are described in Chapter 21. The blades may be covered with plastic or rubber tubing to protect the patient's teeth from damage. As shown in Fig. 11.13, the pieces of tubing should not be so short that they might fall off and be inhaled by the patient. Plastic tubing is more easily threaded onto the blade of the gag if it is first softened by immersion in boiling water; however, the use of plastic tubing may lead to problems with methods of sterilization.

When the gag is being inserted into the patient's mouth it should be held by the blades, as shown in Fig. 11.14a, and not by the handles, since the latter causes the gag to open before it is inserted (Fig. 11.14b).

Instead of a gag, a prop may be used to keep the patient's mouth open. Since the days of Hewitt (1857–1916) the prop has been re-invented many times and a typical set is shown in Fig. 11.15. A prop should be attached to a length of cord or chain to facilitate its retrieval if it slips into the patient's mouth. Conveniently, three or four props of different sizes may be linked together by their chains.

Various forms of throat pack have been produced, including those consisting of absorbent tampons and preformed foam-rubber. Strips of gamgee about 5-cm wide remain the most popular and adaptable. This material comes in rolls, in various thicknesses. It may be pre-cut into lengths which should be not less than 30-cm long. When in use the end of the

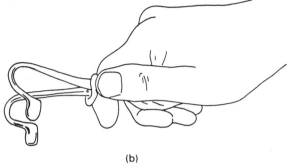

(a)

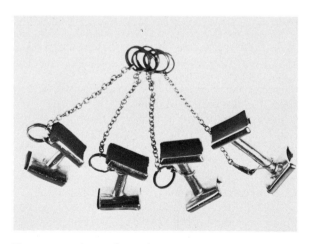

(b)

**Figure 11.14** A mouth gag held (a) correctly and (b) incorrectly.

**Figure 11.15** A set of mouth props.

pack should always remain outside the mouth to facilitate its removal. If one pack is inadequate, a second should be used and the ends of both should be kept outside the mouth.

# Suction Equipment

In the dental operatory suction equipment should be of the high displacement type (see Chapter 19). The high-pressure, low-displacement type, such as that produced by a hospital piped medical vacuum or a good quality portable electrically operated suction pump, may be satisfactory, but low-displacement types such as the foot-operated suction pump or the venturi type working off the water tap give far less than the desirable performance.

The sucker is used most commonly to remove blood and debris from the site of operation, and only seldom to remove regurgitated or vomited stomach contents, or secretions, from the respiratory tract.

It should be remembered, however, that with the low-pressure, high-displacement type of suction equipment, the nozzle should be of wide diameter, between 0.5 and 2 cm, and as short as possible. Long, narrow-bore suction catheters are inappropriate.

# The Dental Chair

The chair itself is justifiably included in this chapter since the ease with which the posture of the patient may be altered and, equally importantly, the security with which he, and his head in particular, may be maintained in the desired position are of paramount importance in the pursuit of safety during dental anaesthesia.

Whether the patient is anaesthetized and subjected to operation in the sitting, semirecumbent or horizontal position is a matter for individual choice. Whichever is preferred there is no argument that the patient who collapses must be placed quickly in the horizontal position — preferably with the legs raised. The anaesthetist should, therefore, be familiar with the workings of the chair and also check before use that any electrical controls are turned on and functioning correctly.

One of the problems of the modern electrically operated dental chair is that it may be slow to operate when the horizontal position is required urgently and in some types there is no manual override to lower the back of the chair speedily if the electrical supply is not energized.

The other disadvantage of modern chairs is that the old 'doughnut' type of headrest, which maintained the position of the patient's head so posi-

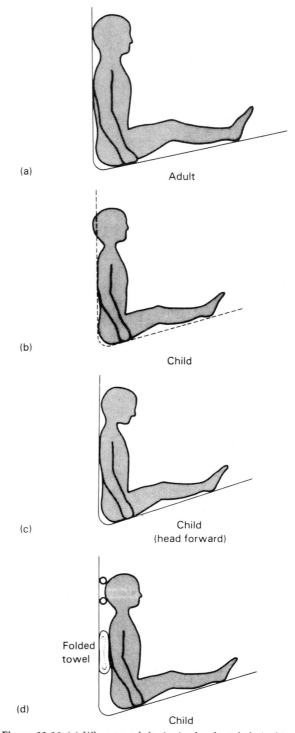

(a) Adult

(b) Child

(c) Child (head forward)

(d) Child — Folded towel

**Figure 11.16** (a) When an adult sits in the dental chair, his occiput is roughly in line with his back. (b) Children tend to have slender necks and prominent occiputs, causing (c) flexion of the neck. (d) A folded towel behind the back and the 'ring of confidence' may help to maintain the head in the correct position.

tively, has been replaced by the flat rest that permits the head of the anaesthetized patient to wobble about. In the case of children this is of even greater importance, since their necks are more slender and the occiput more prominent, making the maintenance of a suitable position more difficult (Fig. 11.16).

Makeshift additions to the headrest include a home-made 'bean bag', consisting of a 3-litre infusion bag filled with rice, designed by J. V. I. Young (personal communication) (Fig. 11.17) and the 'ring of confidence' (Fig. 11.18), which consists of a circular headrest constructed from a discarded length of corrugated breathing tubing.

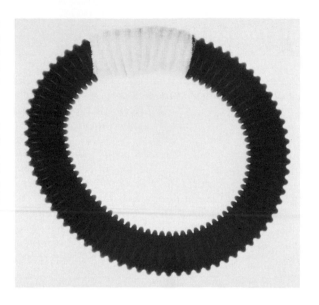

**Figure 11.18** The 'ring of confidence'.

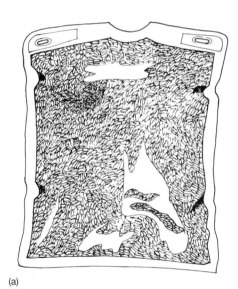

(a)

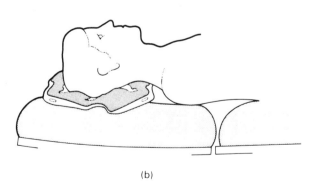

(b)

**Figure 11.17** (a) The 3-litre infusion bag ('bean bag') filled with rice. (b) The 'bean bag' used to hold the patient's head steady during dental chair anaesthesia.

# Piped Medical Gases

The decision as to whether to install a piped gas system in the dental operatory must be influenced by the frequency of use of general anaesthesia and relative analgesia and on the aesthetic aspect of the design of the establishment. Piped gas systems are described in Chapter 4.

Considerable economy of running expenses and time may be achieved by installing large cylinders of nitrous oxide and oxygen instead of small ones mounted on the anaesthetic machine itself. This may be done in several ways.

- A single trolley may carry two large cylinders *and* an anaesthetic machine. This is rather cumbersome, but portable, and may be wheeled, with some effort, from operatory to operatory. The longevity of the cylinder contents is a distinct advantage.
- Two cylinders at the wall of the operatory with regulators and contents gauges attached. These may be secured by a chain or special rings into brackets screwed to the wall. Rubber tubing delivers gases to the anaesthetic machine — and may be detached if non-interchangeable connectors similar to those on the pipeline are used.

# The Itinerant Dental Anaesthetist's Case

## A suggested list of contents

The instrument case has four drawers, the top ones shallow and the lower ones deep.

*Top drawer*
Endotracheal tubes, with connectors
Nasopharyngeal tubes
Bronchoscope blade (to fit laryngoscope handle)
Spare washers for cylinders, vaporizers, etc.
Spare O-rings for bullnose cylinder fittings
Adhesive plaster
Specimen bottles for blood samples
Safety pins

*2nd drawer*
Drugs, including those for resuscitation, and isoprenaline spray
Ampoule files
Sickledex kit
Hawksley haemoglobin scale
Scissors
Airways
Tongue-and-towel forceps
Spencer Wells forceps

*3rd drawer*
Syringes, 5 and 10 ml
Selection of needles
Methohexitone, thiopentone and sterile water
Ampoules of atropine or glycopyrronium bromide (glycopyrrolate)
Miniswabs or cotton wool

*4th drawer*
Nasal inhaler(s)
Vaporizer

Reservoir bag on mount
Check valve (for use in Mapleson A)
Adaptors, McKesson to BOC and New BS, etc.
Bottles of halothane and 70% alcohol skin preparation
Funnel
Cylinder key (ratchet)
Laryngoscope (with batteries removed from handle)
Mouth gag
Straight and angled expiratory valves
Facemask
Catheter mount
Spare laryngoscope batteries and bulb
Spare reservoir bag
Stethoscope
Sphygmomanometer

## Equipment to be kept at the dental operatory

Anaesthetic machine, complete with breathing attachment and preferably a compensated vaporizer
Cylinder key
Throat packs
Mouth gag or props
Suitable headrest
Spare cylinders
Resuscitation equipment (independent of anaesthetic machine and oxygen cylinder)
Pulse-oximeter

## Equipment that may be carried by the anaesthetist

Manual resuscitator
Spare endotracheal tubes and laryngoscope
Cardioscope
Defibrillator
Pulse monitor
Portable suction (standby)

these are sometimes provided by the visiting anaesthetist to minimize capital expenditure on behalf of the dentist.

# 12 Resuscitators and Automatic Ventilators

## Introduction

Three different groups of devices can be used to produce artificial ventilation of the lungs:

1. Manual resuscitators, such as the Ambu and Laerdal systems, and the Oxford inflating bellows.
2. Mechanical ventilators, into which the patient is placed in order to simulate the 'negative' intrathoracic pressure that occurs in spontaneous respiration. This group includes the cabinet type of ventilator such as the Drinker 'Iron Lung' and the Cuirass. These inflate the lungs by an indirect action. These will not be discussed here since they are not normally used in anaesthesia.
3. Mechanical devices that rhythmically inflate the lungs by means of applying intermittent positive pressure to the air passages (IPPV, intermittent positive pressure ventilation).

## Manual Resuscitators

Several manual resuscitators are available from different manufacturers. They are functionally similar and some will be described here.

### Laerdal and Ambu resuscitators (Figs 12.1 & 12.2)

These resuscitators have three components; a self-inflating bag, a system for feeding respirable gas into the bag and a non-rebreathing valve.

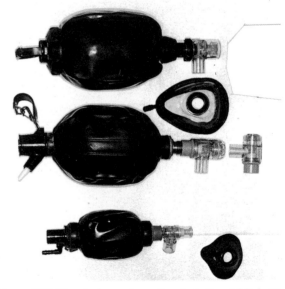

**Figure 12.2** The Ambu system: (top to bottom) Mark III, Mark II, paediatric.

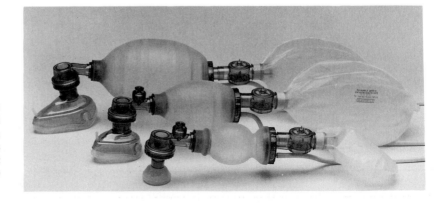

**Figure 12.1** The Laerdal system: (back to front) adult, child and infant sizes. The versions shown all have oxygen reservoir bags attached. The child and infant versions show the overpressure safety valves fitted.

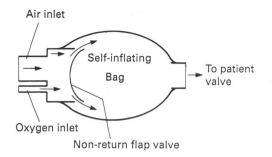

Air inlet

Self-inflating
Bag

To patient
valve

Oxygen inlet

Non-return flap valve

**Figure 12.3** A typical self-inflating bag showing the air and oxygen inlets.

*The self-inflating bag (Fig. 12.3).* This is so constructed (thick foam rubber lining in the case of the Ambu) so that in the resting state it is inflated. It is double ended, housing the respirable gas inlet mechanism at one end and the non-rebreathing valve at the other.

*The respirable gas inlet.* This has three parts. The first consists of a small bore nipple for connection to an oxygen supply and is sited next to a second much wider bore air inlet (see Fig. 12.3). The two are connected to a one-way flap valve which is incorporated in one end of the self-inflating bag. When the bag is squeezed, the gas pressure inside the bag rises, causing this flap valve to close and also preventing escape of this gas back through the inlet device. When the bag is released, its self-inflating characteristic causes fresh gas from the respirable gas inlet to be entrained. This is usually air, unless oxygen is added. In the latter situation, the final concentration of oxygen delivered is a function of the amount of added oxygen and its dilution with entrained air. This, in turn, depends on the ventilatory parameters produced by bag-squeezing (Table 12.1). Both the Ambu and Laerdal systems have a reservoir system that can be connected to the

**Table 12.1**   Oxygen concentrations in a Laerdal resuscitator (with and without the reservoir bag)

(a) **Adult:** Ventilation bag volume 1600 ml; reservoir bag volume 2600 ml

| O$_2$ flow (litres/min) | Tidal vol. (ml) × bag cycling rate per min O$_2$-concentrations (%) using reservoir (without reservoir in brackets) | | | | | |
| --- | --- | --- | --- | --- | --- | --- |
| | 500 × 12 | 500 × 24 | 750 × 12 | 750 × 24 | 1000 × 12 | 1000 × 24 |
| 3 | 56 (37) | 39 (32) | 47 (33) | 34 (29) | 41 (32) | 30 (28) |
| 5 | 81 (52) | 52 (38) | 62 (41) | 42 (33) | 52 (39) | 38 (31) |
| 10 | 100 (73) | 84 (48) | 100 (56) | 65 (42) | 84 (55) | 53 (39) |
| 12 | 100 (84) | 97 (53) | 100 (61) | 74 (45) | 94 (60 | 59 (42) |
| 15 | 100 (89) | 100 (59) | 100 (69) | 86 (48) | 100 (69) | 66 (44) |

(b) **Child:** Ventilation bag volume 500 ml; reservoir bag volume 2600 ml

| O$_2$ flow (litres/min) | Tidal vol. (ml) × bag cycling rate per min | | | |
| --- | --- | --- | --- | --- |
| | 250 × 20 | | 100 × 30 | |
| | O$_2$-concentrations (%) | | | |
| | w/reservoir | wo/reservoir | w/reservoir | wo/reservoir |
| 10 | 100 | 75 | 100 | 90 |

**Infant:** Ventilation bag volume 240 ml; reservoir bag volume 600 ml

| O$_2$ flow (litres/min) | Tidal vol. (ml) × bag cycling rate per min | | | |
| --- | --- | --- | --- | --- |
| | 40 × 30 | | 20 × 40 | |
| | O$_2$-concentrations (%) | | | |
| | w/reservoir | wo/reservoir | w/reservoir | wo/reservoir |
| 4 | 98 | 89 | 98 | 98 |

air entrainment section, so that high concentrations of oxygen (up to 100%) can be given. (Fig. 12.1 shows the Laerdal system with the reservoir bag attached.) However the Ambu reservoir is smaller, so as to be less cumbersome in use, and consequently a higher fresh gas flow is required to maintain the high oxygen concentrations (see Table 12.2).

**Table 12.2** Oxygen concentrations in the Ambu system with reservoir

| $O_2$ (litres/min) | $FIO_2$ (%) | | Tidal volume × frequency |
|---|---|---|---|
| 13 | 85–10 | } | 1000 ml × 15 |
| 4 | above 40 | | |
| 5 | 85–100 | } | 300 ml × 20 |
| 2 | above 40 | | |

*The non-rebreathing valve.* This is housed at the opposite end of the bag to the gas entrainment system described above. It has a number of components that ensure that during the inspiratory phase, gas flows out of the bag and only into the patient port. When the patient exhales, the valve ensures that this exhaled gas escapes through the expiratory port without mixing with the fresh gas stored in the bag. Functionally, most non-rebreathing valves are similar, although there are some differences in their efficiency and their tendency to jam (see below).

### The Ruben valve (Fig. 12.4)

This valve consists of a spring loaded bobbin within the valve housing. In the resting position, the very weak spring holds the bobbin away from the expiratory port and against the inspiratory port, allowing relatively unhindered exhalation via the patient port. This prevents any exhaled gases from mixing with inspiratory gas in the self-inflating bag. When the bag is squeezed, the bobbin is forced across the valve housing, opening and connecting the inspiratory port to the patient port, and at the same time occluding the expiratory port. This manoeuvre allows inspiratory gas to enter the patient's lungs without leaking out through the expiratory port.

The differential resistance of the inspiratory limb (0.7 kPa/0.8 cmH$_2$O at 25 litres/min) and the expiratory limb (0.098 kPa/1 cmH$_2$O at 25 litres/min) allows the valve to function in a similar manner during spontaneous ventilation. In this situation the patient preferentially draws gas from the inspiratory limb, thus forcing the bobbin to

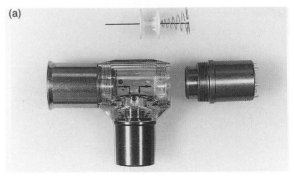

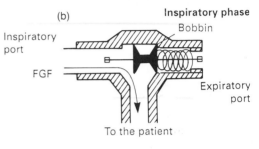

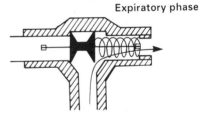

**Figure 12.4** (a) The Ruben valve. (b) Working principles. *Top,* in the inspiratory phase, the bobbin occludes the expiratory port. *Bottom,* during exhalation, the spring causes the bobbin to occlude the inspiratory port.

move and occlude the expiratory port. This valve has a tendency to jam in the inspiratory position (resulting in lung overinflation) if high upstream gas pressures are allowed to develop. For instance, if the valve is used to replace the APL valve in a Magill system during spontaneous ventilation, and the reservoir bag is allowed to over-distend, the valve will jam. In this situation an APL valve upstream of the Ruben valve should always be fitted so as to provide a pressure relief facility if required.

### Ambu valves

*The Ambu 'E' valve (see Fig. 12.5).* In this system, the unidirectional flow of gas is controlled by two labial flap valves. The upstream valve 'A', in the resting position, seals the inspiratory port but leaves the pathway into the expiratory port 'B' open, so that relatively unimpeded expiration can occur. During controlled ventilation the valve 'A' is forced open

(a)

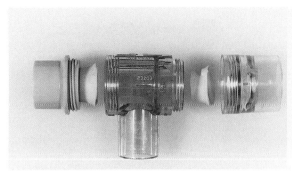

(b)

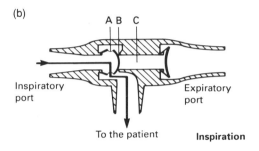

Inspiratory port

Expiratory port

To the patient **Inspiration**

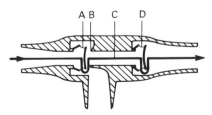

**Expiration**

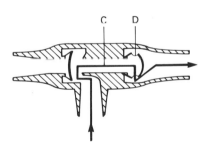

**Expiratory pause**

**Figure 12.5** (a) The Ambu E valve. (b) Working principles. (*Top*) During assisted inspiration. Note that the port B is closed by the pressure of the head of the 'mushroom' valve A. (*Centre*) During expiration. (*Bottom*) During the expiratory pause, excess gases may pass straight through the valve, so preventing excessive build-up of pressure.

and seals port 'B' so that inspiratory gas only enters the patient port. The labial valve 'D' is included to prevent the inhalation of downstream gas should the Ambu valve be used during spontaneous ventilation. This downstream gas may be air when the valve is used as a resuscitator but it could be exhaled gas if used in a circle breathing system.

When this Ambu valve is used for controlled ventilation, a high initial surge of gas is required to produce sufficient movement in valve 'A' to effect a complete expiratory seal. This model is relatively inefficient at lower inspiratory gas flow rates, and in this situation the seal may be incomplete allowing some of the inspiratory gas to pass straight across the valve. This results in lower than expected tidal volumes. In fact, it is possible to occlude totally the patient port and gently squeeze the contents of the self-inflating bag out through the valve! This relative inefficiency greatly decreases the potential for valve jamming. For instance if any high gas pressures were to begin to develop upstream, excess gas would be dumped across the valve. Because of this the Ambu 'E' valve should not be used with automatic resuscitators which do not produce the initial high surge of gas required to produce an effective seal.

*The Ambu-Hesse valve.* This is similar in design to the Ambu E valve described above. However, it provides a lower flow resistance through the valve by using larger valve diameters. This makes it more appropriate for use in anaesthetic breathing systems especially with spontaneous respiration (see Table 12.3).

*The Ambu E2 valve (see Fig. 12.6).* This model contains only the main labial valve (A) seen in the E and Hesse valves. Hence it functions in a similar fashion to these valves when used with controlled ventilation, but behaves differently if used with

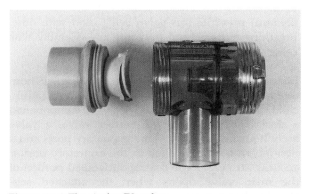

**Figure 12.6** The Ambu E2 valve.

through it. Almost simultaneously the outer disc-shaped portion of the valve is pushed against the apertures in the valve body, thus sealing the expiratory pathway.

EXPIRATORY PHASE. Positive expiratory pressure from the elastic recoil of the patient's lungs causes the duck-billed section of the valve to close thus preventing rebreathing into the bag. It also lifts the outer disc-shaped portion off the expiratory apertures, allowing exhaled gas to escape. Escaping gas also lifts the flaps on a non-return valve in the expiratory port. This is a supplementary valve that prevents air from being aspirated into the expiratory port during spontaneous respiration. This valve is constructed of autoclavable materials and is made in three sizes. All the sizes have a 23-mm external diameter expiratory port and a 22-mm external diameter/15-mm internal diameter inspiratory port so as to minimize the possibility of misconnection. The child and infant models have overpressure safety valves built into the inspiratory port of the valve and which are set to blow off at a pressure of 45 cmH$_2$O. If these pressures ever need to be exceeded, the safety valve can be overridden by finger pressure or a lock clip over the valve.

The self-inflating bag supplied with Laerdal resuscitators has thickened ribs of silicone rubber that provide the rigidity for the self-inflating action. These bags can be supplied with a supplementary reservoir bag (larger than that for the Ambu) for the supply of high oxygen concentrations to patients (see Table 12.1). The reservoir bags are fitted with a double valve (for air entrainment and relief of high pressure) to ensure adequate but not excessive gas pressures in the system.

### The Oxford inflating bellows

The Oxford inflating bellows (Fig. 12.9) is most useful in conjunction with draw-over anaesthetic apparatus. It is surmounted by a knob for easy manual operation, and contains a spring which when unopposed, opens the bellows, drawing atmospheric air. The inlet and outlet are guarded by one way disc valves V$_1$ and V$_2$ so that air is drawn in from the atmosphere and then blown into the patient when the bellows is depressed. Additional oxygen may be added via a tap in the bellows mount. When the patient breathes spontaneously, air may be drawn through without movement of the bellows, and the resistance is therefore low. Since the valves are held on their seats by gravity, the apparatus must be kept upright when in use. Resistance may be lowered even further by placing a magnet on the bracket above the valve in such a way that it attracts the disc and, by holding it up, keeps the downstream valve V$_2$ open. When the Oxford bellows is connected directly to a patient, a non-rebreathing valve must be added, so that during either a spontaneous or controlled inspiration, gas is drawn from the bellows and all exhaled gas leaves via the expiratory port. Note that the disc of V$_2$ should always either be held up or removed altogether when a high efficiency non-rebreathing valve, such as the Ruben (see above) is employed. Failure to do this may cause air to be trapped between the valve V$_2$ and the non-rebreathing valve, causing the latter to jam in its inspiratory mode. This situation prevents the patient exhaling. The subsequent delivered tidal volumes also become trapped in the patient's lungs, which if unrecognized, has resulted in death from barotrauma.

The bellows may be used without a non-rebreathing valve if the facemask is lifted from the patient's face to permit exhalation.

# Positive End-Expiratory Pressure (PEEP)

During the expiratory phase of mechanical ventilation, the expiratory pathway in a resuscitator or ventilator is usually opened to atmosphere, allowing gas to escape, using the energy stored in the elastic recoil of the patient's lungs. In certain clinical situations it is undesirable to allow the gas pressure within the lungs to fall to atmospheric, since this may result in gas trapping, terminal airway closure, micro-atelectasis, etc. These problems can be minimized by prematurely halting the expiratory phase at a pressure above atmospheric, i.e. at a positive end-expiratory pressure, or PEEP.

### PEEP valves

Ideally, a device that can produce this effect should offer no resistance to expiratory flow until the desired PEEP pressure is reached. This is best achieved by an electronically controlled expiratory valve that is activated when the expiratory pressure reaches a given value (Fig. 12.10a). However, such a device is both expensive and rarely portable so a number of purely mechanical devices are available. They usually take the form of a spring-loaded disc valve (Fig. 12.10b) whose spring tension can be varied by a threaded screw, enabling the valve to close when the desired expiratory pressure is attained. This pressure is normally calibrated (in cmH$_2$O) by a marker on the valve body. Simple

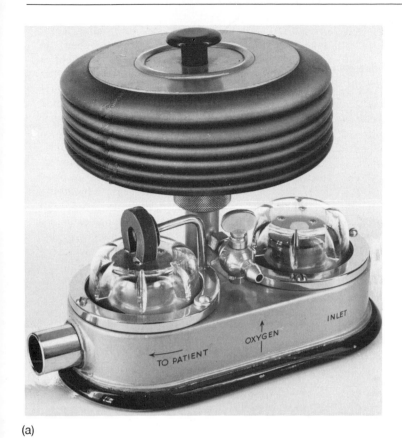

(a)

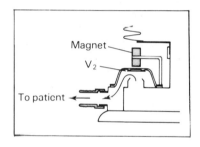

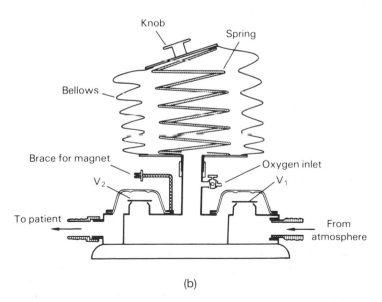

(b)

**Figure 12.9** (a) The Oxford inflating bellows. (b) Working principles. Insert shows gas flow with downstream valve $V_2$ held open by magnet. (See text.)

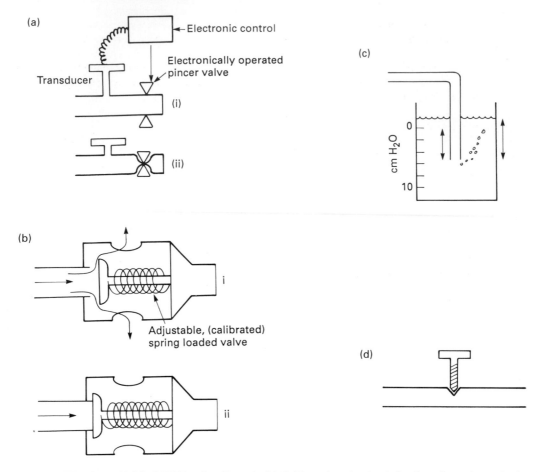

**Fig 12.10** PEEP valves. (a) Ideal PEEP valve (Servo). (b) Calibrated spring-loaded valve. Open in expiration (i) until the desired PEEP pressure is reached then fully closed (ii). (c) Expiratory path under water. The height of the water above the end of the tube determines PEEP. (d) Expiratory flow restrictor.

PEEP devices may also be constructed by immersing a section of the breathing hose at the end of the expiratory pathway under water (Fig. 12.10a). However, they all provide some expiratory resistance throughout the whole of the expiratory cycle, although this is of little practical importance. Note that the device shown in Fig. 12.10d is not truly a PEEP valve. It is in fact an expiratory flow restrictor and will eventually allow expiratory pressure to fall to zero if the expiratory phase is long enough.

Some of these devices plug into the expiratory port of the non-return valves described above. They usually have a 30-mm male tapered connection (if made to ISO standards) to prevent misconnection to the main valve and to fit scavenging devices.

# Automatic Ventilators

In order to inflate a patient's lungs mechanically, the respirable gas in a ventilator or resuscitator, destined for the patient, needs to develop a pressure sufficient to overcome the elastic properties of the lungs (their compliance) and the resistive properties of the airways (their resistance). Compliance and resistance may be normal in healthy patients, requiring the generation of modest (low) pressures for inflation, or may be grossly abnormal in disease, requiring the generation of much higher pressures to overcome them in order to provide the same degree of ventilation. Furthermore, some surgical procedures may make it more difficult to inflate the lungs, e.g. by restricting the movement of the diaphragm, due to posture or internal intervention. An additional factor during anaesthesia is the resistance of the artificial part of the airway, which may increase accidentally e.g. by mucus accumulation or kinking of the endotracheal tube.

## Methods of pressure generation

Respirable gas may attain the required pressure either by being compressed in a ventilator bellows or bag, or alternatively by the adaptation of a suitable source of gas that is already pressurized (cylinder or pipeline supply), in order to power the ventilator. The bellows may be compressed *mechanically* by attaching it to a spring, a weight, a gas-powered piston, or via a cam or gear chain to an electric motor. It may also be compressed *pneumatically* by placing the bellows in a gas-tight canister into which a pressurized gas source is fed (bag in bottle arrangement) or by distending a reinforced rubber bag with the gas and allowing the elastic recoil properties of the bag to provide the driving pressure. The pressure created within the bellows may be *constant* as produced by a weight placed on top of it, or *variable* when produced by some of the other methods. Distensible bags, and bellows attached to springs, produce pressures that steadily decline as the contents are released, whereas those attached to, say, an electric motor that progressively compresses the bellows, produce pressures that gradually increase as the bellows is compressed.

## Classification of ventilators according to their power

Ventilator designs fall into two categories: those suitable only for relatively normal lungs (low powered ventilators) and those that can cope with both normal and abnormal lungs (high powered ventilators).

### Low-powered ventilators (Fig. 12.11a).

Low-powered ventilators generate only the modest gas pressures required to deliver reasonable tidal volumes to lungs with normal and near-normal compliances and resistance. These pressures are often insufficient to overcome the increase in airways resistance and reduction in lung compliance that are seen in diseased lungs. As a result of this, the tidal volume delivered may well be less than the volume anticipated. Their use is therefore limited. When these ventilators are used, the need to monitor lung ventilation must be emphasized.

Either expired minute volume or capnometry can be used to check that ventilation remains satisfactory throughout a procedure. However these ventilators are simpler and more cheaply constructed and are also less likely to cause lung damage than those generating high pressures.

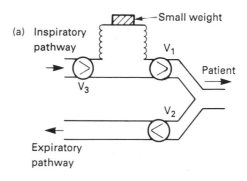

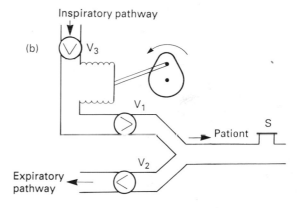

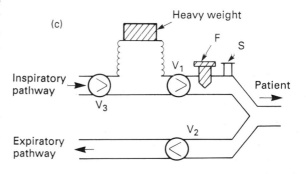

**Figure 12.11** (a) Low-powered ventilator generating constant low pressure. (b) High-powered ventilator generating an increasing pressure. (c) High-powered ventilator generating a constant high pressure. $V_1$, inspiratory valve; $V_2$, expiratory valve; F, flow restrictor; S, overpressure relief valve.

## High-powered ventilators (Fig. 12.11b, c)

In order to prevent changes in ventilator performance in the presence of deteriorating lung conditions, a ventilator needs to be powerful enough to develop a sufficiently high gas pressure, if required, in order to overcome most increases in airways resistance and reduction in lung compliance, but without producing lung damage. Such a pressure (up to 7.8 kPa/80 cmH$_2$O), is high enough to overcome most of these changes with little alteration in desired gas flow. These ventilators may also be referred to as 'flow generators', i.e. gas flow is reliably maintained when applied to a wide variety of lung states. These ventilators are more costly to produce and require the addition of certain safety features to protect patients with both normal and abnormal lungs from excessive pressures. For example, a safety valve is always included in the gas pathway to the patient to release any build-up of potentially dangerous pressures that might damage the lungs. Figure 12.11b shows an example of a typical high-powered ventilator. The pressure-relief valve can either be pre-set (usually at 4.4 kPa/45 cmH$_2$O) or, in more sophisticated machines can be adjustable (up to 7.8 kPa/80 cmH$_2$O) to cope with severe conditions such as asthma and the adult respiratory distress syndrome. The higher the pre-

set safety limit, the narrower becomes the safety margin between safe ventilation and barotrauma.

Those high-powered ventilators that always generate high pressure of gas in the ventilator system prior to its delivery (by using powerful springs, heavy weights or a pipeline gas source) (Fig. 12.11c), require the fitment of a further safety device, a flow restrictor. This reduces the flow to the patient and prevents too rapid a build up of pressure in the lung.

## Inspiratory characteristics of ventilators

Ventilators may produce a variety of pressure waveforms and inspiratory flow characteristics depending on the method of generation of gas pressure and the resistance to flow that the gas meets when the ventilator delivers its intended tidal volume.

## Low-powered ventilators (Fig. 12.12a)

Low-powered ventilators normally generate their power from gas stored under modest pressure in a bellows or distensible bag. Those ventilators exerting a constant gas pressure (weighted bellows) on the patient airway, will have an inspiratory flow rate of gas that is greatest in early inspiration, when

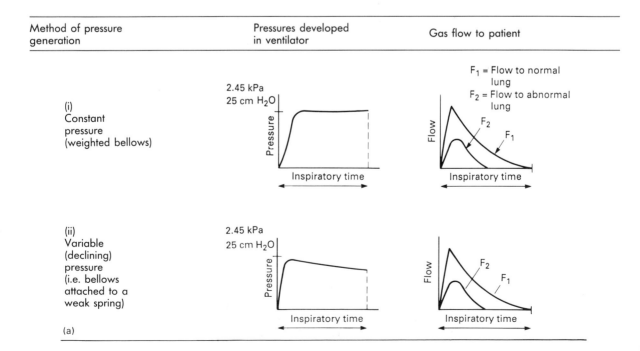

**Figure 12.12** (a) Inspiratory characteristics of low-powered ventilators.

| Method of pressure generation | Pressures developed in ventilator | Gas flow to patient |
|---|---|---|

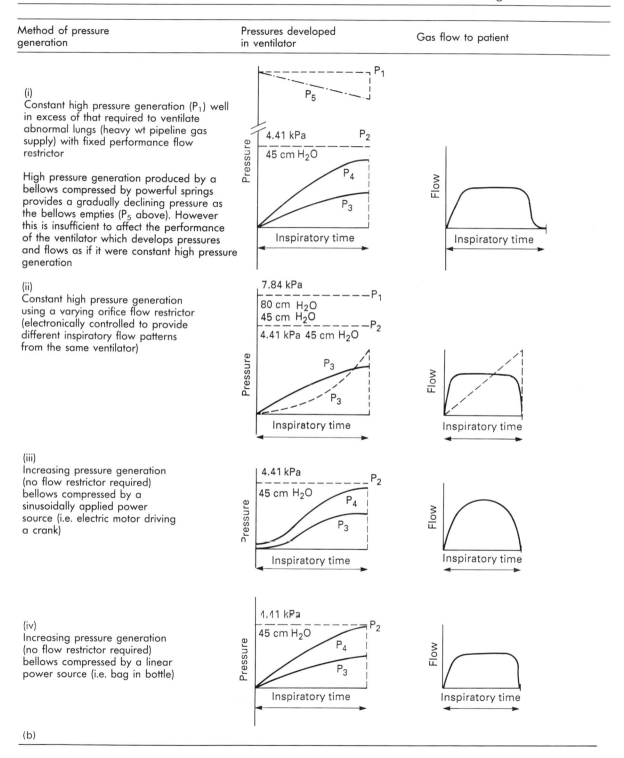

(i)
Constant high pressure generation ($P_1$) well in excess of that required to ventilate abnormal lungs (heavy wt pipeline gas supply) with fixed performance flow restrictor

High pressure generation produced by a bellows compressed by powerful springs provides a gradually declining pressure as the bellows empties ($P_5$ above). However this is insufficient to affect the performance of the ventilator which develops pressures and flows as if it were constant high pressure generation

(ii)
Constant high pressure generation using a varying orifice flow restrictor (electronically controlled to provide different inspiratory flow patterns from the same ventilator)

(iii)
Increasing pressure generation (no flow restrictor required) bellows compressed by a sinusoidally applied power source (i.e. electric motor driving a crank)

(iv)
Increasing pressure generation (no flow restrictor required) bellows compressed by a linear power source (i.e. bag in bottle)

(b)

**Figure 12.12** (*continued*). (b) Inspiratory characteristics of high-powered ventilators. $P_1$ = high constant pressure generated; $P_2$ = safety valve release pressure; $P_3$ = pressure rise downstream of restrictor as a result of flow to normal lungs; $P_4$ = as above but to abnormal lungs; $P_5$ = gradually declining high pressure.

Minute = Tidal volume × rate
volume $\left( \begin{array}{c} \text{insp. flow rate} \\ \times \text{ inspiratory} \\ \text{time} \end{array} \right)$ $\left( \begin{array}{c} 60\,\text{s} \div \\ (\text{insp.} + \text{exp.}) \\ \text{time} \end{array} \right)$

The equation will then be seen to fit all ventilators: e.g. a Penlon Nuffield has controls only for inspiratory time, expiratory time, (both calibrated in seconds), and inspiratory flow calibrated in litres/s. Therefore, tidal volume is derived from inspiratory flow and inspiratory time, and rate is derived from the settings for inspiratory and expiratory time.

The variety and complexity of lung ventilators makes the selection by the anaesthetist of suitable units quite difficult, and it has also lead to long delays in the development of Standards for ventilators. However both European and International Standards are now nearing the publication stage. It is not the intention of these standards to describe a standard ventilator but the aim of both documents is to ensure that manufacturers apply standard tests to their designs and publish the results in a standardized and therefore comparable manner.

It is expected that this will make it much easier to evaluate the respective merits of designs which may be different in many ways.

## Classification of ventilators according to function

There are a number of ways in which a ventilator can be used to inflate a patient's lungs. In an 'open-system' ventilator, fresh gases are delivered to the patient with each inspiration. The expired gas may pass back through the ventilators so that its escape to the atmosphere or through scavenging can be controlled by an expiratory valve, so that PEEP can be applied during the expiratory phase, or so that the expired tidal volume can be measured with a spirometer. However they are always discarded, and none returns to the inspiratory side of the ventilator.

A 'closed-circuit' ventilator takes the place of the anaesthetist's manual squeezing of the reservoir bag of a circle or Mapleson D breathing system. With these systems the fresh gas flow is often smaller than the patient's minute volume, the difference in the latter being made up by recirculating some expired gas which is returned to the bellows. These ventilators usually have provision for only a single hose connection to a breathing system. Provision is also made for the dumping of any excess gas that builds up in the system during the expiratory cycle when the ventilator is in operation.

## Classification of ventilators according to application

The four principle types of ventilator are:

1. 'mechanical thumbs';
2. minute volume dividers;
3. bag squeezers;
4. intermittent blowers.

Types 1, 2, and 4 function as open-system ventilators, i.e. fresh gas is delivered to the patient with each inspiration from the ventilator. Type 3 functions as a bag squeezer, i.e. it replaces the reservoir bag of a Mapleson D or circle breathing system.

Open-system ventilators may be converted to the closed-circuit type by interposing a bag in a bottle arrangement (Fig. 12.13).

## 'Mechanical thumbs'

Figure 12.14a shows a simple T-piece system for spontaneous respiration. In Fig. 12.14b the anaesthetist has occluded the open end of the T-piece with his thumb. The force of the fresh gas flow inflates the patient's lungs until the anaesthetist removes his thumb from the open end, which allows expiration to occur (Fig. 12.14c). By rhythmical application of the thumb to occlude the T-piece, intermittent positive pressure ventilation (IPPV) is achieved. This is, therefore, an 'open-system' ventilator, which operates on the 'mechanical thumb' principle. In ventilators such as the *Sheffield* (Fig. 12.15) and *Amsterdam* (Fig. 12.16), the anaesthetist's thumb is replaced by an electrical solenoid valve, the cycling of which is achieved by an electronic circuit (Fig. 12.14d). A slide-rule or graph is supplied, from which one can calculate the relationships between tidal volume, inspiratory time, expiratory time and fresh gas flow. In past years great advances were made in fluidics which make use of the Coanda phenomenon. Fluidic timing devices have been devised which, requiring the minimum of maintenance, are very reliable and occupy little space. They were ideal for controlling this type of ventilator. Unfortunately they suffered from the drawback that they needed a high flow rate of driving gas and results were not always reproduceable.

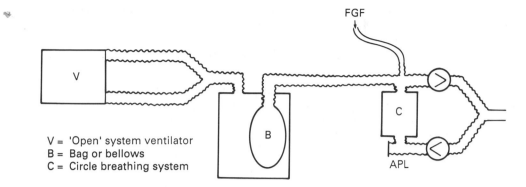

FGF

V = 'Open' system ventilator
B = Bag or bellows
C = Circle breathing system

V

B

C

APL

**Figure 12.13** The 'bag in a bottle' principle. As the driving air is driven into and out of the bottle, the bag, which is connected to the breathing system and contains patient gases, is pneumatically compressed and re-expanded. By this method the patient gases are isolated from the ventilator, which may be powered by and deliver other gases such as compressed air. The 'bag' is often in the form of a bellows, in which case the tidal volume may be indicated.

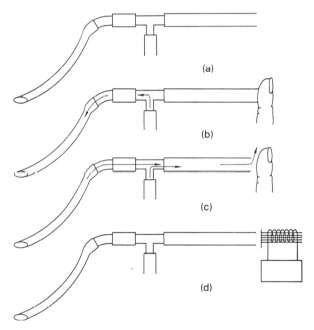

(a)

(b)

(c)

(d)

**Figure 12.14** The T-piece principle and the 'mechanical thumb'. (See text.)

## Minute volume dividers

These ventilators derive their power from the pressure of gases from the outlet of an anaesthetic machine or a similar source. The whole of the driving gas is delivered to the patient and there is no rebreathing. If, for example, the fresh gas flow is 10 litres/min, they deliver the 10 litres to the patient, but it is divided into 'breaths' or doses of varying

volume and frequency — e.g. 10 breaths of 1, 20 of 0.5 or 25 of 0.4 or so on.

The principle behind these ventilators is as follows (see Fig. 12.17). A reservoir R, which is continually pressurized by a spring, a weight or its own elastic recoil, is continuously being filled by the fresh gas flow (FGF). Two valves, $V_1$ and $V_2$, are linked together and operated by a bistable mechanism. When $V_1$ is open and $V_2$ closed, the reservoir discharges gas to the patient, i.e. this is the inspiratory phase. When $V_1$ is closed and $V_2$ open, expiration is permitted and at the same time the reservoir bag is refilled.

Minute volume dividers are simple compared with many other types of ventilator and this makes them attractive to the trainee or non-mechanically-minded anaesthetist. They are also relatively inexpensive to purchase and maintain. Some examples of minute volume dividers are described below.

### The East–Freeman Automatic Vent (Fig. 12.18)

This replaces the APL (expiratory) valve in a Magill breathing system). The reservoir bag is best replaced by one of a heavy-duty material, since it is distended by a considerably greater pressure than occurs in spontaneous breathing. The valve body has three ports. The upstream one I is connected via a corrugated hose to the reservoir bag. Its aperture is occluded by the seating S on the closed end of the bobbin B, which also carries at its centre a small magnet $M_1$. The latter is attracted by another magnet $M_2$, so that in the resting state the port is closed. Note that there is a gap G between the open end of the bobbin and the patient port P, so that the patient may exhale via the expiratory port E.

The fresh gas flow fills the reservoir bag and distends it until the pressure within it is sufficient

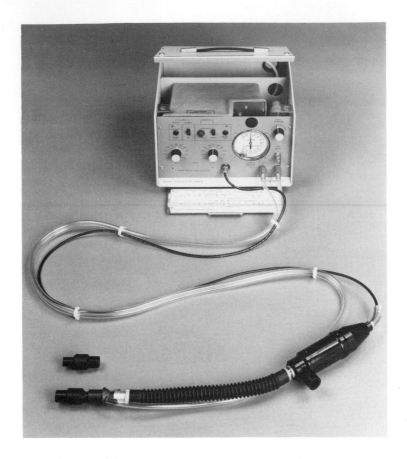

**Figure 12.15** The Sheffield infant ventilator.

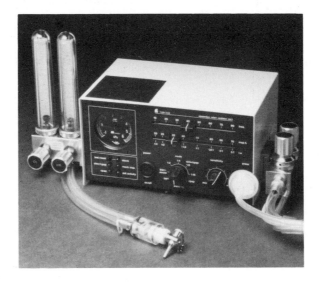

**Figure 12.16** The Amsterdam paediatric ventilator.

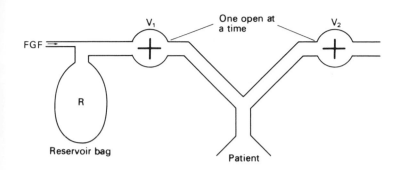

**Figure 12.17** The principle of minute volume dividers. (See text.)

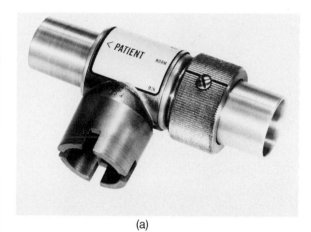

(a)

**Figure 12.18** (a) The East–Freeman Automatic Vent. (b, c) Working principles, I, upstream port; P, patient port; E, expiratory port; B, bobbin; S, seating; $M_1$, $M_2$, magnets; G, gap that allows the exhaled gases to escape via the expiratory port. (See text.)

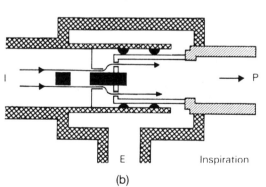

(b)

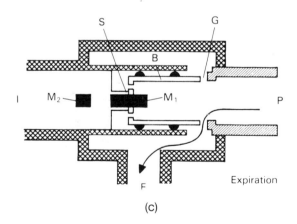

(c)

to overcome the attraction between $M_1$ and $M_2$ and force B off S. B then moves downstream until it closes G. At the same time gases pass from the pressurized reservoir via the hose through holes in the periphery of the closed end of B and thus to the patient. (G being closed, they cannot escape via the expiratory port.)

As the reservoir empties, the pressure falls and the mutual attraction of $M_1$ and $M_2$ returns B to its closed (resting) position. The expiratory phase then starts.

The only adjustments that can be made are to the FGF rate and the separation of the magnets, which can be altered by twisting a ring on the valve body. By altering the strength of the attraction between the magnets, the tidal volume is varied.

The Automatic Vent may be sterilized by cold methods, but care must be taken to avoid the ingress of grit, which could cause it to jam. A smaller reservoir bag should be used when treating children.

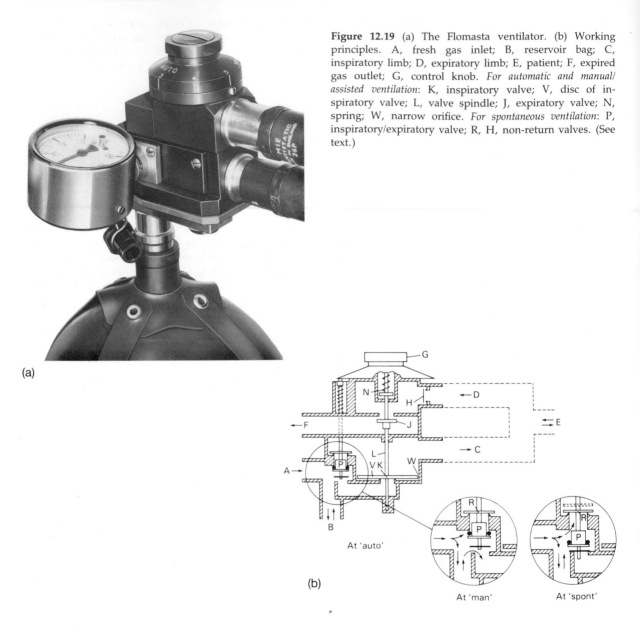

**Figure 12.19** (a) The Flomasta ventilator. (b) Working principles. A, fresh gas inlet; B, reservoir bag; C, inspiratory limb; D, expiratory limb; E, patient; F, expired gas outlet; G, control knob. *For automatic and manual/assisted ventilation*: K, inspiratory valve; V, disc of inspiratory valve; L, valve spindle; J, expiratory valve; N, spring; W, narrow orifice. *For spontaneous ventilation*: P, inspiratory/expiratory valve; R, H, non-return valves. (See text.)

(a)

(b)

At 'auto'

At 'man'    At 'spont'

## The Flomasta (Fig. 12.19)

The Flomasta is a considerably more sophisticated, yet very compact, minute volume divider, which is mounted directly on the outlet of the continuous flow anaesthetic machine. A driving gas pressure of 70–420 kPa (10–60 psi) is required. The single control knob G has a number of settings: the function of the valve in each mode will be described separately. The reservoir bag is enclosed in a net, partly to avoid over-distension and partly to achieve the appropriate volume/pressure characteristics.

During *automatic ventilation* the fresh gases enter

via the inlet A and pass into the reservoir bag B. The pressure within this part of the system rises until it is able to open the inspiratory valve K against the resistance of the spring N. When K opens the gases pass via the inspiratory limb C to the patient, but their escape via the expiratory limb D is prevented by the expiratory valve J (which is connected by the spindle L to the disc V of K), which is closed. The gases therefore pass around V, through a narrow orifice W, and this maintains a relatively high pressure under V until the end of inspiration. As the patient's lungs become distended and the flow through W diminishes, so the pressure difference across V is reduced, and N successfully opposes the upward movement of V. K then closes and J opens, allowing the expired gases to pass to the atmosphere through the outlet F. From here they may be metered by a spirometer or led to a scavenging system. The point at which inspiration ends depends on the tension in N, which in turn is controlled by setting the control knob to one of the 'auto' positions 1, 2, 3, 4 or 5.

During *manual or assisted ventilation* the inspired gases pass through K, raising V and thus closing J. When manual pressure on the reservoir bag is relinquished, K closes and J opens, allowing the expired gases to escape.

During *spontaneous respiration* gases are drawn by the patient through valve P, past the non-return valve R. At this stage he cannot inhale via D because the non-return valve H prevents this. During expiration valve P closes, H opens, and the patient may exhale though the expiratory port.

As optional extras, an airway manometer may be inserted into a small socket that is otherwise occupied by a blanking plug, and a Wright respirometer may be directly attached to the exhaust outlet, which has a cage-mount (23-mm) taper. The Flomasta may be autoclaved, provided that the respirometer and manometer are first removed. The manometer is not likely to become contaminated when in use, since it is in the inspiratory port.

### The Manley MP2, MN2 and MP3

The *Manley MP2* is a minute volume divider ventilator, in which the bistable system operates by a spring and lever and the inspiratory bellows is pressurized by an adjustable weight. There are several improvements of this simple arrangement, as shown in Fig. 12.20.

The main reservoir is a bellows $B_2$. During inspiration since $V_1$ is closed the fresh gas flow (FGF) is accommodated in a second bellows $B_1$, which, when filled to a predetermined but variable volume, trips the bistable system and initiates the expiratory phase. $B_1$ is loaded with a powerful spring so that during the expiratory phase it discharges into $B_2$ the gases that entered it during the inspiratory phase, to which is added the continuing FGF. When $B_2$ has filled to a predetermined volume the bistable mechanism is tripped in the other direction and inspiration starts again.

Valves $V_1$, and $V_2$ and $V_3$ are linked together pneumatically so as to operate as shown below:

| Phase | $V_1$ | $V_2$ | $V_3$ |
|---|---|---|---|
| Inspiration | Closed | Open | Closed |
| Expiration | Open | Closed | Open |

The degree to which $B_1$ fills before tripping controls the inspiratory time, and is determined by the setting of the 'inspiratory phase control'. The 'tidal volume control' may be set to regulate the degree to which $B_1$ is filled before the bistable mechanism is tripped to initiate inspiration. When the ventilator is used in the mode for spontaneous breathing, fresh gases pass directly to the patient, and the expired gases pass through tap $T_2$ to the reservoir bag and finally escape via the expiratory valve E. The inspiratory pressure is dependent on the distance between the weight W and the hinge (or fulcrum). Taps $T_1$ and $T_2$ change the mode of the ventilator between that for automatic ventilation and that for spontaneous or manual ventilation.

The *Manley MN2* (Fig. 12.21a) has a facility for a 'negative' (subatmospheric) expiratory phase, as shown in Fig. 12.21b. An additional bellows $B_3$ is mechanically linked to $B_2$ in such a way that it

**Inspiratory phase**

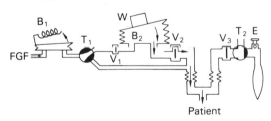

**Expiratory phase: atmospheric**

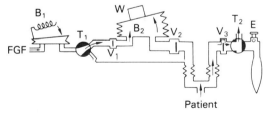

**Manual or spontaneous**

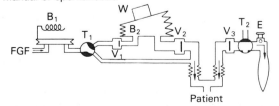

**Figure 12.20** Working principles of the Manley MP2 ventilator, $B_1$, $B_2$, bellows; W, weight; $V_1$, $V_2$, $V_3$, valves; $T_1$, $T_2$, taps; E, APL. FGF = fresh gas flow. (See text.)

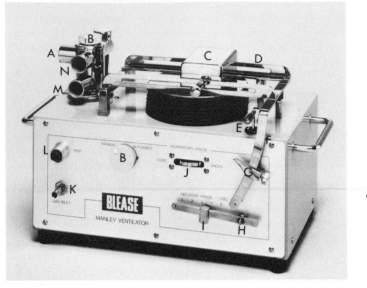

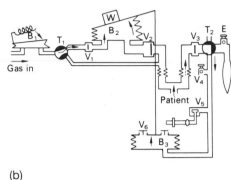

(a)　　　　　　　　　　　　　　　　　　　　　　(b)

**Figure 12.21** (a) The Manley MN2 ventilator. A, to spirometer (not with negative phase); B, control taps; C, sliding weight; D, slide; E, part of bistable mechanism; F, tidal volume selector; G, catch; H, negative pressure control; I, sliding weight; J, inspiratory time control; K, fresh gas inflow; L, to patient; M, from patient; N, to manual bag. (b) Working principles. A 'negative' phase has been added (compare with that shown in Fig. 12.20). $B_1$–$B_3$, bellows; W, weight; $V_1$–$V_6$, valves; $T_1$, $T_2$, taps; E, APL. (See text.)

opens during expiration, drawing air from the patient. An air-inlet $V_5$ also allows the ingress of air once the subatmospheric pressure within $B_3$ has exceeded a level determined by the position of the weight on the control bar. During inspiration, when the bellows closes, the gases within it may escape via a flap valve $V_6$. The negative phase may be isolated by turning tap $T_2$ to an intermediate position. It is only in the latter mode that an expired air spirometer may be attached or scavenging effectively performed. $V_4$ is an expiratory valve through which those gases that do not pass to $B_3$ escape to the atmosphere.

To change the mode between automatic and spontaneous ventilation, *both* taps $T_1$ and $T_2$ must be operated. This is a potential hazard since if they are turned in opposite directions, neither mode is achieved.

Another problem is that this ventilator may not be sterilized easily and quickly. The latter problem has been overcome in its successor, the *Manley MP3* (Fig. 12.22), in which the expiratory unit, complete with a condensation trap, may be detached very easily and autoclaved. This model also has facilities for a higher inspiratory pressure and stroke volume and incorporates an airway manometer. (The *Manley MN3* has a facility for a negative phase.)

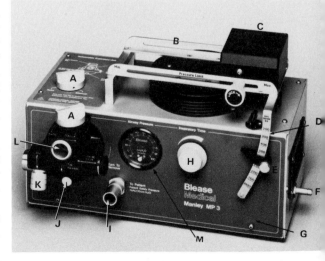

**Figure 12.22** The Manley MP3 ventilator. A, control taps; B, slide; C, sliding weight; D, stroke volume selector; E, catch; F, gas inlet; G, alternative position of gas inlet; H, inspiratory time control; I, to patient; J, tap release knob; K, to bag; L, from patient; M, airway manometer.

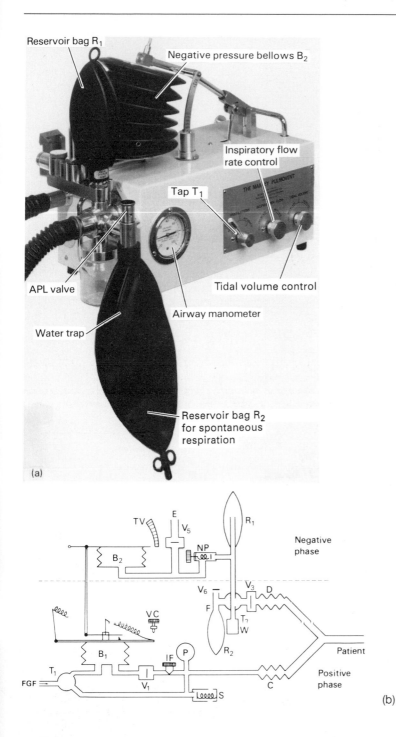

Reservoir bag R₁

Negative pressure bellows B₂

Inspiratory flow rate control

Tap T₁

APL valve

Tidal volume control

Water trap

Airway manometer

Reservoir bag R₂ for spontaneous respiration

(a)

(b)

**Figure 12.23** (a) The Manley Pulmovent ventilator. Superficially this resembles the Manley MN2, MP2 and MP3, but as will be seen in (b) the mechanism is quite different. The first bellows has been omitted and the fresh gas flow enters the main bellows $B_1$ directly. Whereas the MP2 is a low powered ventilator, in which the stroke volume may be influenced by the patient's compliance, the Pulmovent is a high powered ventilator, in which it is the total closure of $B_1$ that leads to the cycling of the ventilator. $B_1$ is closed by a spring, for which there is no adjustment, rather than by an adjustable weight. A negative phase may be added, and is achieved (as in the MN2) by the addition of an extra bellows $B_2$ linked to $B_1$. However, the negative pressure is satisfied during the first part of expiration by the contents of the small reservoir bag $R_1$. Negative pressure is therefore applied only during the expiratory pause. A positive end-expiratory pressure may be achieved by the adjustment of the positive pressure valve NP. Valves $V_1$, $V_3$ and $V_5$ are linked so that when $V_1$ and $V_5$ are open, $V_3$ is closed and vice versa. Taps $T_1$ and $T_2$ must both be turned to change from automatic to spontaneous ventilation, and, in addition, $T_2$ may be turned further to include the negative phase. IF, inspiratory flow rate control; P, airway manometer; VC, tidal volume control; S, overpressure relief valve; C, D, corrugated hose; $R_2$, F and $V_6$, spontaneous breathing system; TV, expiratory tidal volume indicator; E, expiratory port; W, trap for condensed water vapour.

These ventilators produce a power output which depends on the size of the weight used and its position on the slider arm. The MN2 and MP2 with their smaller weights are low-powered ventilators. However the MP3 can develop pressures of 50 cm $H_2O$ (5 kPa) and would probably be regarded as a high-powered ventilator.

## The Manley Pulmovent (Fig. 12.23)

The Manley Pulmovent is another minute volume divider ventilator, but its resemblance to the MN2, MP2 or MP3 is superficial only. The driving gases pass directly to the main bellows $B_1$, which is housed within the cabinet. Cycling is achieved by

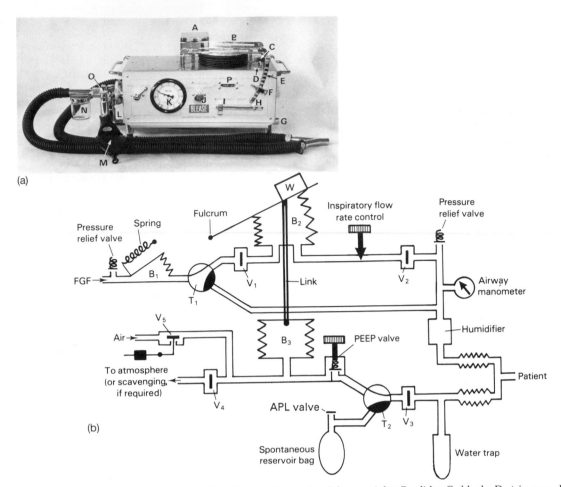

**Fig 12.24** (a) The Blease BM2 Brompton Manley ventilator. A, sliding weight; B, slide; C, block; D, trip arm; E, tidal volume selector; F, catch; G, outlet to atmosphere (or scavenging, if required); H, negative pressure control; I, sliding weight; J, inspiratory flow rate control; K, airway manometer; L, PEEP valve; M, reservoir bag for spontaneous respiration; N, water trap; O, APL valve. (b) Working principles. During automatic ventilation taps $T_1$ and $T_2$ are turned in the direction shown in the diagram. *During the inspiratory phase* the first gas flow (FGF) enters the reservoir bellows $B_1$, which is protected by a pressure relief valve. Valves $V_1$ and $V_3$ are closed and $V_2$ is open. The main bellows $B_2$ is closed by the weight W, and the gases in it pass to the patient via an inspiratory flow rate valve, valve $V_2$ and humidifier (if fitted). In this part of the system there is an airway manometer and a second pressure relief valve to protect the patient.

*During the expiratory phase* $V_2$ is closed and $V_1$ and $V_3$ are open. The fresh gases that had been stored in $B_1$ now pass to $B_2$ via $V_1$, being driven out of $B_1$ by the force of the spring. These gases and the continuing FGF refill $B_2$ to an extent determined by the setting of the catch on the tidal volume selector. The expired gases pass via $V_3$, the PEEP valve and the expiratory valve $V_4$ to the atmosphere or to the scavenging system. The negative pressure bellows $B_3$, which is mechanically linked to $B_2$, may draw expired gases from the patient, but this depends on the setting of the negative pressure control $V_5$. If the weight on the latter is set so that there is no resistance, the ingress of atmospheric air will satisfy the filling of $B_3$ and no negative pressure will be applied to the patient. As the weight on $V_5$ is moved so as to cause loading of $V_5$, negative pressure is generated. Atmospheric air cannot enter via the expiratory valve $V_4$.

A bistable cycling mechanism consisting of a spring and levers opens and closes $V_1$, $V_2$ and $V_3$. As $B_2$ refills during the expiratory phase, the catch on the tidal volume selector impinges on the trip arm, pushing it upwards, causes the cycling mechanism to trip and the inspiratory phase to begin. The next change, from inspiration to expiration, is initiated in *volume cycling* by the catch on the tidal volume selector being positioned so that as $B_2$ reaches the 'empty' position it forces the trip arm down, so tripping the bistable mechanism. Alternatively, in *time cycling*, a lever attached to $B_1$ trips the mechanism when $B_1$ has filled to an extent determined by the setting of the inspiratory time control.

*For spontaneous or manual ventilation*, $T_1$ and $T_2$ are turned so that the FGF passes, via the humidifier, if fitted, directly to the patient, and expired air passes via $V_3$, which is held open, to the spontaneous reservoir bag and escapes via the expiratory valve.

On account of the negative pressure system, accurate measurements with an expired spirometer cannot be made at the outlet.

the stroke volume of the bellows (i.e. bellows excursion) which may be varied by the tidal volume control. This ventilator is, therefore, volume cycled. The main bellows is closed by a powerful spring rather than by an adjustable weight as in previous models, and there is no provision for the adjustment of pressure. It is therefore regarded as a high-powered ventilator. However, there is an inspiratory flow rate control. Again (as in the MN2, MP2 and MP3) there are two controls that need to be adjusted in order to change from the automatic to the manual mode. The bellows $B_2$ surmounted on the top of the cabinet is the expiratory bellows, which may be used to produce a negative expiratory phase, though positive end-expiratory pressure (PEEP) is also available by adjusting the valve NP. Some of the expired gases pass into a small reservoir bag $R_1$, from which they later enter $B_2$ during the early part of the expiratory phase. It is therefore not until the expiratory pause, when $R_1$ has completely emptied, that negative pressure is applied to the patient. The whole of the expiratory system may be removed for autoclaving.

### The Blease BM2 Brompton Manley ventilator

The Blease BM2 Brompton Manley ventilator (Fig. 12.24) is another minute volume divider ventilator resembling the MN2, but it is intended primarily for intensive care, though it may be used equally well for anaesthesia. It may be stood on a flat surface or mounted on a wall rail system. There is a primary reservoir bellows $B_1$, from which gases pass to the main bellows $B_2$, the pressure within which is determined by the position of the weight W. The whole of the expiratory system may be detached, including the negative pressure bellows $B_3$, which, although housed within the cabinet, may be withdrawn from below. Attached to the expiratory system is a water trap, which should be used if humidification of the inspired gases is employed. On the stroke volume arm of the bellows there is a small metal block that can be adjusted in such a way that the bistable mechanism is tripped as soon as $B_2$ is completely emptied. If it has not been adjusted accordingly, and does not strike the tripping mechanism, the inspiratory time is determined by the opening of $B_1$ and may be regulated by adjusting the inspiratory time control. There is also an inspiratory flow control and a manometer. In addition to a negative expiratory phase, there is provision for PEEP. This ventilator may, therefore, be used as a low- or high-powered ventilator (depending on the position of the weight which pressurizes the bellows) and it may be either volume or time cycled.

## Bag squeezers

This type of ventilator is usually employed in conjunction with circle and Mapleson D breathing systems. It relieves the anaesthetist of having to squeeze the breathing bag and, apart from freeing him to do other things, offers the advantages of producing more regular ventilation, with controllable tidal volume and pressure, as well as the application of a negative phase.

The bag or bellows may be squeezed *mechanically* by means of a motor and suitable gears and levers, by a spring, or by a weight which may be adjusted to vary the pressure produced.

In the East Radcliffe ventilator, for example, the bellows is opened by an electric motor operating through a cam, and closed (during the inspiratory phase) by a weight.

In these mechanically driven ventilators it is often impossible to alter the relative lengths of the inspiratory and expiratory phases, and the inspiratory/expiratory ratio is usually somewhere between 1 : 1 and 1 : 2.

However, when the bellows is squeezed *pneumatically* the respiratory pattern can be varied. Examples of these ventilators are discussed below.

### The Cape ventilator (Fig. 12.25)

The Cape ventilator is a mechanical 'bag squeezer' and is easily understood by nursing staff and is used in intensive therapy. For anaesthesia, it is surmounted by an anaesthetic head, with flowmeters and vaporizers, when it is known as the Cape Waine ventilator. Although no longer manufactured, these ventilators still see service in many areas and may do so for many years to come. The working principles of the latter are as follows (see Fig. 12.25a, b).

A flame-proof electric motor drives a crankshaft 1 through a variable speed gear box. This, in turn, operates two cranks, 4 and 5, two cams, 2 and 3, and a tachometer. The rotation of the first crank 4 operates a lever 7 which opens and closes the main (inspiratory) bellows PPB. The extent to which PPB opens depends on the position at which the fulcrum 6 has been set. This is adjusted by the 'volume' control knob. The nearer the fulcrum is to the crank, the greater is the stroke volume. The first cam, 2, operates the inspiratory valve PV1, which permits gases flowing from PPB to pass to the breathing system and the patient. It opens a short while after PPB starts to close, thus causing a temporary rise of pressure, which serves to accelerate the gases and overcome their inertia. The expiratory valve PV2 remains closed during the inspiratory phase. Any

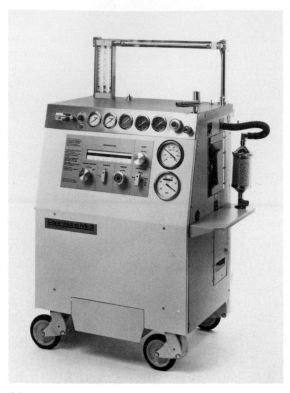

(a)

**Figure 12.25** (a) The Cape Waine (anaesthetic) ventilator. (b) Working principles. 1, crankshaft; 2,3, cams; 4,5, cranks; 6, fulcrum, 7, 8 levers; PPB, inspiratory bellows; NPB; negative pressure bellows; SB1, SB2, reservoir bags; RB, rebreathing bag; PV1, inspiratory valve; PV2 expiratory valve; SV1, SV2, overpressure valves; V1–V6, unidirectional valves; SP1, SPV2, SPV3, APL valves; NCV, negative pressure valve; NSV, relief valve; CSCI, CSC2, CSC3, taps. (See text.)

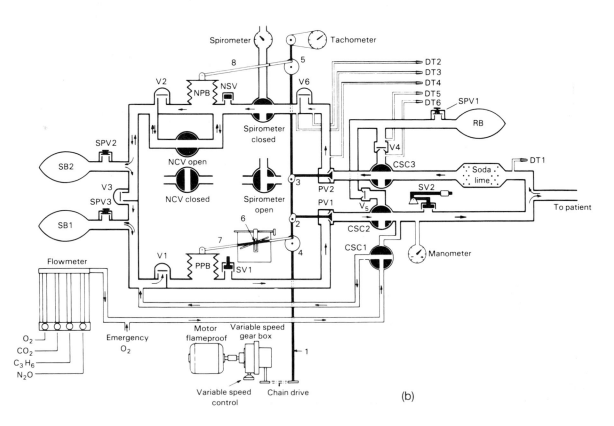

(b)

excess pressure is relieved by an over-pressure valve SV2, the opening pressure of which may be pre-set up to 80 cmH$_2$O. There is a manometer indicating the airway pressure.

During the expiratory phase PV1 closes and PV2 opens, PPB is reopened by 4 and fresh gases are drawn in through a unidirectional valve V1 from the reservoir bag SB1 and the flowmeters. The expired gases pass through the soda lime canister and via PV2 and a unidirectional valve V6 to the first reservoir bag SB2. At the same time the rotation of the second crank 5 operates a lever 8 which opens the negative pressure bellows NPB, but if the negative pressure valve NCV is open, this will draw in gases from SB2 rather than apply negative pressure to the patient. If NCV is closed, negative pressure is applied to the patient, and if this is excessive, air is drawn in through the relief valve NSV. When SB2 is full, gases pass from it through a unidirectional valve V3 to SB1 and will eventually pass again to PPB. The two reservoir bags are surmounted with APL valves SPV2 and SPV3, which allow the escape of excess gases. There is also a valve that may divert the expired gases to a spirometer so that they may be measured. This valve is spring loaded so that it returns to its normal position when it is no longer held open by the anaesthetist. If either SB1 or SB2 is removed and its port left open, air may be drawn in. As the ventilator is intended for long-term use in the intensive-care ward, a filter can be installed within the cabinet of the machine to prevent the ingress of infection or particles from the ambient air.

The rate per minute is indicated by the tachometer, which is also driven by the crankshaft.

Taps CSC1, CSC2 and CSC3 are mechanically linked to operate together. When the control is turned from 'Mech.' to 'Manual', these three taps are turned through 90° counterclockwise from the configuration shown in Fig. 12.25b. The fresh gases then flow directly to the inspiratory limb of the breathing attachment and the expired gases to a bag RB from which they may be rebreathed, passing through valves V4 and V5. There is an APL valve SPV1 on the mount of RB to allow the escape of excess gases. The soda lime canister may be removed, as desired, by the anaesthetist. Water may condense in various parts of the ventilator, particularly when a humidifier is installed, and is drained away by opening the small taps DT1 to DT6, which are located in the cabinet, below soda lime canister.

On the latest version, the control taps (CSC1, CSC2 and CSC3) may be depressed and turned to a third position, in which the fresh gases are diverted from the ventilator and pass directly to a Cardiff

swivel outlet and a Magill attachment. Older models have a separate tap, but may be converted to provide the same facility.

### The East Radcliffe ventilator (Fig. 12.26)

The East Radcliffe ventilator is used for both anaesthesia and intensive care in some areas. It is preferred by many for its rugged and reliable engineering and for its relative simplicity of control. It is driven by an electric motor which runs off the mains supply, but there is a second motor which operates from a 12 V d.c. battery and may be used in an emergency. If all else fails, there is a handle by which the ventilator can be operated manually. As in the Cape Waine, the motor drives a crankshaft

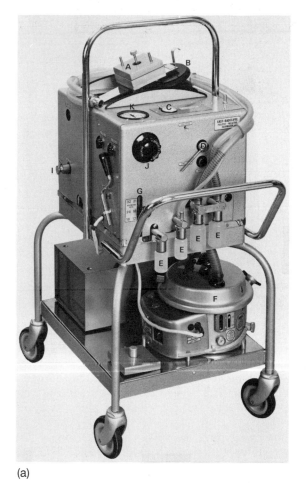

(a)

**Figure 12.26** (a) The East Radcliffe ventilator. A, weights; B, bellows; C, spirometer; D, spirometer control; E, water traps; F, humidifier; G, changeover and rate lever; H, handle for manual operation; I, locking plug; J, negative pressure control; K, airway pressure gauge. (*Continued overleaf.*)

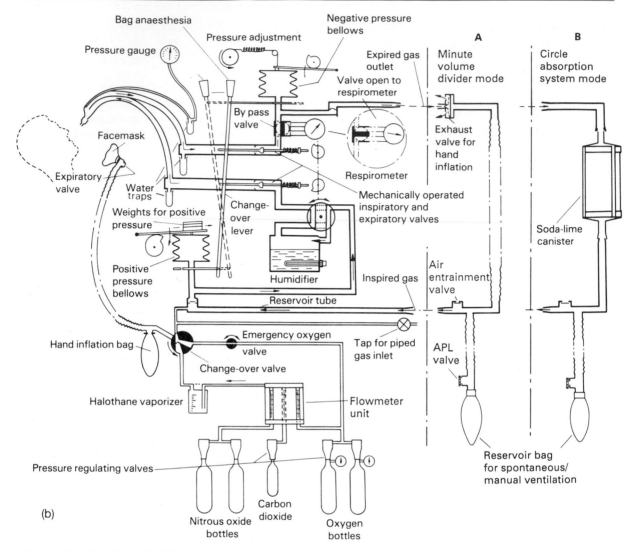

**Figure 12.26** (*Continued*) (b) Working principles. (See text.)

via a gearbox, in this case the Sturmey–Archer gear, which is still commonly used in the pedal bicycle. There are two ranges of speed, high and low; the one required may be selected by the insertion of the appropriate one of two locking plugs that are provided.

The inspiratory (positive pressure) bellows is surmounted by, and fixed to a metal slide, which is hinged at one end and carries a series of adjustable weights. A large plastic snail cam is driven by the crankshaft; this raises the slide, complete with the weights, and because of its attachment to it, the bellows opens, drawing in air or anaesthetic gases, as the case may be. When the maximum diameter of the cam has passed, the slide is free to fall and this compresses the bellows. The gases from the bellows

are unable to pass back through the pathway from whence they came, on account of a unidirectional valve, and pass via the humidifier (if fitted) to an inspiratory valve which is driven by another cam on the crankshaft. When the inspiratory valve is open, the expiratory valve, driven by yet another cam, is closed. The gases therefore pass to the patient. (Note that whereas in the Cape Waine the bellows opens and closes totally come what may, in the East Radcliffe, which is a low-powered ventilator (when used with a small weight), the bellows closes only in accordance with the compliance of the patient. However it may be used as a high-powered ventilator if a heavy weight is employed.)

During the expiratory phase the inspiratory valve closes, the expiratory valve opens and the positive pressure bellows is refilled. The expired gases pass either to the atmosphere or are collected, to be returned to the patient, having passed, if required, through a carbon dioxide absorber.

The ventilator incorporates a spirometer, the control of which is spring-loaded so that it operates only as long as it is held in the 'On' position. There is also a negative pressure bellows which is closed by a cam and opened by a spring whose tension may be adjusted in order to regulate the degree of negative pressure applied.

Provision is made for the connection of a humidifier, and, in order to remove water resulting from condensation, there are water traps at the inspiratory and expiratory ports.

This is another example of a ventilator which, although not commonly used in advanced areas, is still used in many other parts of the world, the great advantage being due to its reliability, simplicity and versatility and it also exemplifies many important principles.

### The Manley Servovent (Fig. 12.27)

Although the Manley Servovent bears a superficial remblance to some of the minute volume dividers described above, it does, in fact, operate on an entirely different principle and is a bag squeezer. The driving gas, which may be compressed air or oxygen at a pressure of 300–400 kPa (45–60 psi), does not reach the patient. Cycling is by a pneumatic logic device with controls for On/Off, expiratory time and inspiratory flow rate. It is therefore time cycled. There is also a tidal volume control which permits a maximum of 1300 ml. During the expiratory phase, the piston P of a pneumatic cylinder is driven by the driving gas and opens the bellows

(a)

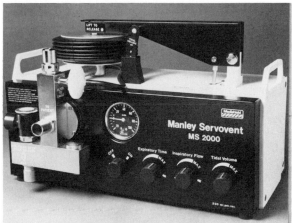

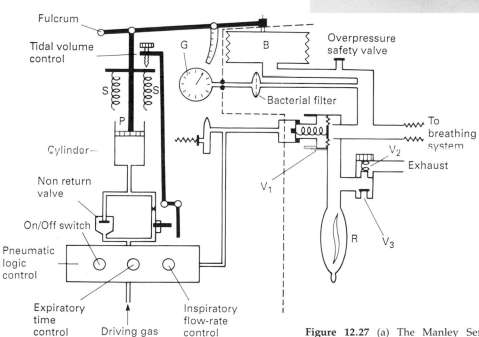

(b)

**Figure 12.27** (a) The Manley Servovent ventilator. (b) Working principles (see text). The portion to the right of the dotted line is detachable for sterilization.

B. During the inspiratory phase, P is returned by a pair of springs S, and B closes, driving the gas to the patient. The inspiratory flow rate control operates by varying a flow restrictor which 'strangles' the exhaust from the cylinder thus slowing down its return movement and determining inspiratory time.

Within the breathing attachment there is a diaphragm-operated valve $V_1$, which is closed during inspiration by pressure from the control unit. Thus, during the inspiratory phase the gases from the bellows can pass only to the patient (or to atmosphere via the safety valve). The airway pressure is shown on a manometer G. As the piston which compresses the bellows is powerful, the ventilator is classified as high-powered. During expiration, $V_1$ opens and the exhaled gases from the patient can pass into the reservoir R. They may be augmented by the fresh gas flow (FGF). As B opens, gases are drawn from R and from the FGF. If there is insufficient volume, air may be drawn in through a non-return valve $V_3$. An excess of pressure in the reservoir is emptied by a relief valve $V_2$. It will be seen, therefore, that during the expiratory phase, and also when the control unit is turned off, the patient is able to breathe backwards and forwards into the reservoir, the gases being augmented by the FGF and excess gases being voided through $V_2$, which must *always* be kept open.

The whole of the breathing attachment, including the bellows, may be detached and sterilized by autoclaving. G is isolated by a bacterial filter, since it is not suitable for this treatment.

The driving gas requirement is fairly heavy (the manufacturers claim an average of 12 litres/min). However, this ventilator may be used in conjunction with a circle absorption system and so the anaesthetic gas flow rate may be low.

## The Oxford ventilator (Fig. 12.28)

The Oxford ventilator is high-powered, time-cycled and may be used for both anaesthesia and intensive care. It is powered by compressed air and controlled by a pneumatic system (Chapter 2). A bellows B containing the aneasthetic gases is operated by a pneumatic cylinder C. The direction of movement of the cylinder is controlled by a spool valve $S_1$. A second spool valve $S_2$ controls a smaller cylinder V which operates the expiratory valve of the breathing system. There is a lever on the piston rod of C which operates a trip valve, $T_1$ or $T_2$, at each end of its movement. The lengths of the inspiratory and expiratory excursion are thereby variable, altering the tidal volume of the ventilator (i.e. that volume of gas expelled from the bellows). The inspiratory and

expiratory flow rates are adjusted by needle valves which 'strangle' the exhaust from the cylinder, thereby slowing its movement. The entire patient gas system may be removed from the ventilator for sterilization and the junction between the expiratory valve and the actuator is magnetic.

## Servo 900 Series ventilator

The Servo 900 Series ventilator is a sophisticated multi-mode ventilator (Fig. 12.29). Many of its functions are more relevant to an intensive care environment and are beyond the remit of this book. However when used to ventilate anaesthetized patients it is most frequently used as a pneumatically driven, electronically controlled minute volume divider.

Fresh gas from the anaesthetic machine is fed into the low-pressure entry port sited on the side of the ventilator and is stored in a spring loaded 2-litre bellows. The spring load can be varied with the front panel key to a maximum working prssure of 11.8 kPa/120 cmH$_2$O (9.8 kPa/100 cmH$_2$O for the now obsolete 900B series) although a much lower pressure of 5.88 kPa/60–65 cmH$_2$O is normally used. If the bellows is overfilled, excess gas is vented through a pressure-relief valve linked to this bellows. This pressurized gas supplies the inspiratory flow to the patient; hence in this mode, the fresh gas flow from the anaesthetic machine should be set slightly (12–15%) in excess of ventilatory parameters set up on the ventilator so that the bellows remain optimally filled.

Alternatively, high pressure gas (420 kPa in the UK) from a blender (nitrous oxide/oxygen) and a special high pressure vaporizer may be fed into the bellows via the high pressure inlet port, which is also sited on the side of the ventilator. Prior to entering the bellows, the gas passes through a demand valve that ensures that when any gas is removed from the reservoir bag it is immediately refilled by gas from the blender and vaporizer. This extends the role of the ventilator from that of a simple minute volume divider to that of a machine that can respond to the extra gas demand caused by a patient breathing spontaneously, either with or between, controlled tidal volumes delivered by the ventilator (synchronized intermittent mandatory ventilation (SIMV) models 900C and E). It also allows a patient's respiratory efforts to be assisted by a variable amount when the 'pressure support' mode is selected (Servo 900C and D).

The ventilator is time cycled and so has a control switch for the cycling *rate* measured in breaths per minute. The inspiratory phase for each cycle is

**Figure 12.28** (a) The Oxford Mark 2 ventilator. Note the electronic digital readout of functions, including inspiratory and expiratory times and respiratory rate. (b) Working principles B, bellows; C, power cylinder; $S_1$, main spool valve; $S_2$, second spool valve; $T_1$, $T_2$, trip valves; V, cylinder controlling expiratory valve. A third spool valve, connected in parallel with the other two, controls the electronic readout facility but has been omitted from the diagram for the sake of clarity. The portion to the right of the diagonal line is detachable for sterilization.

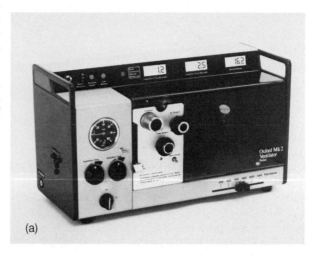

(a)

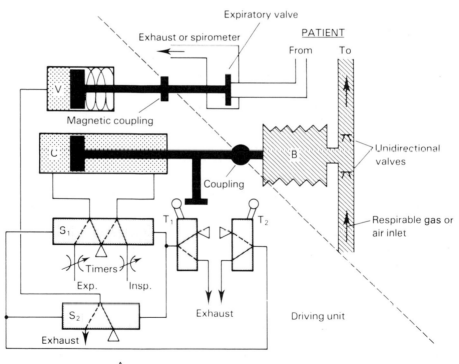

(b)

(a)

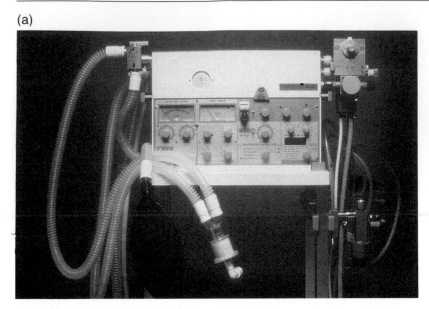

**Figure 12.29** (a) The Servo 900 C Series ventilator. (b) Working principles: A, high pressure gas supply inlet; B, low pressure gas supply inlet; C, demand valve (this is tripped mechanically by the base plate of the bellows to maintain the bellows at two thirds full); D, fuel cell housing; E, non-return valve on the low pressure gas inlet; F, inlet filter housing; G, spring-loaded bellows; H, over-pressure safety valve (set at 120 cmH$_2$O); J, inspiratory pneumotachograph; K, inspiratory pincer valve; L, inspiratory pressure transducer; M, expiratory pneumotachograph; N, expiratory pressure transducer; O, expiratory valve.

(b)

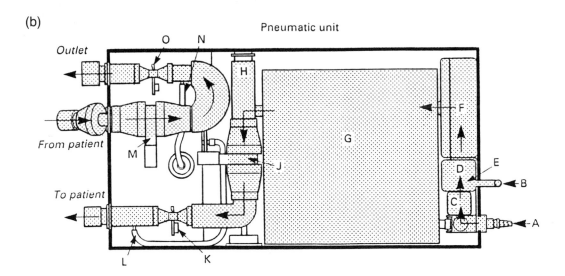

Pneumatic unit

varied by an *inspiratory time* switch which can be supplemented by a variable end-inspiratory pause (*pause time* control switch). As the total cycle time is predetermined, any inspiratory adjustments are made at the expense of expiratory time. The other major parameter that can be adjusted is *minute volume*. The control switch for this is calibrated in litres/min.

The tidal volume delivered during each inspiratory cycle is therefore derived electronically from the settings for minute volume and rate set on the control panel, i.e.

Tidal volume = Minute volume ÷ Rate.

*INSPIRATORY PHASE.* When the electronically operated inspiratory valve (pincer action) opens, gas leaves the bellows and enters the patient's breathing system via a flow transducer. The pincer action of the valve is continuously adjusted via the machine electronics to produce a variety of inspiratory times, flow rates and patterns. The inspiratory flow may be adjusted to provide constant (square-wave), accelerating (ramp-shaped or decelerating (reverse ramp-shaped) patterns depending on the ventilatory mode selected. The flow transducer continuously measures the inspiratory gas flow rate and feeds this information back to the pincer valve control unit. When the desired tidal volume has been delivered, the inspiratory valve closes. If an inspiratory hold facility (variable from 0 to 33% of the initial inspiratory time, on model 900C only) is required, the expiratory valve also remains closed in order to facilitate this.

EXPIRATORY PHASE. The expiratory pathway of the ventilator also contains an electronically operated pincer valve (the expiratory valve), a flow transducer and an airways pressure transducer. Exhalation occurs when this pincer valve opens, allowing gas in the patient's lungs to escape through this pathway. The duration of this expiratory phase is again time cycled. The electronics linked to the flow transducer in the expiratory limb computes expired minute volumes and provides the necessary information to the high and low expired volume alarms.

The airway pressure transducer in the expiratory limb (also linked to a high pressure alarm) is used via the control panel to close prematurely the expiratory valve towards the end of expiration when a PEEP facility is required. It also senses spontaneous respiratory activity and allows the patient to trigger the ventilator to a degree permitted by the settings on the trigger sensitivity control.

*Control panels.* The front panel on the machine is divided into two sections.

PANEL FOR SETTING VENTILATORY PARAMETERS. This main section houses the controls for setting ventilatory parameters as described above; i.e. minute volume, respiratory rate, flow pattern, inspiratory time, inspiratory hold and PEEP.

ALARM PANEL. The various alarms (see above) for high and low airways pressure and expired minute volume are grouped together with visual display meters for these.

The ventilator, in the anaesthetic mode described above is classified as a high-powered ventilator which is used as an inspiratory and expiratory time-cycled minute volume divider.

ALTERNATIVE VENTILATORY MODES. The Servo 900B (now obsolete) and 900C support a number of other ventilatory modes [intermittent mandatory ventilation (IMV), synchronized intermittent mandatory ventilation (SIMV) and pressure support] which increases the capabilities of these ventilators beyond that of a minute volume divider. These are not described here as these modes are mostly used in an intensive care environment and outside the remit of this book. The exception to this is the 'Pressure Control' mode on the 900C model which allows the ventilator to be used in paediatric anaesthesia. In this mode the lungs of the patient are ventilated to a desired pressure irrespective of the size of any deliberate leak caused by the uncuffed endotracheal

tube. The (now obsolete) 900B model does not have this facility but can be easily adapted by (a) reducing the operating pressure in the bellows to the inspiratory pressure required and (b) by setting the minute volume control well in excess of that anticipated. The ventilator will now cycle when the pre-set pressure is reached and will not depend on the anticipated tidal volume set by the ventilator.

*Servo 900D.* The Servo 900D is a scaled-down version of the 900C ventilator, losing some of the sophisticated ventilatory modes, the variable inspiratory wave forms and the variable inspiratory hold facility.

MANUAL VENTILATION/SPONTANEOUS RESPIRATION (ALL MODELS). A manual ventilation mode setting is provided on the control panel. However, in order to function this requires the fitment of a dedicated accessory consisting of bag mount, reservoir bag and a one-way valve to the inspiratory limb of the patient breathing system. In this mode the ventilator supplies gas to the reservoir bag until the pressure within it reaches $0.4 \text{ kPa}/4(\text{cmH}_2\text{O})$ as measured by an inspiratory pressure transducer, at which time gas flow ceases. If the patient makes a respiratory effort, the expiratory valve closes, gas is withdrawn from the reservoir bag and fresh gas enters the lungs. The ventilator senses the pressure drop in the bag and replenishes the lost gas. When the patient exhales, the one-way valve in the bag mount accessory prevents expired gas contaminating the inspiratory limb, and so gas escapes through the expiratory valve, which now opens.

If the bag is manually compressed, the expiratory valve closes in response to the pressure rise and gas in the bag is directed to the patient. When the bag is released, the ventilator senses the pressure drop in the bag and replenishes the lost gas. The sequence of events in expiration is the same as described above during spontaneous respiration.

## Penlon Nuffield 400 Series ventilator (Fig. 12.30)

The Penlon Nuffield 400 is classified as a bag squeezer and is used to power Mapleson D/E and circle systems. It consists of a suspended bellows arrangement within a Perspex canister (the bellows is attached to the top of the canister and travels downwards during filling as opposed to a rising bellows arrangement in which the bellows is attached to the base of its canister and travels upwards during filling). The control unit for the ventilator is also positioned on the top of the bellows and canister. It may be used in either of two modes.

(a)

(b)

Early model
arrangement 6

11

Gases to
breathing
circuit

10

Bellows being
compressed

Spill valve
closed

(c)

Gases from
breathing
circuit

Spill valve
open

Excess
anaesthetic
gas

Bellows
expanding

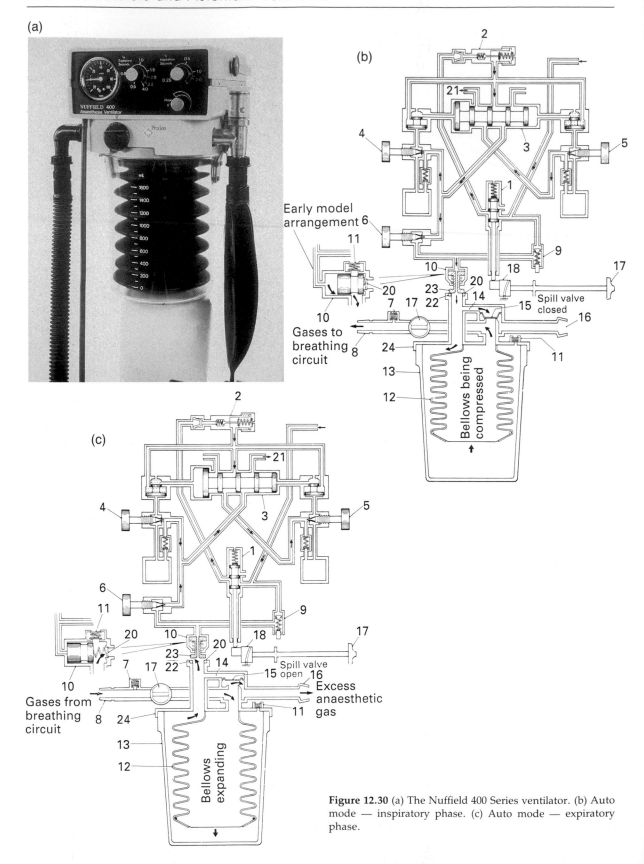

**Figure 12.30** (a) The Nuffield 400 Series ventilator. (b) Auto mode — inspiratory phase. (c) Auto mode — expiratory phase.

*Auto mode.* The drive unit is both powered and controlled pneumatically. When the manual/empty/ auto valve (17) is set to the auto position, this action moves the eccentrically positioned cam (18) to operate a valve (1). This allows driving gas from a compressed gas source at 290–650 kPa (42–95 psi) to enter the drive unit via a pressure regulator (2) and simultaneously supply a spool valve (3) and a logic circuit that controls inspiratory (4) and expiratory timers (5). The spool valve has a bias position in the expiratory phase position when signals are received simultaneously from the inspiratory and expiratory timers. This prevents the spool being stuck in a mid position at any time in the cycle. The adjustable timers provide alternatively pulsed signals to change the position of the spool valve (3) and so control the inspiratory and expiratory phase times.

INSPIRATORY PHASE. Driving gas passes across the spool in the 'open' position to an adjustable flow control (needle) valve (6). From here, it enters the bellows canister through an inflating valve (10). At the same time a piston in the inflating valve is activated by the driving gas and closes the driving gas exhaust port (20). The driving gas entering the canister compresses the bellows, displacing patient gas contained in the bellows out into the patient breathing system connection port (8). The driving gas also acts on a spill valve (15), preventing patient gas from escaping via the exhaust port during this phase. A fixed setting relief valve (4.4 kPa/45 cmH$_2$O) is built into the canister lid to protect the canister against excessive driving gas pressure.

EXPIRATORY PHASE. When the spool is moved to the expiratory position, the driving gas contained in the bellows canister is exhausted to atmosphere via a port (21). The suspended bellows is dragged downwards by a small weight in the bellows base, allowing patient breathing system gas to re-enter the bellows. When the bellows is maximally filled, surplus breathing system gas is dumped through the now opened spill valve (15) to atmosphere.

The ventilator is controlled for rate by the two pneumatic timers, which are calibrated in seconds. Inspiratory tidal volume is controlled by the needle valve (6) and can be read off the calibration scale on the bellows canister.

The ventilator is classified as an inspiratory and expiratory time cycled high-powered ventilator, which functions as a 'bag squeezer'.

*Manual mode.* In the manual mode, the drive unit and bellows arrangement are isolated from the patient breathing system which is now connected directly to a reservoir bag and an optional adjus- table pressure limiting (APL) valve attached to the ventilator.

The suspended bellows arrangement, while allowing convenient placement of the controls at the top of the ventilator housing, has some drawbacks. Prior to connecting a breathing system, the suspended bellows arrangement will be full of air that may need to be purged. An 'empty' setting between the auto and manual modes can be used to compress the bellows and lock the bellows closed in order to purge the system of air.

The suspended bellows uses an internal weight to drag the bellows downwards during the expiratory cycle. If the bellows is split, driving gas could enter the expanded bellows during the inspiratory phase and produce large delivered tidal volumes in excess of those anticipated. Rising bellows arrangements are safer in this respect. However, a bellows leak may be detected by using the 'empty' setting to compress the bellows. A gas-tight bellows remains compressed, but a leaky bellows sucks in air through the leak and gradually expands. This test should be performed as part of the 'cockpit drill' prior to the start of any anaesthetic.

### Penlon AV Series 500 ventilator (Fig. 12.31)

This ventilator, also classified as a bag squeezer, consists of a control unit supplying driving gas to a Perspex canister containing a rising bellows arrangement (as opposed to the Nuffield 400 arrangement, which has a suspended bellows). The driving gas is divided into aliquots by the control unit, and when fed into the gas-tight Perspex container displaces an equal volume of gas from the bellows unit into the patient connection port.

The control unit is pneumatically driven, but controlled both mechanically and electronically. Figure 12.31b illustrates the working arrangement. Drive gas from a 205–410 kPa (30–60 psi) pressure source (1) passes through a 40 µg particulate filter to a pressure regulator (4) reducing the gas supply pressure to approximately 170 kPa (25 psi). This in turn supplies the *main drive gas valve* (5), which is a large orifice pneumatically driven On/Off valve. This valve is controlled by a secondary electrically operated (solenoid) valve (6), the *drive gas pilot valve*, which opens at the beginning of inspiration and uses its own gas supply (taken from the main drive line) to activate and open the *main drive gas valve*. During inspiration, gas from the *main drive gas valve* is delivered to a *variable orifice needle valve* (7), which determines the gas flow to the bellows container. The needle valve is in turn controlled by an electric motor (9), and *valve position feed-back*

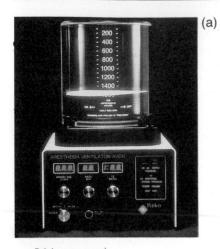

(a)

**Figure 12.31** (a) The Penlon AV 500 Series ventilator. (b) Working principles. (See text.)

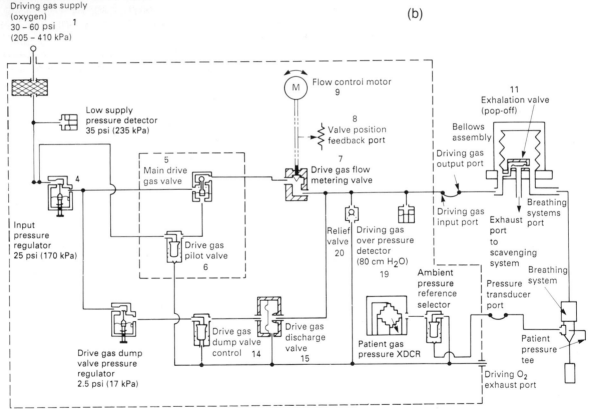

(b)

potentiometer (8). This gas pressurizes the bellows container, closes the *exhalation 'pop off' valve* (11) and causes the bellows to be compressed. This moves the gas contained inside into the attached breathing system. At the end of the inspiratory phase the electrically operated *drive gas pilot valve* closes, shutting the *main drive gas valve*. At the same time the *drive gas discharge valve* (15) opens, venting the driving gas stored in the bellows container to atmosphere. This allows gas from the breathing system back into the bellows.

When the bellows fills completely, excess gas is dumped out through the exhaust port, which is now open. The *drive gas discharge valve* (15) is, of course, shut as it is activated, during the inspiratory phase, by the *drive gas dump valve control* (14). Ventilation settings on the front panel work a microprocessor unit, which in turn controls units (6), (8), (9) and (15) to produce the desired minute volume, rate, and inspiratory/expiratory ratio. The delivered tidal volume can be measured approximately from the calibration on the bellows chamber. A pressure transducer is connected to the patient port in order to monitor breathing system pressure and, via the microprocessor unit, to activate alarms for high and low breathing system pressures. When the high-pressure alarm is activated, the microprocessor also closes the *main drive gas valve* and opens the *drive gas discharge valve*. This prevents further inspiration and allows unimpeded patient exhalation. The value for the high pressure alarm can be set anywhere between 1.96 and 6.86 kPa (20 and 70 cmH$_2$O) via a control on the back panel. Further safety features include a *pressure relief valve* (20) which opens at 8.8 kPa (90 cmH$_2$O) and a *pressure detector* (19) which, via the microprocessor, stops the gas drive if the drive gas pressure exceeds 7.84 kPa (80 cmH$_2$O). The ventilator is thus a time-cycled high-powered ventilator which functions as a bag squeezer.

### The M & IE Carden Ventmaster ventilator (Fig. 12.32)

This ventilator, also classified as a high-powered bag squeezer, consists of a pneumatic control unit intermittently supplying driving gas to a perspex canister containing a rising bellows arrangement.

*Pneumatic control unit.* Driving gas (air or oxygen) (1) at 420 kPa (60 psi) pressure enters the gas power inlet and immediately divides into two, one line feeding the On/Off switch valve (2) and the other feeding the PEEP unit (9) and PEEP control valves (10) (see later). This PEEP facility has been omitted from later versions because of its high gas consumption.

From the On/Off switch the driving gas divides again, one line feeding the main two-way valve (3) which supplies pressurizing gas to the bellows canister, and the second feeding the timing unit operating this valve.

The timing unit consists of a cycle generator (4) generating pressure pulses whose cycling rate is controlled by two pneumatic timers (6, 7) (the inspiratory and expiratory controls). These pressure pulses act in conjunction with a pilot valve to switch the main two way valve on and off. When the valve is switched on, driving gas is diverted to a flow controller (needle valve) (8) which in turn supplies a venturi. The venturi entrains ambient air and accelerates the now combined driving gas through a non-return valve into the spool block. Here it enters the bellows canister and displaces an equal volume of patient gas contained in the bellows into an attached patient breathing system. When the main

two-way valve closes (controlled by the cycle generator), the natural compliance of the patient's lungs pushes breathing system gas back into the rising bellows. When the bellows is full and the pressure therein exceeds 0.20 kPa (3 cmH$_2$O), a weighted one-way valve is lifted and excess gas vented through the exhaust port. The supplementary driving gas supply is connected to an opposing jet in the expiratory port which, when switched on, produces a variable and adjustable amount of PEEP (positive end expiratory pressure).

The above describes the ventilator arranged for use with circle and Mapleson D systems. However, one model is available with a fresh gas input to the bellows which converts it to a Mapleson A arrangement. Exhaled patient gas returns to the bellows to be mixed with fresh gas which allows adjustment of rebreathed carbon dioxide (by increasing or decreasing the fresh gas flow).

This version has a switch arrangement to convert it from a Mapleson A to Mapleson D system, which, regrettably, increases the complexity and potential for inappropriate employment.

A self-inflating bag can also be attached to the system to provide an alternative method of bellows compression when the ventilator is switched off, or if there is a failure of the driving gas.

*Safety features.* The control unit has two mechanical overpressure relief valves fitted to prevent barotrauma to a patient.

### Ohmeda OAV Series model 7710 (Fig. 12.33)

This ventilator consists of a rising bellows arrangement, delivering patient gas to a breathing system, and is driven by a mechanical arm. The movement of the mechanical arm is operated by a two-way pneumatically operated piston to which the gas supply is electronically controlled. The bellows unit is constructed as an easily removable, autoclavable cassette which is available in two functionally different forms.

*The mechanical arm (see Fig. 12.33b).* The mechanical arm is connected to a two-way pneumatic piston, the direction and duration of travel of which is governed by two solenoid valves (5 and 6) controlling the gas supply. The speed of travel however is controlled by two needle valves in the gas suppy (8 and 10). The operation of the solenoid valves is in turn controlled by an electronic control unit.

*Control unit of model 7710 (see Fig. 12.33b).* The mechanical arm is linked through a rack and pinion

(a)

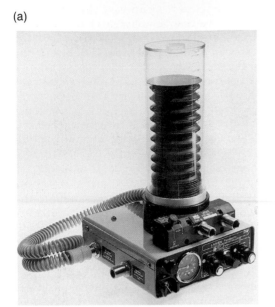

(b)

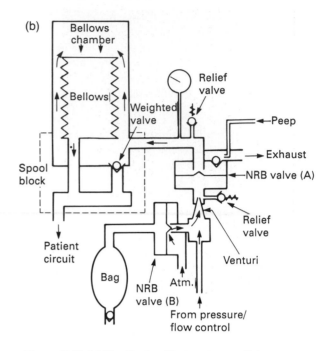

**Figure 12.32** (a) The Carden Ventmaster ventilator. (b) Working principles of the pneumatic control unit (see text). (c) Details of the bellows driving circuit.

(c)

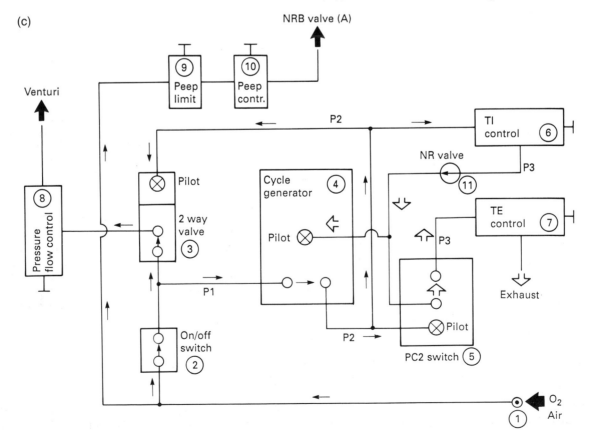

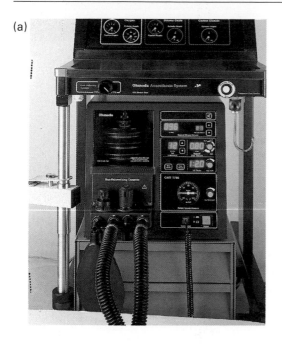

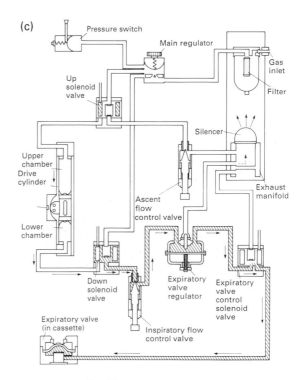

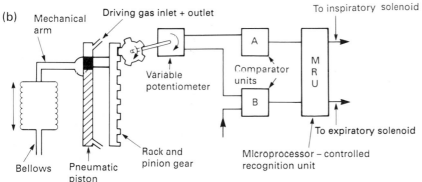

**Figure 12.33** (a) The Ohmeda OAV Series model 7710. (b) The pneumatic circuit controlling the mechanical arm. (c) Schematic diagram of the control unit.

to a variable potentiometer which transmits a voltage signal (depending on the position of the mechanical arm) to two comparator units. Comparator unit B compares the voltage output from the potentiometer when the bellows is fully closed, which a similar reference voltage built into the comparator and which is set at the factory. When the two voltages are the same, the control unit microprocessor recognizes that the bellows is empty. Comparator A receives voltages from (a) the potentiometer when the bellows is ascending and (b) the tidal volume control on the master unit. When these two become equal the control unit microprocessor recognizes that the bellows is now filled with the desired tidal volume and operates the appropriate

solenoids in order to deliver that tidal volume. The control unit also receives information from a respirometer and pressure gauge which are connected to the attached patient breathing system when in use. It evaluates these and subsequently displays values for expired tidal volume, respiratory rate, expired minute volume and inspiratory/expiratory ratio. The unit also includes alarms for high and low pressure and low expired minute volume.

## Ohmeda OAV Series model 7750 ventilator (Fig. 12.34)

This ventilator operates in a similar fashion to the Series 7710 with three exceptions. Firstly, it includes

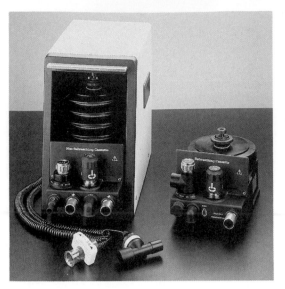

(ai)

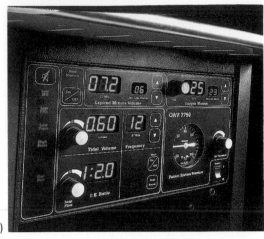

(aii)

**Figure 12.34** (ai) Two versions of the bellows unit for the Ohmeda OAV Series model 7750. (aii) Master control unit. (b) Working principles with rebreathing cassette. (c) Working principles with non-rebreathing cassette. (d) Manual ventilation in non-rebreathing mode. (e) Schematic diagram of the control unit.

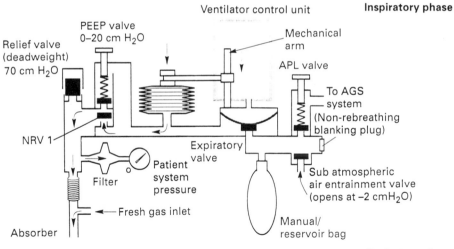

**Inspiratory phase**

Ventilator control unit

Mechanical arm

APL valve

PEEP valve 0–20 cm $H_2O$

Relief valve (deadweight) 70 cm $H_2O$

To AGS system (Non-rebreathing blanking plug)

NRV 1

Expiratory valve

Sub atmospheric air entrainment valve (opens at –2 cm$H_2O$)

Filter

Patient system pressure

Fresh gas inlet

Manual/ reservoir bag

Absorber

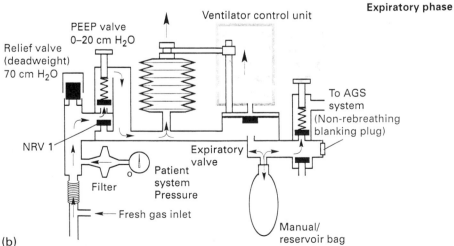

**Expiratory phase**

Ventilator control unit

PEEP valve 0–20 cm $H_2O$

Relief valve (deadweight) 70 cm $H_2O$

To AGS system (Non-rebreathing blanking plug)

NRV 1

Expiratory valve

Filter

Patient system Pressure

Fresh gas inlet

Manual/ reservoir bag

(b)

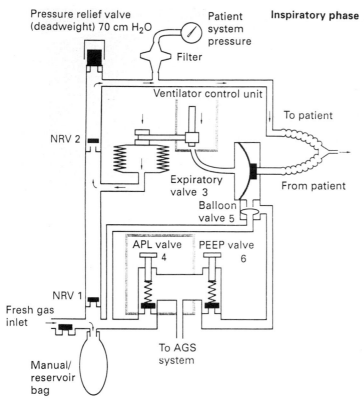

(ci)

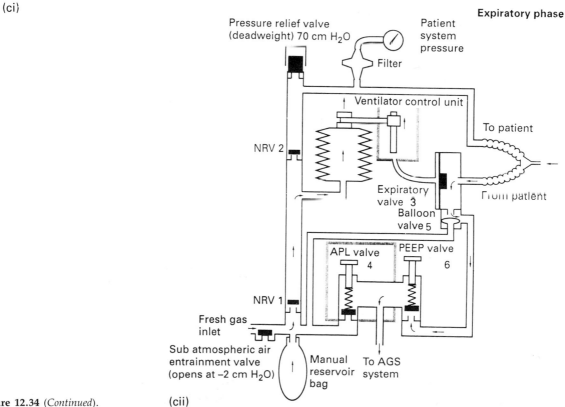

**Figure 12.34** (*Continued*).    (cii)

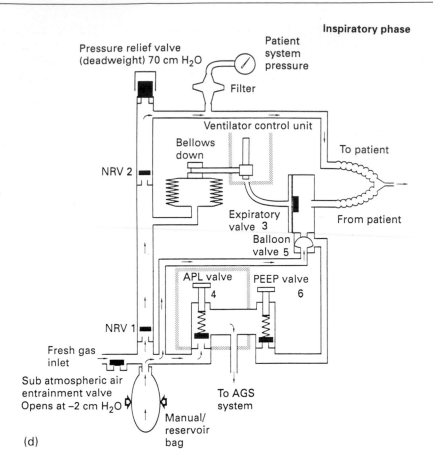

(d)

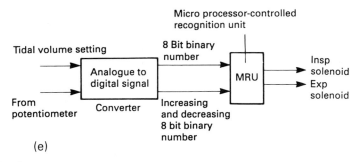

(e)

**Figure 12.34** (*Continued*).

a fuel cell oxygen analyser in the system. Secondly, the bellows unit is physically separate from the master control unit (Fig. 12.34a) and is connected only by an 'umbilical' cable. Thirdly, the comparator units have been replaced by a more sophisticated system for controlling bellows travel. In this system, the potentiometer voltages produced by bellows travel are continuously received by an analogue-to-digital converter (see Chapter 2). This device converts input voltages to a digital set of binary

numbers. The converter also receives the voltage input from the tidal volume control. The digital outputs from the A/D converter are fed into a microprocessor which continuously compares the numbers produced with a factory pre-set reference number for the empty bellows position. The microprocessor in turn activates the solenoid valves which govern the duration and direction of travel of the pneumatic piston.

Because some of the binary numbers are factory

pre-set (zero bellows volume setting) the master unit and the bellows unit must be treated as a matched pair and will not function if either is attached to a different unit. In addition to the displays and alarms seen on the 7710, the 7750 also has a facility for the inclusion of a fuel cell oxygen analyser and display. In fact, if the analyser is not connected to the control unit an alarm will continuously operate and cannot be switched off while the ventilator is functioning.

*Rebreathing cassette (see Fig. 12.34b).* This cassette has a single hose connection to a patient breathing system (Mapleson D/E or circle system), At the beginning of the inspiratory phase, the bellows is compressed by the mechanical arm and delivers the patient gas through a non-return valve (1) into the patient breathing system. The expiratory valve (2) is closed by gas pressure from the control unit. If an inspiratory hold facility on the control unit is selected, the bellows and the expiratory valve are held closed for a further 25% of the initially selected inspiratory time. At the start of expiration, the expiratory valve is released, opening the expiratory limb (including the reservoir bag) and the bellows is driven upwards by the mechanical arm. The elastic recoil of the lungs pushes patient system gas through an opened PEEP valve, back towards the rising bellows, which fills with a mixture of this gas and gas stored in the reservoir bag. At the end of the travel of the bellows, surplus patient system gas initially refills the reservoir bag and any excess leaves via the APL valve (3) to be scavenged.

Safety features include a 6.86 kPa (70 cmH$_2$O) relief dead weight valve (5) and a pressure gauge (6) which is linked to the control unit (see Fig. 12.34d). In this mode the ventilator is a high-powered, time-cycled bag squeezer.

*Non-rebreathing cassette (Fig. 12.34c).* The ventilator can be adapted to operate in a non-rebreathing mode using the appropriate cassette. Fresh gas enters the system and is stored in a reservoir bag (1). When the bellows unit is made to expand, the negative pressure created sucks gas from the reservoir bag through a non-rebreathing valve (NRV 1) into the bellows.

During the inspiratory phase, this gas is pushed out of the bellows and via a non-return valve (NRV 2) into the inspiratory limb of an attached breathing system. At the same time, the control unit pneumatically closes the expiratory valve (3). During this inspiratory phase the continuous flow of fresh gas fills the reservoir bag and any surplus spills over via an APL valve (4) to the exhaust port and

scavenging system. At the end of inspiration, if the inspiratory hold facility is activated, the bellows and expiratory valve are held closed for a further 25% of the initial inspiratory time. At the start of expiration, the expiratory valve is released and the elastic recoil of the lungs pushes gas into the patient system expiratory limb, past the expiratory valve (3) past the balloon valve (5), through the PEEP facility (6), and out through the expiratory port. At any time during the expiratory phase, the patient can breathe spontaneously through the inspiratory part of the system via the reservoir bag and non-rebreathing valves 1 and 2. The inspiratory circuit also houses an air entrainment port so that if fresh gas flow is inadequate, air will be entrained. The safety features include a pressure relief dead weight valve of 6.84 kPa (70 cmH$_2$O) and a pressure gauge linked to the control unit. In this mode the ventilator is a high-powered, time-cycled minute volume divider.

*Manual ventilation (Fig. 12.34d).* This can be achieved by switching the control unit off, partially or fully closing the APL valve, and squeezing the reservoir bag. The balloon valve acts as a subsidiary expiratory valve, which is activated by the reservoir bag during manual ventilation. In the manual mode, the drive unit and the bellows arrangement are isolated from the patient breathing system, the latter being connected directly to a reservoir bag and an optional adjustable pressure limiting (APL) valve which is attached to the cassette.

### Cape TC50 ventilator (Fig. 12.35)

This ventilator consists of a bellows unit whose travel is controlled by a mechanical arm linked to a variable-speed, low geared electric motor (Fig. 12.35b).

*INSPIRATORY PHASE.* The mechanical arm linking the electric motor to the bellows has two components. When the electric motor is switched on, it causes the crank to rotate. The latter pushes the inner rod of the mechanical arm forward until it engages the outer arm. At this stage the mechanical arm starts to compress the bellows. The speed of the electric motor controls the cycle time and is adjusted by a knob on the front panel of the machine. The ventilator can therefore be regarded as time cycled. As the motor is powerful, the machine is capable of generating high pressure (high-powered ventilator) and when connected to a patient breathing system requires the fitment of a safety valve.

*EXPIRATORY PHASE.* At the end of the inspiratory phase, the mechanical arm retreats as a result of the rotary action of the eccentric crank. The bellows is re-expanded by the spring to a point fixed by the tidal volume control which acts as a mechanical stop (see Fig. 12.35b). At this point the two components of the mechanical arm separate, allowing the crank to complete its rotation to be ready for the next inspiration. The mode of operation of the arm is referred to as a lost motion drive.

*INSPIRATORY/EXPIRATORY RATIO.* The inspiratory/expiratory ratio varies according to the tidal volume selected from 1 to 8 at a minimum tidal volume setting, to 1 to 2 at the maximum volume selected. For example, at low tidal volume settings, the inner rod of the mechanical arm has a long 'inspiratory' travel before it picks up the outer arm in order to compress the bellows. This effectively delays the inspiratory phase and prolongs the expiratory phase.

The ventilator is usually supplied with a 'gas entrainment block' for direct connection to the bellows port and this includes an overpressure relief valve (factory pre-set at 45 cmH$_2$O). The block has an outlet port which may then be connected to an appropriate breathing system (see below). As the electric motor is powerful, the ventilator is regarded as being high-powered. The cycling rate is controlled by the speed of the electric motor, which can be varied. It is therefore time-cycled.

*Ventilatory modes.*

● Non-rebreathing system (System A). Bellows

(a)

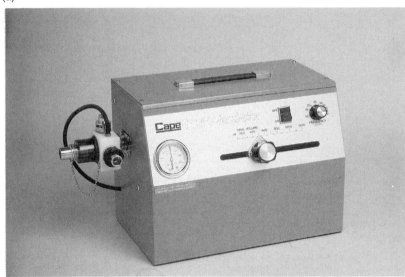

**Figure 12.35** (a) The Cape TC50 ventilator. (b) Working principles (see text). (c) Ventilatory modes: (upper) non-rebreathing system; (lower) Mapleson D system.

(b)

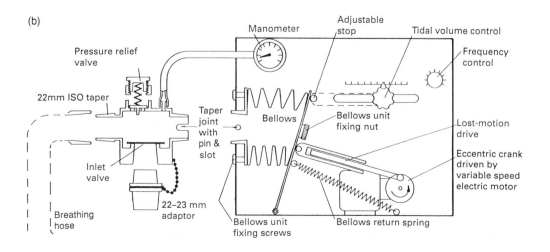

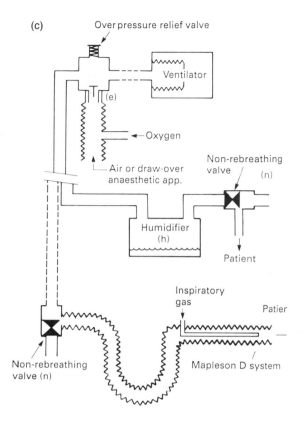

**Figure 12.35** (*Continued*).

excursion entrains respirable gas from the valve inlet (e) and then directs it into the breathing system which has a non-rebreathing valve (n) positioned close to the patient. The respirable gas can either be air, or with a suitable attachment, an air and oxygen mixture, with or without anaesthetic agents from a drawover system (Triservice, see Chapter 24). A humidifier (h) may also be added for intensive care situations. The ventilator with this system in use is popular with the Armed Services for anaesthesia and intensive care applications under battlefield conditions.

- Mapleson 'D' system. The non-rebreathing valve may alternatively be connected directly to the entrainment valve block and then attached via a suitable length of hosing to the reservoir bag port of a Mapleson D system so that it behaves as a 'bag squeezer'.
- Some interesting 'home made' attachments have been described to allow the ventilator to be used in a circle system. These have been mainly for use in developing countries where the availability of volatile anaesthetic agents and compressed gases is at a premium. However there is

no purpose-built device made by the manufacturers.

## Intermittent blowers

These ventilators are driven by a continuous flow of gases or air, a pressure of 300–400 kPa (45–60 psi) usually being required. Part of the driving gas may be delivered to the patient but, by means of an injector, air, oxygen or anaesthetic gases may be added to it.

### The Bird Mark 7 ventilator (Fig. 12.36)

The Bird Mark 7 ventilator is given as an example of an intermittent blower ventilator. It is not suitable for anaesthesia unless it is used in conjunction with a special anaesthesia assistor-controller attachment, which is essentially a 'bag in a bottle' device. It is more useful for the long-term ventilation of patients on oxygen, air or air–oxygen mixtures, and for respiratory therapy. It is driven by medical compressed air or oxygen.

The transparent plastic case C is divided into two

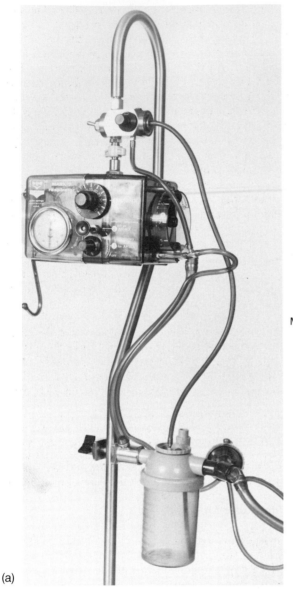

(a)

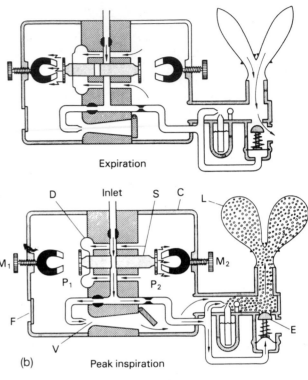

Expiration

Peak inspiration

(b)

**Figure 12.36** (a) The Bird Mark 7 ventilator. (b) Working principles, C, transparent plastic case; D, diaphragm; S, shuttle valve; $P_1$, $P_2$, soft-iron plates; $M_1$, $M_2$, magnets; E, pneumatic expiratory valve; L, lungs; V, venturi; F, air inlet filter. (See text.)

compartments by the diaphragm D. Attached to D is a shuttle valve S, at either end of which are soft-iron plates $P_1$ and $P_2$. By virtue of the attraction of each of these plates to magnets, a bistable mechanism is created. The distance between each magnet and the adjacent plate (and hence the force of attraction between them) can be adjusted by the control knobs $M_1$ and $M_2$ at either end of the case.

During inspiration, air passes from the inlet through S not only towards the patient, through a wide-bore tube (which has been omitted in Fig. 12.36 for the sake of clarity), but also to a second tube by which it closes the pneumatic expiratory valve E. The latter tube may also supply air to a

nebulizer in order to humidify the inspiratory gases.

If required, air may be entrained by the venturi V to provide an air–oxygen mixture. It is drawn from the left-hand side of the case, which it enters through the filter F.

As the airway pressure increases during inspiration, the pressure within the right-hand side of the case rises until its influence upon D produces a force sufficient to overcome the magnetic attraction between $P_2$ and $M_2$. S, being bistable, moves rapidly to the left, $P_1$ being attracted by $M_1$.

Omitted from the diagram, for the sake of clarity, is a smaller chamber bounded by a diaphragm which is reinforced by a spring. This chamber is pressurized during the inspiratory phase, thus moving the diaphragm against the tension in the spring. During the expiratory phase the driving gas is discontinued and the spring drives the diaphragm back to its resting position, at a rate determined by the setting of an expiratory time control needle valve, which allows air to escape from the smaller chamber.

To return to the shuttle valve S, when it moves to the left it interrupts the driving gas supply, the pressure in the right-hand side of the box falls to atmospheric, E opens and the expired gases escape to the atmosphere. As the gas slowly escapes from the smaller chamber, its diaphragm is returned to its resting position and a lever linked to it impinges upon $P_1$. When it does so with sufficient force to distract $P_1$ from $M_1$, the shuttle moves to the right and the cycle recommences.

### The Pneupac and Penlon A-P ventilators (Figs 12.37–12.41)

These range from a small portable resuscitator to an anaesthetic ventilator, but since they all have the same working principle they will be described together. Each consists of a 'control module'* and a 'patient valve', and the difference between them lies in the extent to which their inspiratory and expiratory timers can be altered. For instance, the two Pneupac models for infants and children each have a single knob for tidal volume, which is actually the variable restrictor in the inspiratory timer. (Since the flow rate is constant, the tidal volume varies directly with time.) The Pneupac adult ventilator has no variables. In the Penlon A-P the inspiratory and expiratory times may be altered and there is also an inspiratory flow rate control.

The patient valve (Fig. 12.39) may be connected to the control module by a long narrow-bore tube, as in the Pneupac ventilator, or it may be attached directly to the control module, as in the Penlon A-P. It contains a piston P which in the resting state, under the control of the spring S, closes the inspiratory port and opens the expiratory port to permit exhalation.

During inspiration the pressure of gas from the control module acts on P with sufficient force to overcome S and so close the expiratory port and open the inspiratory port to the patient.

The Pneupac patient valve, in a special metal form, may be autoclaved, but the more commonly supplied plastic version should not be subjected to temperatures above 90°C. It may be sterilized by any cold chemical agent.

*The Pneupac ventilator.* The control module (Fig. 12.40) consists essentially of a spool valve B and two timers, one for the inspiratory phase (I) and the other for the expiratory phase (E). The spool valve has five ports and there is a pneumatic actuator at each end.

---

* The term 'module' is, strictly speaking, an arbitrary unit of measurement used in the building and other industries to describe and standardize the sizes of the various units used. Recently the term has been wrongly employed to describe any units that may be connected together regardless of their size and shape.

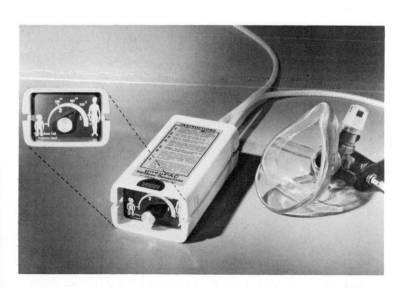

**Figure 12.37** The Pneupac child/adult ventilator.

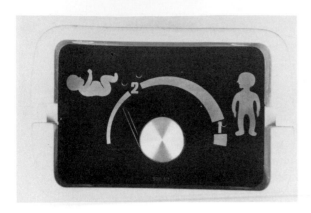

**Figure 12.38** The Pneupac child ventilator.

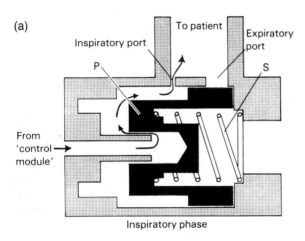

(a)

To patient

Inspiratory port

Expiratory port

P

S

From 'control module'

Inspiratory phase

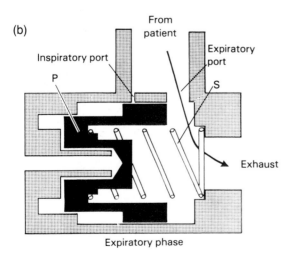

(b)

From patient

Inspiratory port

Expiratory port

P

S

Exhaust

Expiratory phase

**Figure 12.39** Working principles of the Pneupac patient valve. (a) Inspiratory phase. (b) Expiratory phase. P, Piston; S, spring. (See text.)

Each timer contains a piston (P) which is driven by gas that is metered by a flow restrictor and stored in a capacitor (C) until the pressure is high enough to actuate the piston. When this happens, driving gas is delivered to the end of the spool valve, driving the spool to the opposite end.

The driving gas, which may be oxygen, a nitrous oxide–oxygen mixture or compressed air at a pressure of 305–610 kPa (45–90 psi), enters the control module at A, passes through a filter F, a pressure regulator R and then to port 1 of B. When the spool is to the left-hand side of the control module, the gas passes from port 1 to port 2 and then on via a flow controller V to the patient valve. This is the inspiratory phase. From port 2 the gas also passes to the inspiratory timer I, where it is metered by the flow restrictor 8, which, on the inspiratory side, is variable. As the inspiratory flow rate is constant, this control determines the stroke volume. At the end of the time determined by the setting of 8, the timer operates and the gas passes via port 6 to the actuator at the left-hand end of B, driving the spool to the right-hand side of the control module. This is the end of the inspiratory phase. The driving gas entering B at port 1 now leaves by port 3 and passes to the expiratory timer E. The sequence of events now repeats itself, except that there is a fixed restrictor, 9, in the expiratory timer and therefore a constant expiratory time. When the expiratory timer operates, the gas passes to B by port 7, driving the spool back to the right-hand side of the control module, initiating the next inspiratory phase. Trapped signals (Chapter 2) are vented at ports 4 and 5.

In some versions of the control module both timers are variable, and in others both are fixed.

*The Nuffield anaesthesia ventilator, Series 200 (Fig. 12.41).* This is an elaboration of the Pneupac ventilator. Here, the patient valve is connected directly on to the control module and there are variable inspiratory and expiratory timers and a variable inspiratory flow rate control. There is also an airway manometer and an On/Off switch.

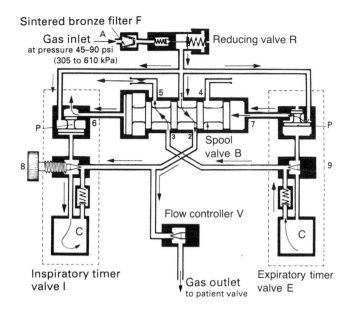

Sintered bronze filter F

Gas inlet A at pressure 45–90 psi (305 to 610 kPa)

Reducing valve R

Spool valve B

Flow controller V

Inspiratory timer valve I

Gas outlet to patient valve

Expiratory timer valve E

**Figure 12.40** The Pneupac control module. A, point of entry of driving gas; F, filter; R, pressure regulator; B, spool valve, with ports 1–5; I, inspiratory timer; 8, variable flow restrictor; 9, fixed flow restrictor; P, pistons; C, capacitors; E, expiratory timer; F, flow controller. (See text.)

**Figure 12.41** (a) The Penlon Nuffield anaesthetic ventilator. (b) Schematic diagram. Key: as Fig. 12.40. The mechanism of this is similar to that of the Pneupac. There are both variable inspiratory and expiratory timers, an airway manometer and a variable flow restrictor that controls the inspiratory flow rate.

(a)

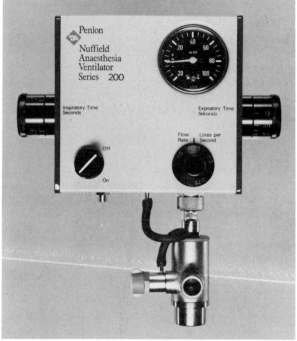

(b)

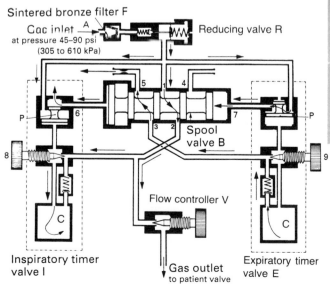

Sintered bronze filter F

Gas inlet A at pressure 45–90 psi (305 to 610 kPa)

Reducing valve R

Spool valve B

Flow controller V

Inspiratory timer valve I

Gas outlet to patient valve

Expiratory timer valve E

## Jet ventilation

There are two ways in which a high-pressure jet of gas may be used to ventilate a patient.

*1. Simple jetting — short term.* For short procedures such as bronchoscopy, a patient may be paralysed and then ventilated by applying an intermittent jet via the bronchoscope (Fig. 12.42). By the venturi effect, air is entrained by the driving gas, which is usually oxygen, at a pressure of up of 420 kPa (60 psi). The jetting may be regulated by hand. Anaesthesia is maintained intravenously.

Alternatively, for procedures such as microlaryngeal surgery, oxygen or a gaseous mixture may be delivered via a Carden tube (see Fig 9.54) which is inserted into the trachea entirely below the larynx. With only the narrow bore catheter passing through the larynx, the vocal cords may easily be seen and operated on by the surgeon. Exhaled gases pass to the atmosphere by the natural air passages.

The Carden jetting device (Fig 12.43) may be run from a 420 kPa (60 psi) pipeline outlet, from a cylinder with an appropriate pressure regulator, or from a blender for oxygen and air or oxygen and nitrous oxide. It includes a variable-pressure regulator and a pressure gauge. It is intended for short-term application only.

*2. High-frequency ventilation.* Conventional intermittent positive pressure ventilation, i.e. at rates of 10–30 cycles per minute and with tidal volumes of 500–1000 ml, frequently depresses, as well as produces fluctuations in cardiac output. During inspiration, the resultant increased alveolar pressure compresses the pulmonary vascular bed and forces the blood contained therein towards the left side of the heart, resulting in a greater stroke volume and a short lived increase in cardiac output. The compressed pulmonary vascular bed subsequently provides an increased resistance to blood flow, a fall in the blood supply to the left side of the heart and a reduction in cardiac output. During exhalation, the resultant reduction in alveolar pressure causes blood to refill the pulmonary vascular bed preferentially rather than supply the left side of the heart, a manoeuvre which further reduces cardiac output.

In the late 1960s, Swedish researchers, conducting a series of cardiovascular experiments in animals, required stable conditions for cardiac output. However the experiments necessitated that the animals were artificially ventilated. To achieve the stable cardiac output required, very small tidal volumes were chosen, along with high cycling rates so as to

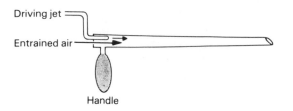

**Figure 12.42** A simple jetting device attached to a bronchoscope.

provide adequate minute ventilation without a significant rise or fluctuation in alveolar pressures. The inspiratory gas was delivered through a catheter placed at the carina (to reduce dead space), via a specially constructed ventilator. The salient features of the latter were that (a) it had a very small internal volume and (b) it developed sufficient pressure to deliver the gas rapidly through a narrow bore inspiratory hose. The design of the ventilator and breathing hose proved to be the most significant factor, as its small internal volume ensured that the very small desired tidal volume was delivered efficiently, and not reduced by being absorbed in the internal volume of the system. (The internal volume of the wide bore breathing hoses of most conventional ventilators partially absorbs inspiratory gas as a 'compression volume', reducing its speed of delivery and its intended volume.) It soon became apparent that, provided the design principles of the equipment were adhered to, the system provided effective ventilation in humans. The technique not only reduced alveolar pressures, minimizing falls in cardiac output, but also produced further benefits over conventional IPPV (see below). Furthermore, it was discovered that the inspiratory gas could be delivered (with some modification), via more conventional methods such as an endotracheal tube, rather than a catheter placed at the carina. Further investigation revealed that the technique was effective over a wide range of both respiratory rates (60–400 cycles per minute) and tidal volumes, mostly lower than the anticipated anatomical dead space. However the mechanism by which gas transport occurs is the subject of much debate and is not within the remit of this book.

*ADVANTAGES OF HIGH-FREQUENCY VENTILATION.* The claimed advantages over conventional ventilatory techniques are an efficient alveolar ventilation but with a substantial reduction in mean airway and alveolar pressures. As previously mentioned, this results in a minimal disturbance of cardiac output, and subsequent renal function. It also minimizes leaks from bronchopleural fistulae, often with an improvement in gas exchange. Furthermore, it also appears to be a more comfortable method of providing ventilatory support for patients in the intensive care unit. The most commonly used method of applying high-frequency ventilation is either to apply a high pressure gas source through a narrow bore catheter, the end of which can be placed either within the trachea, or in a cannula inserted coaxially in an endotracheal tube. Alternatively the gas may be directed into a purpose-built fine bore coaxial tube within the endotracheal tube wall. The term covering the methods described above, is 'jet ventilation'.

*Application of high-frequency jet ventilation in anaesthesia.* The high velocity of inspiratory gas leaving the jet (being turbulent) produces foreward entrainment of adjacent gas (in effect a venturi device). This system therefore does not require a cuffed endotracheal to ensure delivery of the appropriate tidal volume. If the catheter is placed distal to a disrupted airway (for example during a tracheal resection), adequate ventilation may still be achieved. Furthermore, the small bore delivery tubes increase surgical access in both pulmonary and laryngeal surgery. Also, the low delivered tidal volumes reduce lung movement, again improving surgical access as well as reducing alveolar pressures, which in turn reduces the risk of barotrauma and gas leaks from bronchopleural fistulae.

The lower alveolar pressures minimize the adverse effect of positive pressure ventilation on the central venous pressure and cardiac output, with reported benefits in cardiac and neurological surgery.

*Apparatus problems associated with high frequency jet ventilation.*
*INHALATIONAL ANAESTHESIA.* Current jet ventilation systems (the most popular method) do not readily lend themselves to providing inhalaltional anaesthesia. Although nitrous oxide and oxygen mixture can be used with the ventilators (via a high-pressure blender) there are no commerical high-pressure vaporizers available for the addition of inhalational agents. Furthermore, as the jet may

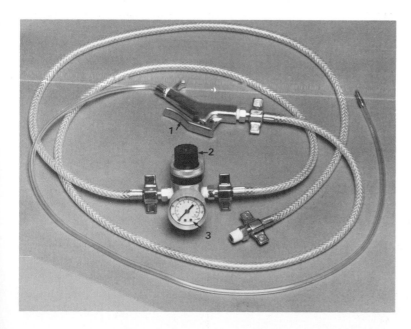

**Figure 12.43** The Carden jetting device. 1, trigger; 2, pressure regulator; 3, pressure gauge.

sometimes act as a venturi, entrained gas in any attached breathing system needs to be of the same composition as the driving gas in order to guarantee a suitably inspired oxygen concentration.

*HUMIDIFICATION.* Conventional hot-water or condenser humidifiers are impractical for use with high-frequency ventilation, as they have too high an internal volume. The small delivered tidal volumes with high-frequency ventilation get 'lost' in the humidifier and are not delivered to the patient. However, purpose-built humidifiers with a very low internal volume have been developed (see Penlon Bromsgrove humidified jet ventilator below).

*MEASUREMENT OF DELIVERED TIDAL VOLUMES.* The high respiratory rates and small tidal volumes make conventional measurement of ventilatory functions (expired tidal and minute volumes, and end tidal carbon dioxide) very difficult. A much higher reliance is placed upon blood gas measurement in this situation.

### Penlon Bromsgrove humidified jet ventilator (Fig. 12.44)

This ventilator and purpose-built humidifier goes a long way to solving the major problems of high-frequency ventilation. It is a purpose-built ventilator which is pneumatically driven but electronically controlled.

High pressure (420 kPa in the UK) respirable gas, either from a blender or a pipeline supply, is used to power the ventilator. The gas initially passes through an input solenoid (1, Fig. 12.44b) that acts as a On/Off switch as well as a safety device, since it switches off the supply under adverse conditions. The latter include excessively high gas supply pressures, excessive jet driving pressures or failure of the jet drive solenoid (4). Drive gas from this input solenoid then passes through a variable drive pressure regulator which determines the size of the jetted gas volume that is to be delivered.

The accumulator (3) downstream acts as a reservoir minimizing pressure fluctuations caused by the high instantaneous gas demand during the active jet phase. The restrictor (3a) downstream from the accumulator ensures that its contents are dispensed evenly when the jet drive solenoid (which controls the duration of the jet phase) opens. The nebulizer (5) (see Fig. 12.44) is a compact (15-ml capacity) precision Bernoulli device with a ball anvil to regulate the droplet size. The humidifying liquid is fed from a reservoir chamber (8-ml capacity) into a co-axially placed line within the stream of the jet. The working jet actively aspirates the liquid from this line (Bernouilli effect) and drives it against the ball anvil, producing water droplets between 1 and 20 μm in size. The driving gas, now suitably humidified, is dispensed downstream to the patient connection.

*Ventilator controls.*

*RATE.* This is electronically controlled and displayed on a digital indicator as cycles per minute.

*INSPIRATORY TIME.* This control governs the inspiratory time and therefore indirectly determines the I/E ratio.

*JET DRIVE PRESSURE.* This control adjusts the drive pressure and so controls the volume of jetted gas per cycle, the pressure of which is continuously registered on the gauge.

As there is no single control for delivered tidal volume, the anticipated tidal volume is therefore derived from the drive pressure, the ventilatory frequency and the inspiratory time.

*DISPLAY SELECTOR SWITCH.* This has six possible settings and displays their values via an LED. The first selects a stand-by mode which enables the user to enter the required ventilation parameters prior to using the machine. The second is a test position, and the others in order are jet drive pressure and minimum mean peak airway pressures.

*Safety features.* Patient airway pressures are monitored by a transducer via a sampling line in the patient's airway and the information is relayed to the alarm system. If the pressures exceed the user's set values, the input and jet solenoids are deactivated preventing further gas delivery until normal airway pressures are restored. The ventilator itself is protected against inadvertently high delivery pressures by a transducer in the drive pathway which deactivates the same solenoids as above when factory adjusted values are exceeded. Both systems are provided with audible and visual alarms. There is also a high inspiratory time alarm and a ventilator-inoperative alarm. The airways pressure line is intermittently purged (purge system, 9 in Fig. 12.44b) with gas during the expiratory cycle to prevent potential occlusion. The ventilator is extremely versatile providing delivered tidal volumes from 5 to 500 ml, respiratory rates between 4 and 200 cycles per minute, inspiratory times from 10 to 60% of the total cycle time and levels of humidity up to a maximum of 90 mg/litre.

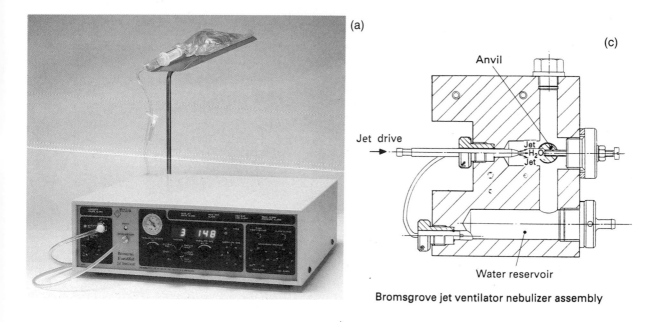

Bromsgrove jet ventilator nebulizer assembly

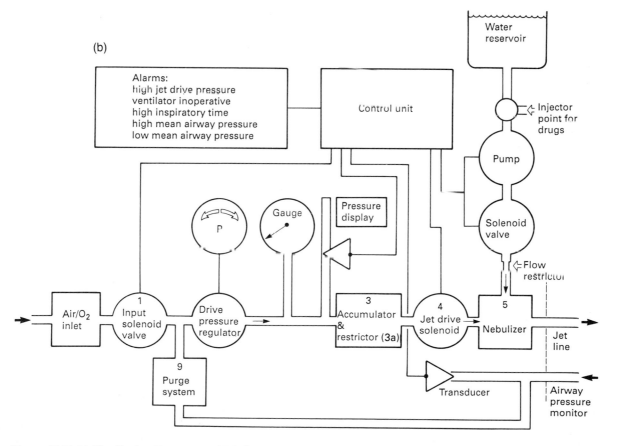

**Figure 12.44** (a) The Penlon Bromsgrove high-frequency jet ventilator. (b) Working principles (see text). (c) Schematic diagram of the nebulizer assembly.

# Accessories That May be Used in Conjunction with Ventilators

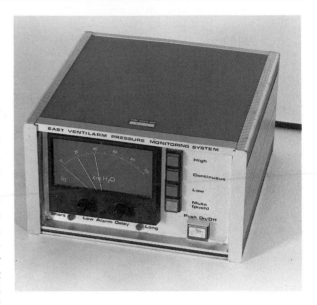

**Figure 12.45** The East Ventilarm airways pressure alarm.

It is imperative that the performance of a ventilator be monitored during its use. Failure to notice a breathing system disconnection or power failure when it is in use on a paralysed or anaesthetized patient has all too often resulted in either severe cerebral damage or death from the resultant hypoxia. The adequacy of the intact and working system also requires careful monitoring to ensure that the patient receives an appropriate minute ventilation and is protected against excessive pressures generated in his or her airways. Most modern ventilator systems are fitted with measurement devices that are capable of providing an audible and/or visual alarm if the fluctuations that they measure fall outside predetermined limits. They may also, for instance, in the presence of excessive airways pressures, override the ventilator controls so as to prevent harm to the patient.

These devices are also available individually and can be attached to older ventilator systems that were not provided with them when manufactured. However, they normally provide only a warning signal and cannot alter the function of the ventilator. The various types of accessories are listed below.

*Airways pressure alarm.* This is a multipurpose accessory which senses, and on some models displays, the pressure in the breathing hoses of a ventilator system. It is usually fitted with an audible and/or visual alarm for high and low airways pressure. The values for these may either be pre-set by the manufacturer (typically 45 cmH$_2$O for the high alarm limit and 5–8 cmH$_2$O for the lower) or may be adjusted by the user. There is a time delay on the lower alarm to allow the normally low pressures at the end of an expiratory phase to occur. This device acts as an apnoea alarm, a breathing system disconnect alarm and a warning of high airways pressure. On sophisticated ventilators this accessory is an integral part of the system and, by overriding the ventilator controls, prevents pressures higher that those set on the alarm from occurring. Figure 12.45 shows a typical airways pressure alarm. The device should be independently powered (battery back-up if it is an integral part of a mains electricity-operated ventilator), so as to detect a mains power failure.

*Spirometer.* The minute ventilation settings on many ventilators are usually only an approximate guide to their output. Also, there may well be losses due to leaks around the endotracheal tube or from any other part of the breathing attachment. Furthermore a ventilator system that uses a large reservoir bellows filled at atmospheric pressure, along with distensible breathing hoses, may well 'lose' 20% of the intended tidal volume during compression of these gases prior to their being delivered. A spirometer measures the flow of gases and therefore is capable of determining the eventual tidal volume delivered. Ideally, the device should be placed as near to the patient's airway as possible so as to avoid measuring the 'compression' volumes mentioned above. Furthermore only the patient's *exhaled* gases should be measured, as these were the ones actually delivered despite any leaks. It is not always practicable to site these devices close to the patient. Some ventilators house them in the expiratory pathway within the machine. In this position they may well measure a small amount of gas that was compressed in the hosing during inspiration but never reached the patient.

Spirometers measure the flow of gas either by using a turbine (Wright respiration monitor, see Figs 5.8 and 5.9) pressure differentials across a fixed resistance (pneumotachographs, see Chapter 5), or by ultrasonic methods. The signal produced by these devices can be used to activate alarms for high and low measured volumes.

Spirometers may also be used to detect ventilator failure, apnoea and breathing system disconnection, as well as small leaks undetected by the pressure alarm. However, they may not detect high airways pressures (depending on the method used) and should be used in conjunction with a pressure alarm.

*Ventilation rate meter.* This indicates the frequency, in cycles per minute, of the ventilator and in conjunction with measurement of tidal volume, using a spirometer, gives an indication of the minute volume.

# 13 Humidifiers

## Introduction

Humidity is the term used to describe the amount of water vapour present in air or in the gases concerned. The amount of water that a gas can carry depends upon its temperature. The graph in Fig. 13.1 shows the maximum amount of water that can be carried in air and how it varies with temperature.

For the rest of the chapter, unless otherwise stated, the humidity of *air* will be considered, but the same considerations apply to anaesthetic gases.

## Definitions

The *absolute humidity* is the mass of water vapour *actually* present in a unit volume of air. It is usually measured in grams per cubic metre ($g/m^3$).

The maximum mass of water vapour that *can* be carried in a cubic metre of air at a particular temperature will be referred to in this book as the *humidity at saturation* (Fig. 13.1).

The *relative humidity* is the ratio between the absolute humidity and the humidity at saturation at the same temperature. It is usually expressed as a percentage.

Some examples will be considered to elucidate the important implications, since these are not always understood.

(1) Suppose that the temperature of air in a room is 15°C and that it has a relative humidity of 50%. From Fig. 13.1 it can be seen that the humidity at saturation at this temperature is about 13 $g/m^3$; the actual amount of water vapour in the air is therefore 50% of this, i.e. 6.5 $g/m^3$.

At body temperature (37°C), the humidity at saturation is about 43 $g/m^3$. Therefore, when the temperature of the air in the same room is raised to body temperature, its relative humidity is (6.5/43) × 100%, i.e. approximately 15%. If the air is to be saturated with water vapour within the body, the

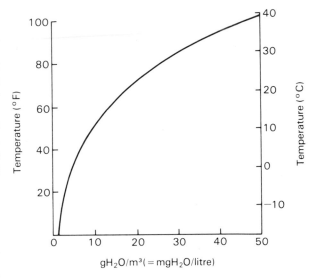

**Figure 13.1** Graph showing the mass of water that is carried at saturated vapour pressure in terms of grams of water per cubic metre of air.

respiratory epithelium must vaporize 43 − 6.5 = 36.5 g of water per cubic metre of room air inhaled. Since 1 $m^3$ is 1000 litres, 36.5 mg of water are required per litre of inspired air.

(2) If a humidifier saturates air at room temperature and then the air is warmed to body temperature, the absolute humidity is unchanged but the relative humidity falls to only about 30%.

(3) If air is saturated with water vapour at body temperature, i.e. in a 'warm' humidifier, and is then allowed to cool to room temperature before it reaches the patient, some of the water vapour will condense out and become liquid again. When the air is eventually re-warmed in the patient's respiratory tract, the relative humidity again will be only 30%. From this it will be seen that if the inspired air is required to have a relative humidity of 100% at body temperature, it will either have to be supersaturated at the lower temperature or will have to be maintained at body temperature after humidification. Supersaturation is achieved by adding to

the air a mist or fog of minute droplets of water, which vaporize when the relative humidity falls.

It should be understood that humidification refers to the addition to the air of water in the form of either vapour or nebulized droplets. The addition of excessive amounts of water in the form of droplets to the inspired air may lead to overloading of the lungs with water.

# The Importance of Humidification

Air or anaesthetic gases need to be humidified for the following reasons.

- Medical air, oxygen and nitrous oxide supplied either by pipeline or cylinder are dry gases. As already mentioned, this is to protect against corrosion, condensation and frost in cylinders, pipes, valves, etc.
- The upper respiratory tract normally acts as a heat and moisture exchanger (HME) increasing the relative humidity of inspired air to 100% at 37°C. This may be bypassed by endotracheal tubes or tracheostomies.

The atmosphere of the operating theatre, for which there is usually air conditioning, should be kept at a suitable level of relative humidity. This should be between 50 and 70%. Too high a humidity results in a most uncomfortable and tiring atmosphere for the staff, and too low a humidity can increase the risk of explosion due to static electricity. Ventilation and humidifying equipent used in operating theatres does not come within the scope of this book.

## Consequences of under-humidification

- The latent heat of vaporization of water is 2.43 MJ/kg. This energy will be used by the patient to saturate dry inspired gas. Yet more energy will be used to raise its temperature to 37°C. This may amount to up to a third of a neonate's basal heat production, with the possible fall in core temperature of more than 1°C per hour of ventilation with dry gases.
- There is a net loss of water from the patient in exhaled saturated gas.
- Dry gases cause the tracheal mucosa to become dry, inflamed and ulcerated and ciliary movement and mucus flow may also cease. Lung compliance will fall.

## Disadvantages and risks of humidification

The potential risks of humidification include infection, water intoxication, mucosal cooling, mucosal heating, increase in dead space, and increased resistance to gas flow.

## Classification of humidifiers

The various humidification devices used may be classified in three ways. First, they may be classified according to whether they produce water vapour or droplets of water, however small. The latter are generally referred to as nebulizers: the term humidifier refers strictly to the former only. There is a great deal of variation in the size of droplets produced by nebulizers and this will be discussed later. A second classification depends on the source of energy. This may be either electric power, as in humidifiers and the ultrasonic nebulizer, or the power of a jet of air or gas in the venturi type, which may be used to humidify oxygen from the cylinder or pipeline. The 'bubble bottle', in which the gas is simply bubbled through water, is an example of a passive humidifier, as is the 'artificial nose' or heat and moisture exchanger (HME), which will be described below. The third classification is based on whether they are hot or cold. Those that are heated can produce air at body temperature or even higher, that is saturated with water vapour. Needless to say, caution must be taken to prevent scalding of the patient by air that has been heated to a temperature above that of the body. Some cold nebulizers produce such a profusion of droplets that even when the air has been warmed in the body to body temperature, the droplets are sufficient in mass to produce 100% humidity.

Nebulizers may also be used to administer drugs as an aerosol into the patient. However, unless the droplet size is very small, the drugs may not reach the alveoli as required, but be deposited in the bronchial tree and thus may be ineffectual. The scope for this type of administration of drugs is therefore limited unless there is close control of droplet size.

The four most commonly used humidifiers are:

- ambient temperature water vapour supplier. This usually consists of a water reservoir through which the gas is bubbled, e.g. use of a Boyle's bottle vaporizer;
- heated water vapour supplier or humidifier;
- nebulizer;
- heat and moisture exchanger.

The approximate efficiency of each of these systems is shown in Table 13.1.

**Table 13.1** Efficiency of humidification systems

|  | Cold water | Hot water | Nebulizer | HME |
|---|---|---|---|---|
| Temperature (°C) | Ambient | 36–38 | 23–36 | <35 |
| Relative humidity (%) | <100 | 100 | >100 | <<100 |
| Absolute humidity (mg/litre) | 15–20 | 42–47 | 177–1536 | 27–36 |
| Compliance | Low | Moderate to high | Low | Low |

# Examples of Humidification Equipment

(1) A simple bottle humidifier (Fig. 13.2), such as a Boyle's bottle, may be used on an anaesthetic machine. If the air passes over the surface of the water, a modest amount of vaporization takes place. Unless there is a very large surface area of water and a very low flow rate of gas, however, the air is by no means saturated with water vapour. Improvements to this type of humidifier may be made by either bubbling the air through the water or increasing the surface area with wicks immersed in the water, in the same way as in vaporizers for volatile anaesthetic agents (Fig. 13.3). To increase humidification further, the bottle may be housed in a heated jacket

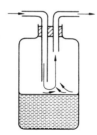

**Figure 13.2** A simple bottle humidifier.

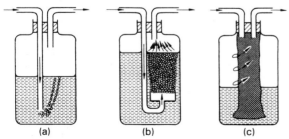

**Figure 13.3** Methods of increasing humidification. (a) Bubbling gases through water, in (b) using a sintered filter, which breaks up the air into a very large number of small bubbles to maximize the rate of vaporization; (c) by immersing a wick.

or may even contain an electric heating element (Fig. 13.4).

In the case of heated humidifiers, the temperature of the water must be thermostatically controlled. In general two thermostats in series are used, so that if one thermostat were to fail the other would still cut off the electricity supply before a dangerous temperature was reached. After use, this type of humidifier may be sterilized by intentionally boiling the water inside it using a bypass switch to override the thermostats. The outlet and delivery tube from a heated humidifier should be lagged if possible, to reduce the cooling that would result in condensation of some of the water vapour. Some heated water humidifiers even have a coaxial electric heater wire in the attached breathing hose to maintain the temperature. Ideally, a temperature sensor should be installed at the patient end of the delivery tube, in order to allow the maintenance of maximum efficiency without the risk of scalding the patient.

Where the gases are bubbled through water, provision should be made to prevent the accidental reverse connection of the bottle, which would cause the water to be forced along the delivery tube to the patient. Two precautions are generally taken to prevent such an accident: a 'trap' or empty bottle B of the same capacity as the 'bubble bottle', A is interposed between the latter and the patient (Fig. 13.5) and the humidifier is always kept at a lower level than the patient, so that, in the event of an accident there is no risk of water running down the tubes and scalding, or even drowning, the patient.

(2) Water vapour or steam may be produced simply by boiling water. This is not a satisfactory method for use in conjunction with anaesthetic apparatus, but may be useful in the treatment of a patient, especially in his own home, by humidifying the whole atmosphere of the room. Simple steam therapy achieved by boiling water is not appropriate in hospitals and the danger of scalding the patient should be remembered.

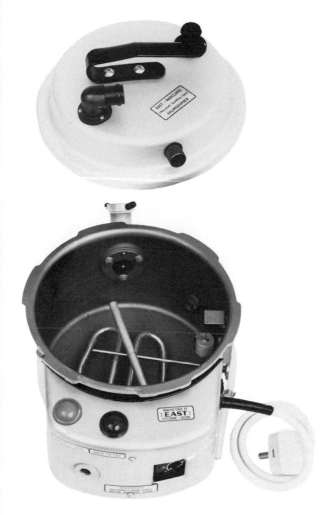

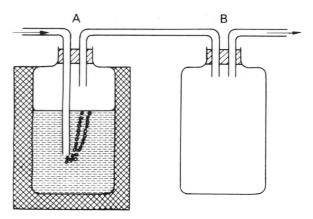

**Figure 13.5** A 'trap bottle' **B** is interposed between the 'bubble bottle' **A** and the patient to prevent water reaching the patient in the event of accidental reverse connection of the bubble bottle.

**Figure 13.4** The Marshall Spalding humidifier, which incorporates an electric heating element. This humidifier may be sterilized by intentionally boiling the water inside it. Note the appropriate warning lights.

(3) A jet of air or gases may be used to entrain water drawn up from a reservoir (Fig. 13.6). As the water enters the jet it is broken up into a large number of droplets, i.e. it is nebulized. This principle is used in simple sprays for administering topical analgesics and is also used to humidify the inspired air in some ventilators. Such nebulizers create large droplets, but if these are made to impinge on a solid 'anvil' they are broken up into smaller ones.

(4) The water may also be broken up into a large number of small droplets by causing a fine jet to impinge upon one or more objects, such as pins, while subjected to a moving air stream. This system is used in the air-conditioning plants for operating

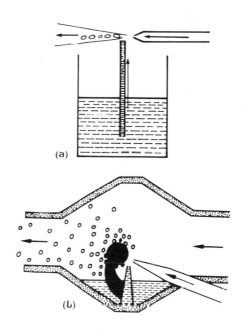

**Figure 13.6** The principle of a nebulizer. (a) Employing the Bernoulli effect, a jet of air may be used to draw a liquid up a small tube from a reservoir and to entrain it as droplets. (b) The droplets may be made to impinge on an 'anvil', so causing them to be broken up into still smaller droplets.

theatres, and also in some medical nebulizers.

(5) In ultrasonic nebulizers (Fig. 13.7), water is broken up into droplets or fine particles by a continual sonic bombardment generated by a high-frequency resonator.

(a)

(b)

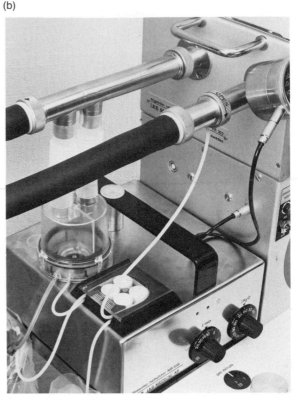

**Figure 13.7**    (a) A cloud of droplets emerging from an ultrasonic nebulizer. (b) The delivery of the correct volume of water by a peristaltic pump in the NB 108 nebulizer.

When considering nebulizers, thought must be given to the size of the particles of water. Too large a droplet will fall out of the 'mist' and be deposited on the breathing tube rather than passing down to the patient's lungs, while too fine a particle will be carried right down almost to the alveoli but will not sufficiently humidify the patient's tracheal and bronchial mucosa.

Ultrasonic nebulizers are useful for the dispersal of antiseptics when sterilizing anaesthetic machines and ventilators and some may be connected directly to the breathing system. However, problems have been experienced when using them for the humidification of gases, because the amount of water nebulized was excessive and virtually drowned the patient.

Two types of ultrasonic nebulizer require further comment. In one, a drop of water is allowed to fall on a vibrating 'transducer' and is broken up into small droplets (which one manufacturer claims are of uniform size, around 1 μm). In the other, the transducer is submerged and droplets of a variety of sizes, usually in excess of 1 μm, are produced. Since the volume of a sphere is proportional to the third power of the radius, it will be appreciated that a 2-μm droplet is eight times as heavy as a 1 μm one, and will therefore 'fall out' far more quickly. If the 'submerged' type of transducer is allowed to run dry, it may be irreparably damaged. Various measures to prevent such damage are incorporated in some models.

(6) In the 'hot-rod' humidifier, water is fed on to a heated surface. The heater is electrically energized, and may be surmounted by a block of material such as porcelain, which increases the surface area and has a large heat capacity and thus ensures immediate vaporization. The volume of water may be metered so as to ensure the production of, say, 75% relative humidity at 37°C. Thus if the incoming gases are fresh and unhumidified, or if they are merely room air with some pre-existing humidity, the output will be adequately, but not excessively, humidified. The reservoir of water may be in the form of a plastic infusion bag, as shown in Fig. 13.8. The breathing attachment may be coaxially arranged so that the expired gases in the outer portion help to prevent cooling of the inspired gases within the inner tube. The tubing may be detached for sterilization by autoclaving.

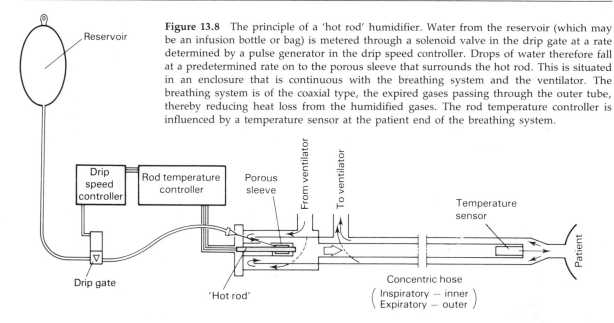

**Figure 13.8** The principle of a 'hot rod' humidifier. Water from the reservoir (which may be an infusion bottle or bag) is metered through a solenoid valve in the drip gate at a rate determined by a pulse generator in the drip speed controller. Drops of water therefore fall at a predetermined rate on to the porous sleeve that surrounds the hot rod. This is situated in an enclosure that is continuous with the breathing system and the ventilator. The breathing system is of the coaxial type, the expired gases passing through the outer tube, thereby reducing heat loss from the humidified gases. The rod temperature controller is influenced by a temperature sensor at the patient end of the breathing system.

(7) Heat and moisture exchangers (HMEs) are of three types: condenser, hygroscopic and hydrophobic. The purpose of the HME is to conserve the patient's own heat and moisture without external energy or water supply. The earliest type, the condenser HME, consists of a wire mesh screen in the path of the respiratory gases, as close to the mouth as possible. On exhalation, water vapour condenses on the wire mesh and this then evaporates again during the inspiratory phase. Hygroscopic HMEs are more efficient, as a greater proportion of expiratory water vapour is adsorbed into its element. This element may consist of paper coated with calcium chloride, glass fibre, or polypropylene coated with lithium chloride. The latest HMEs are of the hydrophobic type, which has a folded ceramic fibre element.

Both the hygroscopic and the hydrophobic types are much more efficient than the condenser type, which also suffers from the disadvantage that it provides no microbiological barrier. The hygroscopic and the hydrophobic types both provide some bacteriological protection, although the hydrophobic is said to be more efficient.

The construction of a typical HME is shown in Fig. 13.9.

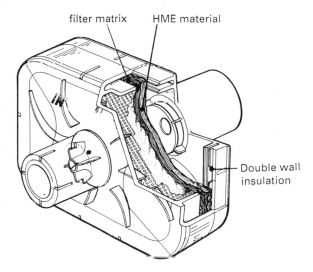

**Figure 13.9** A typical heat and moisture exchanging filter.

# 14 Equipment for Paediatric Anaesthesia

## Introduction

Various items of equipment required for paediatric anaesthesia have already been described in the appropriate chapters. It is important to understand the reasons why these differ from those employed for anaesthetizing adults. When selecting apparatus for paediatric anaesthesia, account must be taken of the respiratory physiological, anatomical and mechanical factors involved, which differ from those that present when adults are being anaesthetized.

### Difference in respiratory physiology between adults and children

Respiration in infants and neonates has a more sinusoidal pattern than in adults. The absence of an expiratory pause decreases the time in which fresh gas is able to flush away alveolar gas which is present at the end of expiration in all partial rebreathing systems (Mapleson A, D, E and F). This renders them all relatively less efficient during spontaneous respiration than in adults.

Tidal volumes are small in infants and neonates so that any increased apparatus dead space may well become a high proportion of the tidal volume, with a significant effect on carbon dioxide elimination, oxygenation and the resultant increased work of breathing. Furthermore, any resistance to airflow caused by turbulence in breathing systems and angled connectors also increases the work of breathing. If the volume of the breathing system is high, this requires considerable kinetic energy expenditure in repeatedly reversing the direction of air flow within it.

Thus a system such as the Magill breathing system (Mapleson A) with high internal volume, relatively large apparatus dead space (see Fig. 14.1) and an APL valve providing expiratory resistance is inappropriate in neonates and small infants. In fact, a number of adult breathing systems, even if scaled down, may not necessarily be suitable for infants and less so for neonates.

### Anatomical differences between adults and children

The anatomy of the upper airway of an infant or small child is different from that of an adult. In the

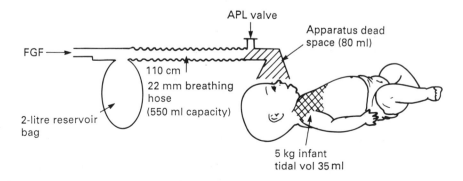

**Figure 14.1** A typical adult breathing system (Mapleson A system). APL = adjustable pressure limiting valve.

**Table 14.1** Dimensions of rubber and Portex endotracheal tubes. (Mean and ranges from five tubes of each size)

| Nominal size (mm) | Type | ID (mm) | OD (mm) |
|---|---|---|---|
| 2.5 | Rubber | 2.55 (2.5–2.65) | 4.4 (4.2–4.5) |
|     | Portex | 2.5  (2.45–2.55) | 3.5 (3.45–3.55) |
| 3.0 | Rubber | 3.0  (2.95–3.10) | 5.1 (5.0–5.2) |
|     | Portex | 3.0  (2.95–3.05) | 4.2 (4.15–4.25) |
| 3.5 | Rubber | 3.5  (3.45–3.55) | 5.4 (5.3–5.45) |
|     | Portex | 3.5  (3.45–3.55) | 4.9 (4.85–4.95) |

infant, the narrowest part is at the cricoid ring and not the larynx as in an adult. Hence tubes that pass easily through the larynx may well be too tight a fit at the cricoid ring.

The diameter of the laryngeal and cricoid inlet of an infant is narrow and if intubation is to be carried out the tube will further reduce the effective diameter of this airway. A small reduction in the airways diameter of an already small air passage will greatly increase the resistance to flow (Poisseuille law, see Chapter 1) and may provide too great a resistance to spontaneous respiration. Many anaesthetists would thus electively ventilate an infant who is intubated with a small endotracheal tube (2–3.5-mm internal diameter).

A similar situation arises when a tube that was too tight a fit is removed from a small airway. The resultant mucosal oedema and small reduction in airway diameter may be enough to cause severe respiratory embarrassment.

For these reasons, tube material and design assume far greater importance in small children than adults. For instance, plastic tubes have a greater internal diameter (due to thinner walls) than red rubber tubes of similar external diameter and are therefore preferred when small tubes are required (Table 14.1). Similarly, plain tubes also provide greater internal diameter than cuffed tubes of the same external diameter. This is because cuffed tubes have thicker (stronger) walls in order to reduce the possibility of inward herniation of the tube wall underneath the cuff site when the cuff is inflated. Plain tubes are thus almost always chosen when tubes of 6-mm internal diameter or less are required. In any case, the cricoid ring, being near-circular in a child, provides a better fit, obviating the need for a cuff.

# Mechanical Factors for Consideration in Paediatric Anaesthesia

## The anaesthetic machine

A continuous flow machine is needed: intermittent flow or draw-over machines require too much inspiratory effort by the patient and are therefore unsuitable for small children. The single exception is that in dental-chair anaesthesia of short duration varying flow machines, such as the McKesson intermittent flow machine, the AE or the Walton Five, may be used provided that the 'pressure' control is advanced sufficiently to give an adequate fresh gas flow (FGF) rate.

The vaporizer should be of a type that gives an accurate percentage of vapour, even when low flow rates are used. Nevertheless, in most instances a relatively high FGF rate is employed.

There should be a pressure relief valve at the end of the back bar, particularly where the regulated pressure is high (i.e. 420 kPa (60 psi)).

## Breathing systems

Breathing systems for use with very small children should ideally:

- have minimal functional/apparatus dead space;
- be either valveless or fitted with very low resistance valves;
- have small internal gas volumes;
- be constructed in such a way as to minimize gas turbulence and subsequent flow resistance.

In practice, Mapleson D, E and F systems (see Chapter 9) are the most commonly used as they most closely meet the criteria for an ideal paediatric system.

### The T-piece system

Mapleson D, E and F systems are based on modifications to Ayre's original T-piece system. The most commonly used of these is the Mapleson F (Jackson Rees Modification) which includes a T-piece with a reservoir hose and a bag (Fig. 14.2). It is suitable for both spontaneous and controlled ventilation. The absence of conventional valves, which inevitably present resistance, and its simplicity, make it the preferred system. Fresh gas enters the system via a T-piece which is situated as close to the patient as possible. One arm of the T-piece is

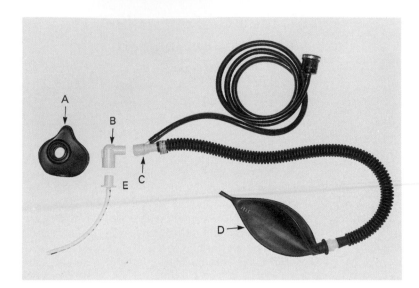

**Figure 14.2** Recent version of Jackson Rees modification to Ayre's T-piece paediatric breathing system. A, Rendell–Baker paediatric facemask. B, Right-angle connector. C, T-piece. D, Reservoir bag. E, 15-mm ISO standard endotracheal connector.

attached to a reservoir system consisting of a corrugated breathing hose and distensible bag with an exit hole in the tail. The other arm is attached to the patient's airway. This latter connection constitutes the apparatus dead space and should be made minimal by siting the T-piece as close to the patient as possible. The capacity of the expiratory limb is important when used without a reservoir bag as was originally intended. If it is less than the patient's tidal volume, then air entrainment is possible at low fresh gas flow rates, and in the extreme when the expiratory limb presents mainly as an orifice, then the fresh gas flow rate should be equal to the peak inspiratory flow rate to prevent air entrainment and dilution of inhaled anaesthetic gases.

Furthermore, the necessary fresh gas flow rate required to prevent rebreathing not only varies with the size of the patient and metabolic state but also with the respiratory rate, and whether this is spontaneous or controlled.

Recent work has shown that the respiratory rate plays an important part in deciding the fresh gas flow rate in T-piece systems both for controlled and, more importantly, spontaneous respiration. A longer expiratory phase allows a greater time for fresh gas to flush downstream the expired gas entering the reservoir limb. This reduces the potential for exhaled carbon dioxide to be present in the initial portion of the subsequent inspiratory mixture. One formula which takes this into account is:

FGF (fresh gas flow rate) (ml/min)
= 15 × weight (kg) × respiratory rate (per min)

i.e. a 10-kg infant with a respiratory rate varying between 20 and 30 breaths per minute requires a fresh gas flow rate of between 3000 and 4500 ml/min.

## Modifications to Ayre's T-piece arrangement

Several methods of reducing the apparatus/functional dead space even further than Ayre's original T-piece have been described.

*The Cape Town attachment* (Fig. 14.3a). This directs fresh gas into the endotracheal/facemask connection. The functional dead space of this system has been shown to be less than the apparatus dead space due to the continuous flushing action of the fresh gas.

*Coaxial arrangement* (Fig. 14.3b). A coaxial arrangement of the gas delivery tube, as in a Bain system, acts in a similar manner to the Cape Town attachment. It is worthy of note that the Bain breathing system is functionally similar to the T-piece. Only the resistance in the expiratory valve (when present) for spontaneous respiration and the increased compliance of the long outer limb (for intermittent positive pressure ventilation (IPPV)) make it functionally marginally inferior for use in infants. When the valve is used as part of the system, it should not be used in children weighing less than 20 kg.

*The Y-piece* (Fig. 14.3c). Fresh gas entering a Y-piece reduces the functional dead space by utilizing the Coanda effect (see Chapter 2).

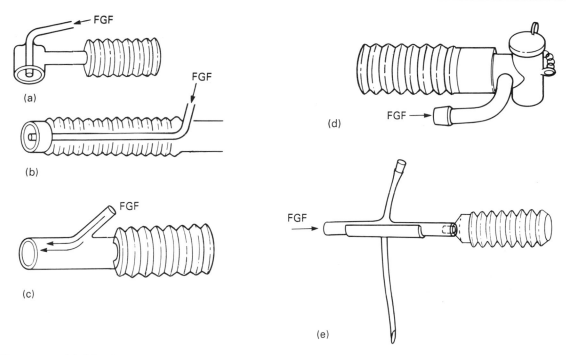

**Figure 14.3** Modifications to Ayre's T-piece arrangement. (a) Cape Town arrangement. (b) Coaxial arrangement. (c) Y-piece. (d) Bethune T-piece. (e) Jackson Rees T-tube. FGF = fresh gas flow.

*The Bethune T-piece* (Fig. 14.3d). In this system, the fresh gas flow enters the breathing system closer to the patient than in a traditional T-piece.

*Jackson Rees T tube* (Fig. 14.3e). The T-piece is incorporated within an endotracheal tube. However the increased resistance to flow across the respiratory limb has reduced the popularity of this design.

Many of the modifications described above are included in the Stellenbosch Universal T-piece system (Fig. 14.4). This is an anaesthesia kit with certain interesting refinements for use in children up to the age of about 5 years and includes connections for both facemask and endotracheal methods. It includes a modification of the Ayre's T-piece and also of the Jackson Rees modification of that system. The T-piece itself has been redesigned in such a way that the fresh gas entry is directed towards the patient so that the fresh gas stream remains separated from the expired stream. It may be connected directly to a modified Magill endotracheal connector or may be attached to a right-angled facemask mount. A port on the facemask

mount is normally occluded by a bung, but could be used for suction, though it may be used for the introduction of the fresh gas inflow so as to reduce dead space as in the Cape Town attachment. If this is done, the port on the T-piece should be occluded by the same bung.

The facemask mount has an external diameter to fit a facemask and an internal diameter to fit an endotracheal adaptor. The expiratory limb consists of a 12-mm internal diameter plastic tube of 500 mm length and 15-ml capacity. It terminates in a 15-mm male plastic connection which accepts a double-ended bag of capacity between 500 and 1000 ml. Alternatively, it may be connected to a ventilator. The tail end of this bag is connected to a special outlet which, if left unattended, will allow excess gases to escape. If a thumb is placed over an aperture in the plastic attachment to this bag, it will occlude the outlet and facilitate artificial ventilation by squeezing of the bag. The attachment may therefore be used in several methods of administering anaesthesia to children up to about 5 years of age. It also includes a scavenging system that can be attached to the expiratory end of the T-piece system complete with double-ended bag.

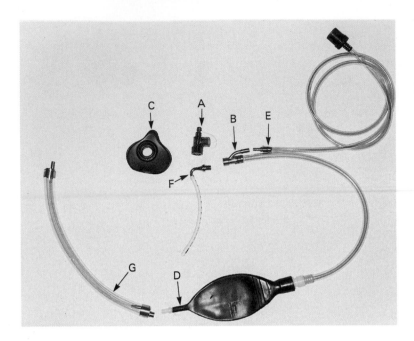

**Figure 14.4** Stellenbosch Universal T-piece system. A, Cape Town arrangement (with FGF port sealed off). B, Y-piece. C, Rendell–Baker paediatric facepiece. D, Reservoir bag. E, fresh gas source for connection to either A or B. F, Modified Magill endotracheal connector. G, Scavenging attachment.

### The Digby–Leigh system

The Digby–Leigh system (Fig. 14.5) positively prevents rebreathing and may be used for spontaneous ventilation in patients of up to 2 or 3 years of age. There are two unidirectional valves which, being constructed of mica, are fragile but nevertheless very light and present very little resistance. The fresh gases enter the distal end of the reservoir bag, and the delivery tube continues through almost the whole length of the bag, so that the freshest gases pass through towards the patient, thus accelerating any change in their composition that the anaesthetist might make. From the reservoir bag the gases pass to the patient via the inspiratory valve, which cannot be observed since it is situated within a metal enclosure. There is no spring or adjustment to either the inspiratory or the expiratory valve disc and the only means of closing the expiratory valve is by pressure from a finger — taking great care not to damage it. This attachment is, therefore, inappropriate for IPPV. The expiratory valve is very sensitive and if not correctly orientated will not operate properly. The valve body ends in a female taper into which either a facepiece mount or an endotracheal connector may be inserted.

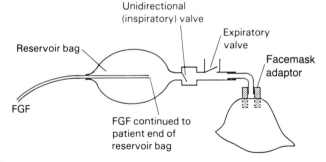

**Figure 14.5** The Digby–Leigh non-rebreathing system. FGF = fresh gas flow.

In spite of the mechanical difficulty mentioned above, the Digby–Leigh system is popular with many anaesthetists for techniques employing spontaneous ventilation in infants and small children.

Some manufacturers produce compendia of fittings that may be connected up by the anaesthetist to form a variety of breathing systems. If these are used, it must be ensured that they are suitably assembled and that the basic principles, such as the reduction of dead space and the prevention of rebreathing without carbon dioxide absorption, are observed. They are capable of being assembled incorrectly, with dangerous consequences.

## Mapleson A systems

The efficiency of this system in children depends not only on its ability to function as an A system (see Chapter 9) but in the ability of various commercial designs in minimizing the apparatus dead space, as well as decreasing the resistance to flow in any mechanical expiratory valve used. The Magill configuration with the APL valve housing between the patient and the fresh gas flow increases the apparatus dead space (40 ml) and should not be used in children weighing less than 20 kg. However, systems such as the Lack and the A configuration of the Humphrey ADE (see Chapter 9) deposit fresh gas much closer to the patient's airway (apparatus dead space 1.8 ml) and are consequently more effective. The Humphrey A system modified to use 15-mm breathing hose has been used in paediatric patients weighing under 15 kg during spontaneous respiration. Fresh gas flow of approximately 123 ml/kg/min from the system has been shown to prevent rebreathing compared with 386 ml/kg/min for a traditional Mapleson F arrangement of the Ayre's T-piece.

In all versions of the Mapleson A system, if the standard 2-litre bag is replaced by a 1-litre one, then respiratory movements will be more easily observed in small patients. This does not necessarily mean that the system becomes more efficient, however. Mapleson A systems should not be used for controlled ventilation in children because the required fresh gas flow to prevent rebreathing is high and unpredictable.

## Mapleson B systems

A refinement of the Mapleson B system for paediatric use is the Rendell–Baker system. Dead space is reduced by introducing the fresh gas through a chimney arrangement as near as possible to the patient (see Fig. 14.6). Expired gas is vented via a second chimney to a smaller and lighter APL valve than would conventionally be used. Fresh gas flow rates for spontaneous respiration should be set at 2–3 times the anticipated minute ventilation (i.e. more than for a Mapleson A but slightly less than that required for a Mapleson D system).

## Systems utilizing carbon dioxide absorption

In the days when cyclopropane, which is explosive and costly, was commonly used there was a preference for these systems. 'To-and-fro' absorption systems with a Waters' canister of similar device did not prove altogether satisfactory. This is because there was a large dead space, which

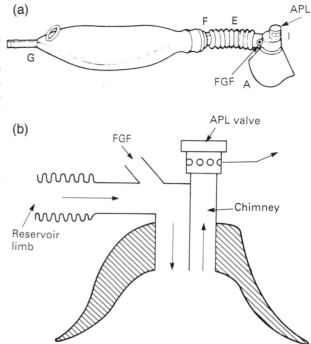

**Figure 14.6** (a) Rendell–Baker system. (b) Working principles showing the 'chimney' and paediatric facemask which reduce the apparatus dead space.

increased as the soda lime at the patient end of the canister became exhausted, because of the possibility of the inhalation of soda lime dust, and because of the cumbersome arrangement when the absorber had to be placed close to the patient's head.

Adult circle absorbers can be used for children, but it is preferable to use breathing systems with scaled-down components and tubing, in order to overcome the inertia of large volumes of gases. Special facemask mounts overcame the problems of weight and, by incorporating a chimney, reduced the dead space. More modern, lightweight plastic tubing and components, in which the need for antistatic precautions has been obviated by the use of non-explosive anaesthetic agents, lend themselves to more suitable breathing attachments for paediatric work. With the increasing awareness of atmospheric pollution and the use of scavenging systems, there may be a return of the popularity of low flow systems. The work done in breathing would be reduced and the efficiency of the system would be considerable increased by the employment of a Revell's circulator, or Jorgensen's venturi circulator (Chapter 9).

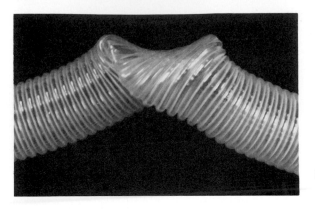

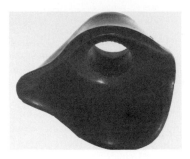

**Figure 14.8**　A paediatric facemask.

**Figure 14.7**　A lightweight corrugated hose may become twisted along its long axis and as a result become obstructed. This is because it is not flexible around its long axis.

# The Components of a Breathing System

(1) RESERVOIR BAGS. These may be smaller than the usual 2-litre bag used for adults, 0.5- or 1.0-litre bags being the most popular. The capacity of the bag must be not less than the patient's tidal volume. The material of which it is constructed must not be too stiff.

(2) CORRUGATED HOSE. The new plastic hoses available are considerably lighter than the old rubber or neoprene ones. They therefore drag far less on the facemask or endotracheal tube. They may also be of smaller diameter. 15 mm Smooth bore hosing is now available with a reinforcing spiral attached to its outer surface. The smooth inner lining produces less resistance to flow when compared with corrugated hose of similar diameter. Also the lack of corrugation makes it easier to clean and less likely to harbour infection. Some plastic hoses have the disadvantage that although they may be easily coiled up they offer resistance to twisting along their long axis (Fig. 14.7). This leads to movement of the hose being transmitted to the facemask or endotracheal tube, which is undesirable.

(3) APL (EXPIRATORY) VALVES. The Heidbrink valve may offer too much resistance for an infant. There are several smaller, lighter valves, such as the Rendell–Baker (Fig. 14.6) made of plastic and having a chimney to reduce dead space.

(4) FACEMASKS. Facemasks for neonates and infants, an example of which is shown in Fig. 14.8 (see also Chapter 9), are usually anatomically moulded to fit the face as closely as possible. Considerable experience in the selection of a facemask of exactly the right size is required to achieve a good fit but without obstructing the nares. Flaps and inflated pads are not used, as the smooth, round and soft tissues of the patient's face usually facilitate a good fit.

For larger infants and children a facemask with a flap, such as the Everseal, may be used. The dead space is often reduced by employing a relatively large facemask, into which the face fits, rather than a small one which perches on top of it (Fig. 9.39). It will be noted that the entry from the breathing attachment is positioned immediately over the airway.

(5) FACEMASK MOUNTS. The 'chimney' used with the Revell's and other circulators is described in Chapter 9.

(6) ENDOTRACHEAL CONNECTORS (see also Chapter 9). Endotracheal tubes are usually connected (in the UK) to a catheter mount either by a one-piece connector (i.e. Magill oral or nasal, Metal Cardiff or Worcester, or a connector which comes in two halves (Portex Cardiff, Knight, Bennett).

Prior to any standardization, connector sizes were left to individual designs. Hence Magill connectors were 13 mm, Worcester 12 mm, Metal Cardiff 12 mm, Knight 9 mm and Bennett 14 mm. However a 15-mm connection size was standardized which, although suitable for adults and large children, was too cumbersome for infants and neonates. More recently, a number of manufacturers have produced 8.5-mm connectors for endotracheal tube sizes of 2–6 mm internal diameter with adaptors to connect to the 15-mm standard if required.

The Portex Mini-Link system shown in Fig. 14.9 is an example of this new system.

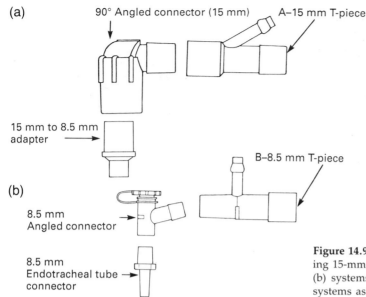

(a)

90° Angled connector (15 mm)     A–15 mm T-piece

15 mm to 8.5 mm adapter

B–8.5 mm T-piece

(b)

8.5 mm Angled connector

8.5 mm Endotracheal tube connector

**Figure 14.9**   Paediatric breathing system connectors showing 15-mm ISO standard (a) and 8.5-mm Portex Mini-Link (b) systems with adaptors for interconnection of the two systems as required.

Choice of the appropriate size of endotracheal tubes for infants and neonates is very important. Tubes must be of a size which, when inserted, allow a small leak when tested with positive-pressure ventilation. A tube that is big enough to compress the tracheal mucosa may well produce mucosal oedema and a reduction in the airway size on extubation. Mucosal oedema of 1 mm in a neonate will effectively reduce the tracheal airway by 60%! An air leak is therefore essential to demonstrate that the tube is not too large. The leak should be detectable at inflation pressures of less than 25 cmH$_2$O. The length of the tube is also important so as to prevent the tube slipping down a main bronchus and causing unilateral ventilation. Tube sizes and lengths are shown in Tables 14.2 and 14.3.

Cuffed endotracheal tubes are undesirable for use in children under 10 years. The cuff and the thicker wall construction of the tube (designed to prevent internal herniation of the tube when the cuff is inflated) effectively reduce the internal diameter of these tubes, compared to plain tubes of the same external diameter.

**Table 14.2**   Diameters of endotracheal tubes for various ages

| Age of patient | Internal diameter of tube (mm) |
|---|---|
| Preterm | 2.5 |
| At birth | 3.0 or 3.5 |
| 6 months | 4.0 |
| 1 year | 4.5 |
| Over 1 year | According to formula: $$\frac{\text{Age in years}}{4} + 4.5$$ |

From Jackson Rees, G. and Cecil Gray, T. *Paediatric Anaesthesia—Trends in Current Practice*. London: Butterworths (1981).

**Table 14.3**   Endotracheal tubes: correct lengths for given diameters

| Nasal | | Oral | |
|---|---|---|---|
| Diameter (mm) | Length (mm) | Diameter (mm) | Length (mm) |
| 2.5 | 13.0 | 2.5 | 10.5 |
| 3.0 | 13.0 | 3.0 | 10.5 |
| 3.5 | 14.0 | 3.5 | 11.0 |
| 4.0 | 14.5 | 4.0 | 12.0 |
| 4.5 | 15.0 | 4.5 | 13.5 |
| 5.0 | 16.5 | 5.0 | 14.0 |
| 5.5 | 17.0 | 5.5 | 14.5 |
| 6.0 | 17.5 | 6.0 | 15.0 |
| 65 | 18.5 | 6.5 | 16.0 |
| 7.0 | 19.0 | 7.0 | 17.5 |
| 8.0 | 19.5 | 8.0 | 18.5 |

From Jackson Rees, G. and Cecil Gray, T. *Paediatric Anaesthesia—Trends in Current Practice*. London: Butterworths (1981).

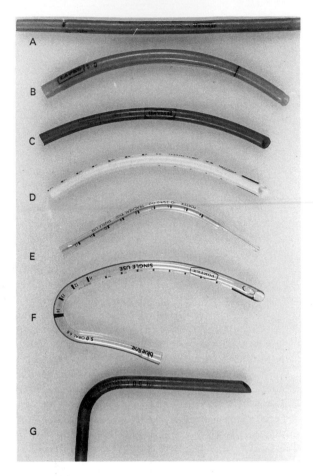

**Figure 14.10** Paediatric endotracheal tubes. From top: Armoured latex tube (orotracheal); Enderby orotracheal tube; Magill pattern red rubber orotracheal tube; plastic Magill pattern orotracheal tube; Cole pattern orotracheal tube (plastic); RAE pattern orotracheal tube; Oxford pattern red rubber orotracheal tube.

## Endotracheal tube types

(a) ARMOURED TUBES (Fig. 14.10A). The armour is provided by a nylon or wire spiral embedded in the wall of the tube which prevents it from kinking when the tube is acutely angled. The inevitable thickness of the tube is often too great for neonatal use. Formerly, armoured tubes were constructed of latex or red rubber, which perishes rapidly, but recently silicone rubber armoured tubes have been developed.

(b) ENDERBY TUBES (Fig. 14.10B). The Enderby tube is not only armoured but also tapered. The distal portion is a snug fit at the larynx and cricoid ring, whereas the wider proximal part offers less resistance. The consequent extra capacity does not pose measurable problems in terms of increased dead space.

(c) MAGILL PATTERN. Magill tubes (Fig. 14.10C, D) are curved, parallel-sided and bevelled at the tip from left to right so that they would, if too long, pass down the right main bronchus. They are probably the most commonly used tubes and are supplied long, requiring cutting to length. They can be made of red rubber or thermoplastic and can be passed either nasally or orally.

(d) COLE PATTERN TUBES (Fig. 14.10E). The body of a Cole pattern tube is relatively large, culminating in a shoulder leading to a small intratracheal section. The design minimizes the possibility of endobronchial insertion as the body is too large to pass through the larynx. However, the flow resistance of these tubes is greater than that of the parallel sided variety due to turbulence at the shoulder. Furthermore, laryngeal damage caused by pressure from the shoulder can occur and the tube is not now in common use.

(e) RAE (RING, ADAIR AND ELWIN) PATTERN TUBES (Fig. 14.10F). These are supplied as oral and nasal varieties that have pre-formed curves and are supplied cut to length. The proximal portion of these tubes is designed to be longer than other tubes so that the endotracheal connector is thus sited some distance from the patient's airway to provide easier surgical access. However, the oral version of the tube in the smaller sizes has been known to kink at the point of maximum curvature, especially when used with a Boyle–Davis gag. Furthermore, tubes with internal diameters of 3 mm or less have appreciably more resistance to flow than equivalent-sized Magill pattern plastic tubes and should perhaps be used only with controlled ventilation.

(f) OXFORD PRE-FORMED TUBES (Fig. 14.10G). These are shaped in a right angle (90°). The body of the tube is usually made from a thicker material than a Magill pattern tube so as to resist kinking and crushing in the pharynx with any neck flexion manoeuvre. However, the wall at the tip of the tube is tapered at the point at which it is designed to enter the larynx in order to maximize the effective internal diameter of that tube.

The bevel is cut from back to front at the tip of the tube. The tubes are supplied in different sizes and are all pre-cut to length.

## Nasotracheal intubation

Where intubation is to be prolonged, as in the

Intensive Care Unit, nasal tubes may be preferable. Not only are they less restrictive of access to the mouth, e.g. for tube feeding, they are also less prone to movement within the trachea and thus to traumatizing the delicate mucosa in that area since they are splinted by the nose and nasopharynx.

# Resistance to Gas Flow in Breathing Systems

*Endotracheal connectors* (Fig. 14.11). Most connectors for neonates have been shown to create turbulent flow at flow rates seen in clinical practice. Curved

**Table 14.4**  Resistance of tracheal tube connectors ($cmH_2O$/litre/s)

| Connector | Smallest ID (mm) | Fresh Gas Flow (litre/min) | | |
|---|---|---|---|---|
| | | 1 | 3 | 5 |
| Cardiff | 2.6 | 9 | 20 | 30 |
| Magill | 2.8 | 12 | 22 | 32 |
| Oxford | 2.5 | 12 | 24 | 36 |
| Oxford | 3.0 | 5 | 10 | 15 |
| Penlon 15-mm cone | 2.5 | 21 | 30 | 44 |
| Portex 15-mm cone | 2.7 | 13 | 24 | 33 |

From Hatch, D. J. (1981) *British Journal of Anaesthesia.*

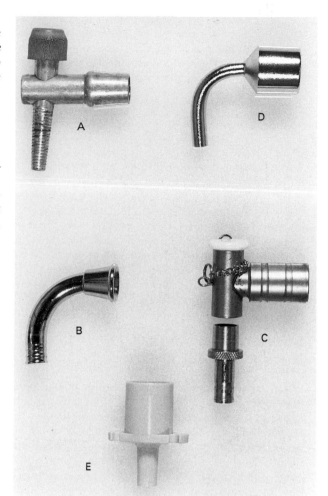

**Figure 14.11**  Paediatric endotracheal tube connectors. A, Cardiff. B, Magill. C, Oxford. D, Penlon. E, Portex.

**Table 14.5**  Resistance of endotracheal tubes without connectors ($cmH_2O$/litre/s)

| | Flow (litre/min) | | |
|---|---|---|---|
| | 1 | 3 | 5 |
| 2.5-mm | | | |
| Portex | 19 | 21 | 23 |
| Rubber | 15 | 17 | 20 |
| JR | 45 | 74 | 106 |
| 3.0-mm | | | |
| Portex | 8 | 11 | 12 |
| Rubber | 12 | 15 | 17 |
| JR | 24 | 35 | 47 |
| 3.5-mm | | | |
| Portex | 4 | 5 | 7 |
| Rubber | 7 | 9 | 11 |
| JR | 18 | 26 | 30 |

JR = Jackson Rees.

connectors were always thought to be better at creating lamina flow and reducing flow resistance, although, as can be seen from Table 14.4 this is not necessarily the case. Curved connectors (Magill) perform no better than an angled Cardiff connector. Fifteen-millimetre connectors (ISO Tapers, Portex and Penlon cones) have higher resistances to flow even though they do not have a bend in them. This is caused by turbulence at the junction with the taper used for attachment to an endotracheal tube.
*Endotracheal tubes.* Plastic tubes (Portex) have been shown to have thinner walls than equivalent tubes of similar construction and of the same internal diameter. It may therefore be possible to use plastic tubes half a size larger than red rubber ones, with a corresponding reduction in flow resistance (Tables 14.1 and 14.5).

The resistance of Jackson Rees tubes when measured between one side of the wide-bore cross arm and the tracheal limb (with the suction port and the other side of the wide-bore cross arm occluded) was substantially greater than that of equivalent-sized Portex tubes.

## Laryngoscopes

When compared with an adult, the neonate has a more anteriorly placed laryngeal inlet that is more easily obscured by a relatively larger and more floppy epiglottis and tongue. The intubating view is improved by using laryngoscopes with either straight blades or less curved blades than those of an adult Mackintosh laryngoscope. The choice of paediatric laryngoscope and blades is extensive and selection is largely a matter of user preference. Some examples of laryngoscope blades are shown in Fig. 14.12.

## Suction Equipment

When treating neonates and infants, a relatively low-power vacuum should be used in spite of the fact that a very narrow catheter may be needed to aspirate viscous secretions. Too high a vacuum could result in pulmonary atelectasis. Damage to the delicate mucosa could result from the employment of a catheter with an inappropriate termination by performing a 'suction biopsy'. Paediatric suction catheters should have a limiting pressure vent in the handle that can be occluded or partially occluded by a thumb to control suction pressure as well as having a tip with multiple side holes so that the suction tip does not attach itself to the tracheal wall.

## Ventilators

Chapter 12 describes ventilators in general and includes automatic ventilators that may be used for children, infants and neonates. However there are some practical points that might well be considered here.

### Neonates

The simplest way to achieve IPPV in infants and neonates is to employ a T-piece system and intermittently occlude the expiratory limb with a thumb. The disadvantage of this system is that the

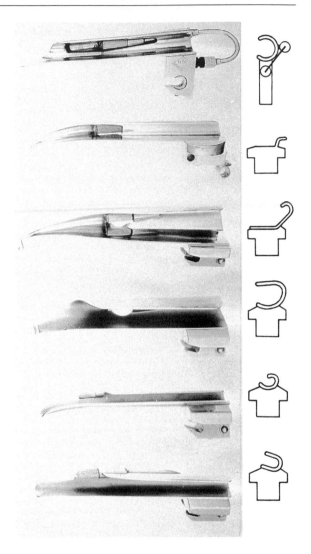

**Figure 14.12** Straight laryngoscope blades for use in infants. From top: Anderson–Magill, Seward, Robertshaw, Oxford, Miller, Wisconsin.

inspiratory flow rate is limited to the FGF (fresh gas flow rate). This is suitable for neonates and infants, but is a great waste of fresh gas in children above 20 kg. T-piece occluders such as the Sheffield, Vickers and Amsterdam are therefore of limited value in the older child.

### Children

Adding a bellows or bag to the expiratory limb as in the Jackson Rees modification of the T-piece, allows much higher inspiratory flow rates. This is because FGF rate is augmented by gases that have been displaced from the expiratory limb as a result of the 'bag' being squeezed. A number of 'bag squeezer' ventilators have the ability to substitute the adult bellows with a paediatric version with a much smaller volume (e.g. Carden, Penlon Oxford and OAV 500 ventilators).

The Newton valve (see below), which can be driven by a number of low-compliance ventilators (Nuffield 200) provides a gas piston in the Jackson Rees T-piece expiratory limb to similar effect. These ventilators allow the T-piece system to function more efficiently, providing normocarbic conditions at FGF rates of 120–150 ml/kg/min.

### The Newton valve (Fig. 14.13)

This is an ingenious device which consists of a patient port, ventilator input port, and fixed orifice gas outlet. The valve is connected via the patient port to the expiratory limb of a T-piece with the reservoir bag removed (Mapleson E). At low ventilator gas flow rates the pressure developed inside the valve (as a result of continuous leakage from the fixed orifice outlet) only partially dams the expiratory limb of the breathing system, and so acts as a partial 'thumb occluder', providing very small tidal volumes. At these tidal volumes the 'internal volume' of the valve (and hence compliance) is relatively high in relation to the delivered tidal volume and the performance of the ventilator may well be more variable than expected when used in infants with low or changing compliance.

As the flow rate of driving gas into the valve increases, the valve becomes effectively a 'thumb occluder' when the gas into the valve equals the gas leaving the valve via the fixed orifice outlet. When the ventilator delivers an even greater flow into the valve, part of this gas enters the expiratory limb of the T-piece, driving patient gas backwards in the system, thus acting as a 'bag squeezer' delivering relatively larger tidal volumes. In the latter mode, however, it is heavily consumptive of driving gas (15–30 litres/min), which may be important in situations where cylinders only are used.

A further solution is to use a ventilator with a low internal compliance that accurately measures inspiratory tidal volumes in a conventional, unidirectional breathing system (Servo series B & C). Paediatric (15-ml) breathing hoses are required to reduce the potential compressible volumes of respiratory gases to a minimum.

## Paediatric Scavenging Systems

The absence of an APL (expiratory) valve in most paediatric breathing attachments precludes the use

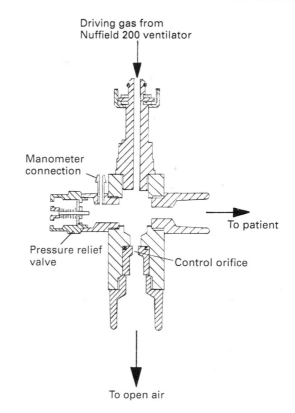

**Figure 14.13** Newton valve, sectional view.

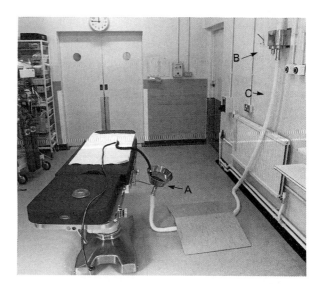

**Figure 14.14** Howarth–Great Ormond Street collecting system. A, Collecting dish with sieve base. B, Junction with air-break system leading to extractor fan. C, Wide-bore collecting hose.

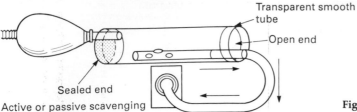

Transparent smooth tube

Open end

Sealed end

Active or passive scavenging

**Figure 14.15**  Diagram of a Stellenbosch collector.

of adult-type collecting systems for scavenging. However, alternative systems do exist.

(1) The Howarth–Great Ormond Street Hospital collecting system consists of a funnel arrangement (Fig. 14.14) into which the double-ended bag is placed. The base of the funnel, which has a plate with multiple perforations, is connected to a very wide-bore extraction hose that ducts the expired gas to a vacuum unit. This type of system would be classified as a high-volume, low-vacuum active gas scavenging unit. The very wide-bore extraction hose allows a high gas extraction rate (750 litres/min) at low gas velocities with a very low noise level.

(2) A number of arrangements for shrouding the double-ended bag have been described. One of the most elegant is the system that is supplied with the Stellenbosch kit (Fig. 14.15).

# 15 Monitoring of Gases

## Introduction

The term monitoring means the continuous assessment of one or more variables, whereas measurement implies a single assessment at a discrete time.

Monitoring technology used in anaesthesia may be classified as the monitoring of equipment function and the monitoring of physiological parameters. Physiological monitoring may be further classified as either invasive or non-invasive depending upon whether the patient's microbiological barrier is crossed by any component of the monitoring system. Monitoring techniques included in this chapter will cover monitoring of equipment function. Non-invasive monitoring such as would be applied during routine anaesthetic practice is discussed in Chapter 16.

## Inspired Oxygen Concentration

Inspired oxygen concentration is most commonly measured by one of three methods. Two of these are electrochemical: the galvanic cell, more commonly referred to as a fuel cell, and the polarographic cell. The third method is physical, relying on the paramagnetic property of oxygen.

The galvanic or *fuel cell*, Fig. 15.1a, is similar to the cell of a primary battery but the potential difference between the anode and cathode is proportional to the oxygen concentration to which it is exposed. A typical fuel cell consists of a gold-mesh cathode separated from the gas under test by a gas-permeable plastic membrane. The anode is made of lead and the electrolyte is potassium hydroxide.

Oxygen is consumed at the cathode, the reaction being

$$O_2 + 4e^- + 2H_2O \rightarrow 4(OH^-)$$

At the anode electrons are released by combination of hydroxyl ions, from the potassium hydroxide electrolyte, with lead:

$$Pb + 2(OH^-) \rightarrow PbO + H_2O + 2e^-$$

As the fuel cell is temperature sensitive, compensation has to be provided, usually in the form of a thermistor. The oxygen concentration may be displayed by a simple voltmeter calibrated in percentage of oxygen.

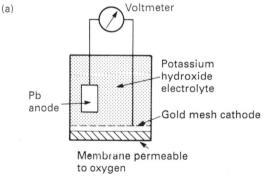

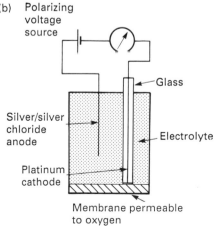

**Figure 15.1** Working principles of (a) galvanic oxygen fuel cell, (b) polarographic oxygen analyser.

The *polarographic oxygen cell* is of the same type as is used for the analysis of oxygen in blood. The construction is shown in Fig. 15.1b. A fine platinum cathode is separated from the gas under test by a thin layer of electrolyte and contained by a Teflon membrane which is permeable to oxygen gas. A polarizing voltage of about 0.6 V is applied between the cathode and a platinum anode, which is also immersed in the electrolyte solution. Oxygen diffuses through the membrane into the electrolyte solution at the cathode. Electrons combine with the oxygen at the cathode and reduce them to hydroxyl ions. A current thus flows which is proportional to the oxygen concentration. The current is very small and therefore requires amplification. Unfortunately, the polarographic analyser is sensitive, sometimes very sensitive, to nitrous oxide.

Both galvanic and polarographic oxygen cells have a limited life.

*Paramagnetic oxygen analysers* rely on the unusual magnetic property of the oxygen molecule called paramagnetism, whereby it is attracted by a magnetic field, in contrast to most other gases, including nitrous oxide, which are weakly diamagnetic and are therefore repelled. Conventional paramagnetic oxygen analysers, for example the Servomex (Fig. 15.2), consist of a small chamber into which is drawn the gas mixture under test. In the chamber are a pair of nitrogen-filled non-magnetic spheres, in a dumbbell arrangement, supported in a non-uniform powerful magnetic field by a hair-spring balance. A gas mixture containing oxygen in the chamber will be attracted to the magnetic field thus displacing the spheres. The amount of displacement will be dependent upon the concentration of oxygen. Movement of the dumbbell arrangement about its axis is detected by directing a small beam of light onto a mirror on the dumbbells and thence to photocells. Any deflection of the beam causes an increase or decrease in current through a feedback coil that is part of the dumbbell assembly. The current is varied until the dumbbells return to the null position. The current required to do this is also directed through a meter that is calibrated in percentage of oxygen. The Servomex oxygen analyser is commonly used to check oxygen pipelines and air–oxygen mixers, and to test the output of anaesthetic machines and check the calibration of fuel cells.

Another oxygen analyser based on this principle has been developed by Datex (Fig. 15.3). A small sample of gas mixture is continuously drawn through a capillary tube at the same rate as a gas of known constant oxygen concentration (air). A powerful pulsed magnetic field is arranged over the junction of the two capillary tubes. This causes a

(a)

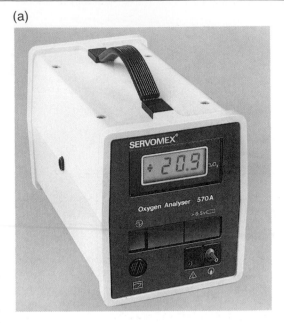

(b)

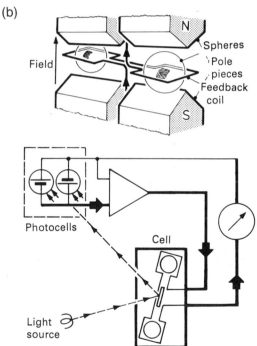

**Figure 15.2**   (a) Servomex paramagnetic oxygen analyser. (b) Working principles.

pulsed pressure difference to occur between the two tubes if there is a difference in the oxygen concentration between the two tubes. The pressure difference is measured with a semiconductor transducer, and the resultant electrical signal is displayed as oxygen concentration and used for controlling alarms and even gas mixing valves.

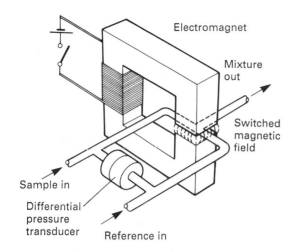

**Figure 15.3** Datex paramagnetic oxygen analyser.

# Nitrous Oxide and the Volatile Agents

Until recently, the only measurement technique capable of measuring oxygen, nitrous oxide, the volatile anaesthetic agents and any other gas, was mass spectrometry which is outside the scope of this text. The mass spectrometer has been used in routine anaesthetic practice but it is very expensive and complicated and requires continuous attention from highly trained staff. A technique new to anaesthesia, Raman spectroscopy, is almost as versatile and will be described. Many other physical techniques have been developed for the measurement of individual anaesthetic agents, although most of them are not agent-specific. Techniques include interferometry, surface absorption, ultraviolet and infrared absorption spectroscopy, and photo-acoustic spectroscopy.

### The Riken gas indicator

The Riken gas indicator (Fig. 15.4) is an *interferometer* (interference–refractometer). It depends for its operation on the fact that there is a difference between the refractive index of clean air and that of air containing another gas. Light from a small lamp bulb is condensed into a beam, which is split into two parallel beams by prisms. Each parallel beam then passes through a chamber, one of which contains clean air and the other the sample of gas to be analysed. There is a difference in the effective length of the paths taken by the two beams, which, when they are brought together again, causes the

appearance of an interference fringe that includes two characteristic dark lines, one of which is taken as the reference. The position of the reference line may be moved by a control knob until it falls on a reference point on the scale when the sampling chamber is filled with air. By means of a small manual aspirator, the sample of gas is then drawn into the sampling chamber and this causes a change in the position of the reference line on the scale. The displacement is proportional to the concentration of the gas. There is a vernier scale for more precise reading.

The interferometer may be calibrated for any required gas or vapour: one calibrated for halothane in oxygen may be used for other vapours by reference to a conversion table. Although it is not convenient for repeated or continuous measurements during anaesthesia, the Riken gas indicator is a most satisfactory and portable instrument for

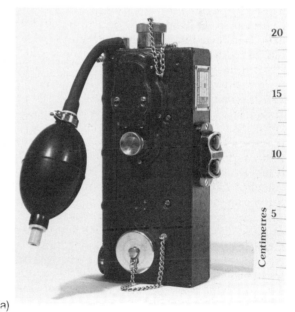

(a)

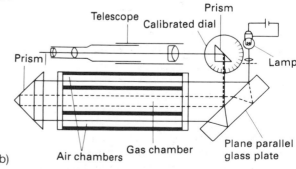

(b)

**Figure 15.4** (a) The Riken gas indicator. (b) Working principles.

checking the calibration of vaporizers for any known anaesthetic agent and is far less costly than most other instruments. The battery and bulb are easy to replace.

Large bench-type interferometers are used by vaporizer manufacturers for calibration purposes (see page 73).

### The Dräger Narcotest halothane indicator

The Dräger Narcotest halothane indicator (Fig 15.5) is a relatively simple device which depends on the effect that the volatile anaesthetic agents have on silicone rubber. The gases containing the vapour circulate around strands of the rubber under tension and alter its length by changing its modulus of elasticity. A bimetallic strip compensates for changes in environmental temperature. A clamp may be used to secure the pointer during transport. The Narcotest has the advantage that it requires no electrical power and may be kept continuously in-line during anaesthesia.

The disadvantages include its maximum span of up to 3% halothane; its non-specificity, although calibration factors enable it to be used for other agents, and the fact that it is markedly affected by nitrous oxide in the carrier gas. Since the operation of this device is dependent upon rubber/gas and oil/gas solubility coefficients, it has been suggested that it approximates to a 'MAC meter'.

### The Engström Emma anaesthetic vapour analyser

A number of materials exhibit a marked piezo-electric effect. When quartz crystals are mounted between electrodes and are accurately cut to shape, they may be made to oscillate at a specific frequency. The transducer of the Engström Emma (Fig. 15.6) contains two such crystals, one of which is coated with a layer of silicone oil that can absorb or release halogenated anaesthetic molecules. When a carrier gas containing halogenated vapours passes through the transducer, molecules of the agent are absorbed onto the silicone oil, changing the mass of the oil-coated crystal, and hence its fundamental frequency with respect to the uncoated reference crystal. The measurement of vapour concentration is

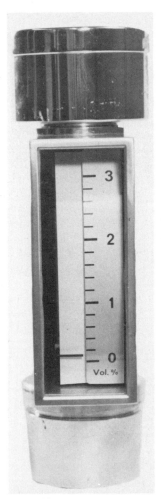

**Figure 15.5** The Dräger Narcotest halothane indicator.

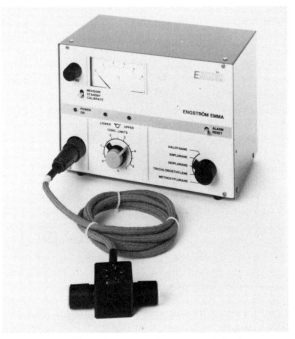

**Figure 15.6** The Engström Emma anaesthetic vapour analyser.

made by comparison of the frequencies of the two crystals. The oil is permanent and should not need replenishing or servicing.

Nitrous oxide produces a small change in calibration, at worst less than 0.2% on the meter scale. If one is using nitrous oxide mixtures, the device can be re-zeroed for the proportion of nitrous oxide in use. Carbon dioxide has no appreciable effect in clinical concentrations. A change of transducers requires simple adjustment of calibration.

The transducers need to be matched to the analyser. On each transducer there is a disc showing a scale, which, having been set to one particular number, is fixed by a screw. In order to make a new transducer compatible, the analyser is switched to 'Calibrate', and if the scale reading does not coincide with the setting on the disc, the electronics of the analyser should be brought into line by adjusting a small screw located in a hole in the right-hand panel of the apparatus.

It is advisable not to use ether with this analyser, since there is a heater in the transducer head, and this could ignite the vapour. The response time of the instrument is 0.1 s.

There are audible alarms for upper and lower limits. There are also visible alarms. A function switch may be set to 'Standby', thus maintaining the heat in the transducer head, but with the alarms switched off.

The frequency of the oscillator is about 9 kHz, and may be interfered with by surgical diathermy.

One of the advantages of this analyser over, for example, the Hook and Tucker, is that it does not merely take a small sample from the gas flow — the entire gas flow passes through the transducer head — and there are therefore fewer problems with inaccuracies due to streaming, etc.

If the transducer is installed in the expiratory limb of a breathing attachment, water vapour may be absorbed by the non-oily crystal and produce a low reading.

The Engström Emma measures the concentration of any substance that is absorbed by the silicone oil and since all volatile anaesthetic agents are oil-soluble, they can be detected. However, it is incapable of distinguishing one agent from another. This device should be regularly calibrated, preferably each time that it is used.

## Infrared absorption spectroscopy

Asymmetric polyatomic molecules absorb infrared (IR) radiation. Carbon dioxide, nitrous oxide and water vapour absorb strongly, whereas helium, argon, hydrogen, oxygen and nitrogen do not.

Molecules that absorb IR convert the IR energy into vibrations at frequencies dependent on molecular mass and atomic bond strength. Hence different compounds absorb IR radiation at different frequencies. Thus, it is possible to determine what a compound is and also its concentration.

The Beer–Lambert law shows the relationship between the absorption of energy and the concentration of gas under test:

$$A = \log \left[ \frac{I_0}{I_1} \right] = \varepsilon l c$$

where $A$ = absorption, $I_0$ = incident intensity, $I_1$ = exit intensity, $\varepsilon$ = molar extinction coefficient, $l$ = path length of cell, $c$ = concentration of sample.

At IR wavelengths, absorption may also be effected by the so called 'pressure broadening' of the molecular frequencies by certain carrier gases, especially helium, argon or hydrogen.

The principles of a typical infrared analyser are shown in Fig. 15.7. Infrared radiation from a nichrome wire filament is directed through a test cell via a chopper wheel which has a number of windows. The windows in the chopper wheel are composed of narrow-bandwidth filters of the wavelength of the absorption peaks of the gas or gases of interest. In the case of the capnograph, the filter passes only energy of wavelength 4.26 μm. In the multigas analyser, 3.3 μm is the common absorption peak for enflurane, isoflurane and halothane as they all absorb at this wavelength, and 4.5 μm for nitrous oxide. Thus, discrete pulses of IR energy at a series of different wavelengths, appropriate to the gases under test, pass through the test cell. The IR detector receives the IR signals which, after amplification and processing, are displayed as the concentrations of each of the component gases or vapours under test. The main advantages of this system are that it rapidly measures the concentration of nitrous oxide, end-tidal and inspired carbon

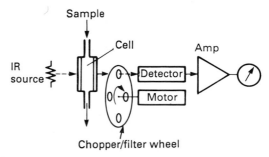

**Figure 15.7**  Components of a typical infrared analyser.

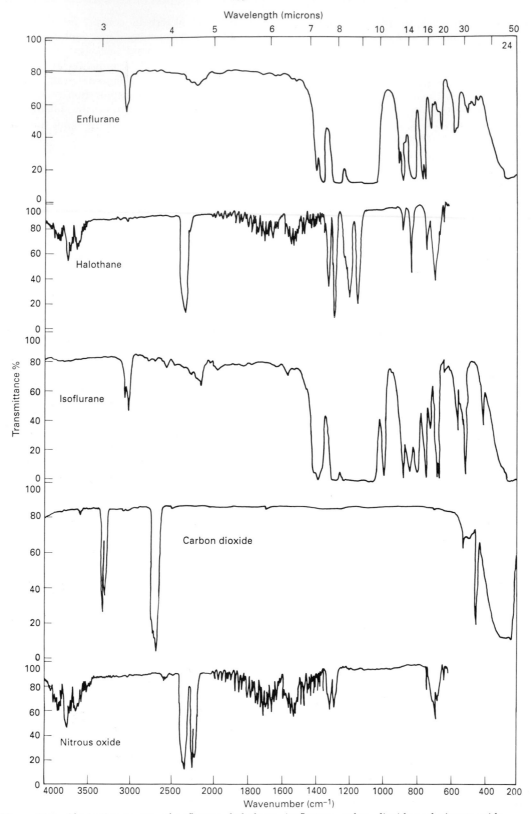

**Figure 15.8** Absorption spectra of enflurane, halothane, isoflurane, carbon dioxide and nitrous oxide.

dioxide, and the volatile agents. However, in the near infrared range, as the absorption peaks of most of the volatile anaesthetic agents are identical at 3.3 μm (Fig. 15.8), it is impossible to distinguish between them. It is necessary to select the correct calibration for the expected vapour and mixtures, or the wrong vapour concentration will be displayed. It is also necessary to remove water vapour, as it is a strong absorber at this wavelength. A similar problem may occur with interference between carbon dioxide and nitrous oxide. It has recently been observed that high levels of blood alcohol may interfere with the calibration when exhaled gas is sampled (or analysed). Most IR multigas analysers also include either a fuel cell or a paramagnetic oxygen analyser as well.

## The Miran infrared spectrophotometer

The Miran (Fig. 15.9) is a high-quality infrared spectrophotometer that is often used for testing the calibration of vaporizers, and also in the assessment of environmental pollution in the operating theatre by anaesthetic agents. A heated nichrome wire IR source is directed through a variable interference filter which is calibrated in wavelength. This filter may either be set at a wavelength that is a known absorption peak of an agent, or may be continuously varied to scan through the near IR spectrum, in order to analyse gas samples. The beam of IR energy then passes through a chamber, of known path length, to the detection system. Two chambers are provided, one with a very short path length, for the measurement of gases and vapours at anaesthetic concentrations, and the other with a long path length, for analysing environmental gases in the parts-per-million range.

## Brüel and Kjaer anaesthetic gas monitor

Acoustic techniques for the analysis and measurement of gas and vapour concentrations may be based on the physical property that, if energy is applied to a gas or vapour, it will expand, causing an increase in pressure.

The Brüel and Kjaer anaesthetic gas monitor (Fig. 15.10) utilizes photo-acoustic spectroscopy. Nitrous oxide, carbon dioxide and the halogenated anaesthetic vapours absorb specific wavelengths in the infrared region. If these gases and vapours are irradiated with pulsatile IR energy, of a suitable wavelength, then a sound wave is produced which can be detected by a microphone.

The schematic representation in Fig. 15.11 shows the principle of the measurement system. The gases

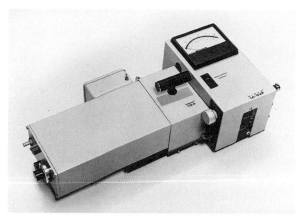

**Figure 15.9** Miran variable-wavelength variable-path-length infrared spectrophotometer, capable of measuring gas concentrations in the percentage range or the parts-per-million range.

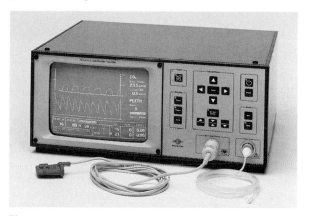

**Figure 15.10** Brüel and Kjaer's anaesthetic gas monitor type 1304.

under test are drawn through a small measurement chamber which is irradiated by an IR source. The radiation is 'chopped' by a rapidly rotating wheel. In order to differentiate between nitrous oxide, carbon dioxide and the volatile agents, the IR beam is chopped at three different frequencies. To do this, the chopper wheel has three concentric bands of holes, and this causes the IR energy to pulsate at three different audio frequencies. Each part of the now divided beam passes through a narrow-band filter appropriate to the absorption of carbon dioxide, nitrous oxide, or the halogenated hydrocarbon anaesthetic vapours. The absorption of the IR energy causes each gas to expand and contract at its relevant audio frequency.

This periodic expansion and contraction produces a pressure fluctuation of audible frequency which can be detected by a microphone. As oxygen does not absorb IR energy, it cannot be measured by

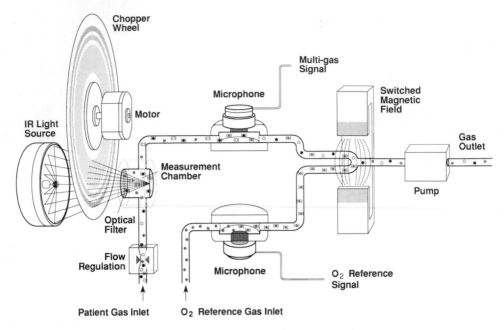

**Figure 15.11** Working principles of the Brüel and Kjaer's anaesthetic gas monitor.

photo-acoustic spectroscopy, but an alternating magnetic field applied to the gas mixture will induce an audible signal in the oxygen by making use of its paramagnetic property.

The multigas signal from the microphone is electronically filtered into its four component parts: oxygen, nitrous oxide, carbon dioxide and halogenated hydrocarbons. As the halogenated anaesthetic vapours in use all have similar IR absorption spectra, photo-acoustic spectroscopy is unable to distinguish between them.

There are a number of important advantages in photo-acoustic spectrometry over conventional IR absorption spectrometry. Firstly the photo-acoustic technique appears to be extremely stable, with virtually no zero drift, and its calibration remains constant over much longer periods of time. The second major advantage is the very fast rise and fall times, giving a much truer representation of any change in gas concentrations. When reading the specification of a gas analyser, it is important to note the conditions under which such things as the rise time are measured. Rise time is usually quoted from the input to the measuring device. However, Brüel and Kjaer quote the rise time when a step change in concentration is made at the patient end of the monitoring catheter.

## Raman scattering

This new technique for gas monitoring makes use of

**Table 15.1** Raman frequency shifts with radiation from an argon laser

| Gas | Frequency shift Wave no. (cm$^{-1}$) | Wave length (nm) |
|---|---|---|
| Carbon dioxide | 1285 | 520.6 |
| Carbon dioxide | 1388 | 523.4 |
| Enflurane | 817 | 508.3 |
| Halothane | 717 | 505.7 |
| Isoflurane | 995 | 512.9 |
| Nitrogen | 2331 | 550.6 |
| Nitrous oxide | 1285 | 520.6 |
| Nitrous oxide | 2224 | 547.4 |
| Oxygen | 1555 | 528.1 |
| Water | 3650 | 593.8 |

a property similar to fluorescence. When gas molecules are bombarded with energy of a discrete wavelength, they may scatter energy at very low levels at a different wavelength. The difference or 'shift' is characteristic of the species of molecule.

Intense monochromatic energy from an argon laser (plasma tube) of wavelength 488 nm irradiates a cell which forms part of the laser (Fig. 15.13). The gas under test is aspirated through the cell. Energy is scattered by the gas molecules. The filters absorb the scattered light of the same wavelength as the laser, that is the 'unshifted' laser wavelength. Any 'shifted' wavelengths pass on through a rapidly rotating filter wheel with narrow-band pass filters appropriate to each of the gases and vapours of interest. The very low levels of light are then detected with a photomultiplier tube. In the Rascal (Fig. 15.12) a separate channel is provided to measure carbon dioxide.

Raman scattering is a new technique in gas analysis with exciting possibilities for multigas analysis, and with the advantages that it is cheaper and more reliable than mass spectroscopy and more versatile than infrared absorption spectroscopy.

## Position of Sampling

The sampling of the respiratory gas may be done in one of two ways, namely *sidestream* or *mainstream*. Because of their methods of analysis, mass spectrometers and Raman spectrometers use sidestream sampling, as do most IR instruments. Only the precise tubing recommended by the manufacturer should be used, and only of the recommended length. Typical IR instruments sample at a flow rate between 50 and 150 ml/min. The problems encountered with sidestream sampling include:

- water-vapour condensation;
- distortion of the respiratory waveform by too high a flow rate, the capillary tube being too long, or the capillary tube diameter being too large.

It is also important that the tip of the sampling tube should always be as near as possible to the patient's trachea, but the sampled gas mixture must not be contaminated by inspired gas during the expiratory phase. This is a definite risk if the sample is extracted near the patient end of a coaxial

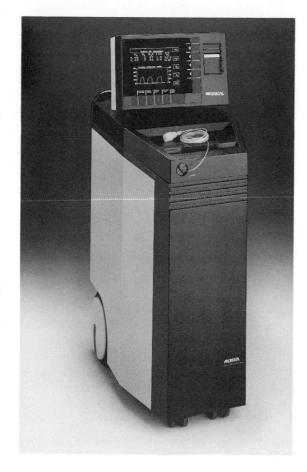

**Figure 15.12**   Rascal anaesthetic gas monitor.

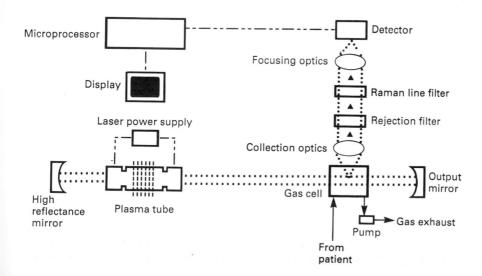

**Figure 15.13**   Working principles of the Raman anaesthetic gas monitor.

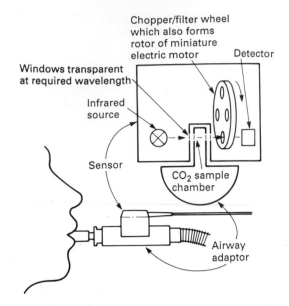

**Figure 15.14** The principle of the Hewlett-Packard mainstream carbon dioxide gas analyser.

Mapleson D breathing system and may give rise to erroneously low end-tidal readings. With sidestream sampling, sometimes the gases should not be returned to the breathing system, because sometimes they are denatured by the measuring technique.

Mainstream sampling, although more cumbersome, does have advantages over sidestream monitoring. The gas to be analysed never leaves the respiratory attachment. Windows, that are transparent to the IR wavelengths in use, form part of an adaptor or even the catheter mount, and a miniature IR source, filter-wheel, motor and detector are attached over the windows (Fig. 15.14). The advantages of mainstream sampling are that there is no delay in the rise and fall times of gas composition changes, no gas is lost from the attachment, no mixing occurs along a capillary tube before analysis, and there are fewer problems with water vapour condensation.

# Breathing Attachment Disconnect Alarms

Breathing disconnect alarms use one of two principles: detection of exhaled tidal volumes, or pressure changes in the breathing attachment. Both of these methods are related to time. With the tidal volume method, a pre-set exhaled tidal volume must recur at greater than a minimum pre-set frequency whereas with the pressure method the airway pressure must exceed a certain pre-set level and then reduce to below that level rhythmically at greater than a minimum pre-set rate. The tidal volume method is applicable to both spontaneously breathing and ventilated patients and usually forms part of a respirometer. The pressure method is applicable only to ventilated patients. It usually incorporates an alarm for excessive inspiratory pressure due, for example, to kinking of the endotracheal tube, but gives no indication of decreased tidal volume with, say, deteriorating compliance.

# Measurement of Respiratory Volumes

The measurement of inhaled and, more importantly, exhaled respiratory volumes during anaesthesia is normally carried out by one of the following techniques:

- turbine respirometer (Wright's);
- positive displacement (Dräger);
- calibrated bellows;
- hot-wire anemometry (*not* with flammable agents);
- vortex shedding.

These techniques measure *flow* and the respiratory volumes are the result of integration with respect to time.

The principles of these techniques are discussed in Chapter 5.

# 16 Non-invasive Patient Monitoring

## Introduction

The physiological monitoring discussed in this chapter includes only non-invasive equipment that would normally be applied to every patient to whom general anaesthesia was administered. Thus only the devices recommended by various 'Standards' of anaesthetic practice are described.

## Electrocardiogram

The electrical signals generated by the beating heart may be detected by placement on the surface of the body of electrodes connected to a high-gain amplifier and may then be displayed on an oscilloscope. As measured at the body surface, typical amplitudes are 1–5 mV with a frequency range of 0.1–100 Hz. This frequency range does *not* imply that the heart rate is of this range but that the PQRST complex may be broken down by Fourier analysis into components made up from the addition of frequencies in this range. This means that to produce a faithful representation of the electrical events, the ECG amplifier must have a bandwidth covering this range, in other words, it should amplify by a constant amount over the range of 0.1–100 Hz. The greater the bandwidth of an amplifier, the more accurately the output will be a function of the input, but also the greater will be the unwanted interference. This interference may be biological, mainly due to noise generated by muscle (electromyogram, EMG) or environmental noise due to power cables, electrical instruments, transformers or surgical diathermy equipment that becomes electrically or magnetically coupled to the body or monitoring leads. For this reason, bandwidth is limited to a compromise between the quality of the ECG signal and the acceptable level of interference. For diagnostic purposes, ECG pre-amplifiers usually have a bandwidth of 0.05–100 Hz, but for monitoring in electrically noisy environments, as in the operating theatre, the bandwidth is limited to 0.5–40 Hz. The effect of this narrower bandwidth is to 'round-off' slightly the sharper peaks and troughs of the QRS complex and markedly reduce interference while making it still quite possible to assess arrhythmias and ischaemia. A band-pass rather than a low-pass filter is also necessary to eliminate the approximately 25 mV of d.c. skin potential that exists at the interface between the recording electrode and the skin. This 25 mV is due in part to the potentials generated by the epidermal layers of the skin, and in part due to the electrochemical cell ('battery') formed by the skin–electrolytic gel–metallic electrode combination.

The tissues of the body have a relatively high electrical resistance and the ECG signal is said to be a high-impedance source; it is therefore necessary to use a high-quality amplifier with a high input impedance. Electrical noise is also generated by the components of the amplifier itself, but careful design can minimize its effect. Safety is a prime consideration, as recording or monitoring the ECG is one of the few techniques in which direct electrical connection is deliberately made to the human body. The patient must therefore be protected from (a) faults that may occur in the monitoring system and (b) an unwanted earth pathway for surgical diathermy or a fault condition leading to an unwanted earth pathway in another piece of apparatus connected to the patient. The monitoring equipment is also protected from damage by high voltages from RF surgical diathermy and even defibrillator pulses.

Figure 16.1 shows the components of a modern ECG monitor. A simple amplifier would have a single input terminal and its output would be a function of the potential difference between that input terminal and the ground reference. Any *electromagnetic interference* (EMI) which would be coupled to the input lead, either inductively or

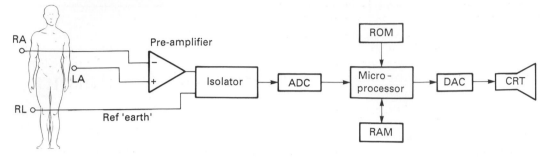

**Figure 16.1** Block diagram of a modern ECG monitor.

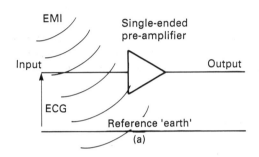

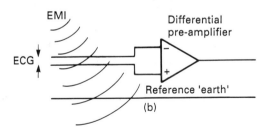

**Figure 16.2** Effect of electromagnetic interference (EMI) on the ECG signal. (a) Single-ended pre-amplifier. Note that the difference in interference to 'input' and 'reference earth' is amplified. (b) Identical EMI affecting (−) and (+) inputs of differential amplifier is cancelled out, as the amplifier amplifies the *difference* between the two inputs.

capacitively, (Fig. 16.2a), would be unlikely to couple to both the input lead and the ground reference to the same extent, and therefore the interference — which may be of much greater amplitude than the ECG signal itself — will also be amplified. Even the simplest of ECG monitors therefore make use of a differential or balanced pre-amplifier (Fig. 16.2b). The reference earth lead is connected to the patient; this lead is often marked 'Right Leg' or 'RL'. However, the ECG is detected as the difference between inverting (−) and non-inverting (+) inputs to the pre-amplifier, which is

designed to have a high common mode rejection ratio (CMRR). The CMRR is a measure of the ratio between the wanted and interfering signals; the higher the value of the CMRR the better the quality of the amplifier. Thus any EMI affecting the input leads will be of the same polarity in both leads and will therefore be cancelled out and only the ECG signal will be amplified.

The pre-amplifier is electrically isolated from the rest of the monitor by either transformers with a high degree of insulation between primary and secondary windings or by *optical isolation*, where the amplified signal is converted to light by a light-emitting diode, which is insulated from a photo-detector that converts the signal back into an electrical one. The very high power of RF surgical diathermy equipment may overwhelm the simple techniques described thus far.

High-quality ECG monitors for use in operating theatres may use *adaptive noise filtering*, a complex digital electronic technique in which the EMI is detected separately from the ECG signal and then subtracted from the ECG+EMI, thus leaving a clean ECG trace without the EMI.

Early ECG monitors used the so-called 'bouncing dot' type of scan on a cathode-ray tube which had a long-persistence output phosphor. It takes a lot of practice to make a diagnosis from this type of display and it is impossible to 'freeze' a frame for further examination as the only 'memory' was the persistence of the phosphor. Today's ECG monitors, and displays of other analogue traces, make use of a microprocessor memory technique. The analogue signal is converted to a digital one by an analogue to digital converter (ADC). Sufficient ECG data, now in digital form, is stored in the semiconductor random access memory (RAM) to fill the width of the display screen. As the latest information is stored, so the oldest is erased, thus ensuring that the most up-to-date 5 or 10 s are stored in the RAM. Simultaneously, the entire RAM is read out very rapidly through the microprocessor and a digital to analogue converter (DAC) to a cathode-ray tube (CRT) display. Thus a 'rolling' display of the previous 5–10 s is displayed and may be 'frozen' for closer examination. If a liquid crystal dislay (LCD) is used it may be driven digitally directly from the microprocessor. ECG monitors for use during anaesthesia may have an alarm that operates when the heart rate goes outside pre-set limits, but further sophistication is usually not provided unless the machine has been designed for use in intensive care situations.

## Pulse Monitoring

The character of the arterial pulse, its rate and its rhythm have always been important, not only to the mystic of medicine but also to scientific diagnosis, and no more so than in the practice of anaesthesia. Although the greatest amount of information may be gained by palpation of the radial pulse, it is usually inconvenient to do this throughout a long surgical procedure. For this reason several non-invasive methods have been developed for electronic monitoring of the arterial pulse. Pulse-plethysmography, as the technique is called, also forms the basis of two modern monitoring techniques: pulse-oximetry and continuous non-invasive blood pressure monitoring described below.

Pulse-plethysmography is based upon the measurement of the increase in the volume of an extremity, usually a finger or an ear lobe, during or shortly after systole. The earliest electronic pulse-plethysmographs consisted of a flexible capsule containing carbon granules which was firmly applied to a finger. As the finger increased in volume with systole, so the capsule was compressed and the electrical resistance of the mass of carbon granules decreased. In the simplest pulse monitor this is detected with a moving-coil meter and a dry battery forming a simple circuit.

All pulse-plethysmograph devices now use the technique of photo-plethysmography (Fig. 16.3). A low level of electromagnetic energy is passed through the extremity. Most of the energy, which must be at a wavelength to which the part is partially translucent, is detected by a semiconductor sensor or photodetector suitable for that wavelength. An increase in volume of the part is then detected as an increase in the absorption of the incident light during systole. The signal from the photodetector is then amplified and may be displayed on a cathode-ray oscilloscope. This tech-

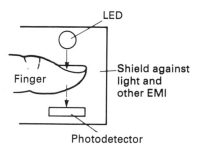

**Figure 16.3** Schematic diagram of the probe of the photoplethysmographic pulse detector.

nique may be so sensitive that the dichrotic notch is easily visible. The 'light' used is usually not at visible wavelengths as it is customary to use near infrared, because it is then possible to use a detector that is sensitive only to these wavelengths, thus eliminating artefacts caused by ambient light.

## Pulse-oximetry

*In vivo* oximetry has a long history since it has long been regarded as of great importance, especially in respiratory physiology and anaesthesia. This history, although fascinating, is unfortunately out of place in this volume and so it is possible only to describe the technique of pulse-oximetry.

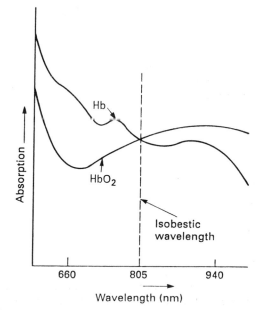

**Figure 16.4** Absorption spectra of oxygenated and deoxygenated HbA.

If the absorption spectrum of a whole finger were plotted with the arterial blood totally saturated with oxygen, and also with it totally unsaturated, the difference in the spectra would be very difficult to see. The absorption spectra of haemoglobin alone is shown in Fig. 16.4, in both the saturated and unsaturated states and the difference in absorption at the various wavelengths is obvious. The pulse-oximeter is able not only to separate the absorption due to haemoglobin from that due to the other constituents of the finger, but also to separate the arterial haemoglobin oxygen saturation from that of the haemoglobin in capillaries, venules and veins. This was not possible before the advent of light-emitting diodes (LEDs) and microprocessors.

Conventional pulse-oximeters transmit through an extremity, usually a finger, energy of two wavelengths: red 660 nm and near infrared 940 nm, alternately and at a frequency between 700 Hz and 1 kHz. This frequency is fast enough for a pulse-photo-plethysmogram to be sensed by a single semiconductor detector as shown in Fig. 16.5. The ratio between the amounts of absorption at the two wavelengths varies almost linearly (Fig. 16.6) with haemoglobin oxygen saturation. The absorption of the two wavelengths by the non-arterial blood and other tissues is eliminated by the simple electronic technique of removing the component of the signal due to them by high-pass filtering. This is because their absorption changes only very slowly, if at all, when compared to the change in absorption due to systole in the arterial absorption (Fig. 16.7). The arterial a.c. component is about 1–2% of the total absorption (a.c. + d.c.) but even this very small amount cannot be caused by the very small change in volume of the arteries during systole. Study of the fluid mechanics of blood flow in small arteries shows that, in systole, a greater proportion of erythrocytes have their diameter perpendicular to the vessel wall than during diastole when they tend

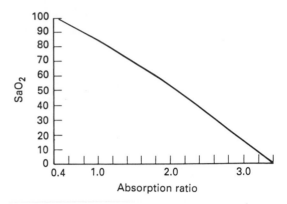

**Figure 16.6**   Theoretical ratio of absorption of red (660 nm) and infrared (940 nm) light energy related to $SaO_2$.

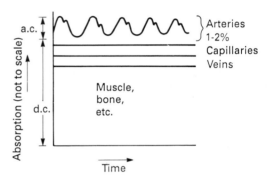

**Figure 16.7**   Composition of the absorption signal as detected by photoplethysmography (not to scale).

to lie parallel to the flow. This would account for the greater than expected increase in absorption during systole.

It is more important with the pulse-oximeter than with almost any other monitor to understand the limitations of the technique so that its results may be used safely.

The most serious limitation of pulse-oximetry is

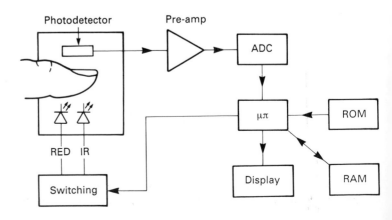

**Figure 16.5**   Schematic diagram of main components of a pulse-oximeter. μπ: micro-processor's central processing unit.

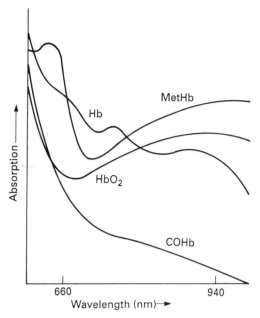

**Figure 16.8** Absorption spectra of two of the interfering dyshaemoglobins: carboxyhaemoglobin (COHb) and methaemoglobin (MetHb).

the errors caused by abnormal substances in the arteries with absorption spectra that interfere with that of normal adult haemoglobin. The most common of these substances are the dyshaemoglobins carboxyhaemoglobin and methaemoglobin, the absorption spectra of which are shown in Fig. 16.8. Increasing, but still very low, concentrations of carboxyhaemoglobin make the pulse-oximeter reading tend towards 100%, whereas increasing concentrations of methaemoglobin make the readings tend towards 85%. Because currently available pulse-oximeters use only two wavelengths, it is impossible for the software of the microprocessor to detect dyshaemoglobins, so the user will therefore be unaware of the error in the reading. Certain injected dyes will adversely affect the accuracy of the indicated oxygen saturation. The operation of a pulse-oximeter may also be effected by the RF diathermy, extraneous light, nail varnish, hypothermia and poor perfusion. In each of these cases, the malfunction is indicated by an alarm.

# Non-invasive Blood Pressure Monitoring

Arterial blood pressure may be estimated non-invasively with an accuracy suitable for clinical purposes. A pneumatic cuff of the appropriate size is applied to the upper arm and is inflated to greater than the expected systolic pressure, thus occluding arterial flow. The cuff is then slowly deflated and some method of arterial blood-flow detection is used to estimate the cuff pressure at which arterial flow *just* begins (systolic pressure) and when arterial flow is totally unimpeded (diastolic pressure). In its simplest form, a mercury manometer or aneroid gauge displays the cuff pressure, whilst flow is detected by auscultation of the Korotkoff sounds with a stethoscope. The stethoscope may be replaced by a microphone, allowing electronic amplification of the sounds. The flow may even be detected by a Doppler ultrasonic flow detector. Arterial blood pressure during anaesthesia is most commonly measured using the oscillometric principle. If one examines carefully the meniscus of the mercury in a mercury sphygmomanometer as the cuff pressure is slowly reduced, small fluctuations, sychronous with heart rhythm, may be seen on the manometer when the cuff is inflated at pressures between systolic and diastolic pressures, with a maximum amplitude at mean arterial blood pressure.

These fluctuations may be detected by a double-cuff device known as an oscillotonometer (Fig. 16.9). A double pneumatic cuff is applied to the upper arm as shown in Fig. 16.9a. The instrument itself consists of two aneroid capsules one of which is coarse (A) and the other very sensitive (B) inside a sealed case and they are connected by a lever mechanism and a rack-and-pinion to a pointer, as shown in Fig. 16.9b. Capsule A is sealed and responds to changes in pressure in the case. Capsule B is connected to the distal cuff. The valve lever is biased to position 1 where the release valve is occluded and there is free communication between the two sides of capsule B. Manual inflation of the system with the bulb causes an increase in pressure equally in both cuffs, and the case of the instrument and this pressure is indicated on the scale as the capsule A decreases in volume. When the pressure is in excess of the expected arterial pressure, inflation is ceased and the lever is moved to position 2. A small-bore aperture is now interposed between the inside and outside of capsule B and air is allowed to leak slowly from the system through the pressure release valve. Pulsations occurring in the distal cuff are indicated by fluctuations of capsule B only. As the pressure in the system is released, oscillations will first occur at systolic blood pressure, reach a maximum at the mean pressure, and should finally disappear at the diastolic pressure.

The oscillotonometer gives only a useable clinical

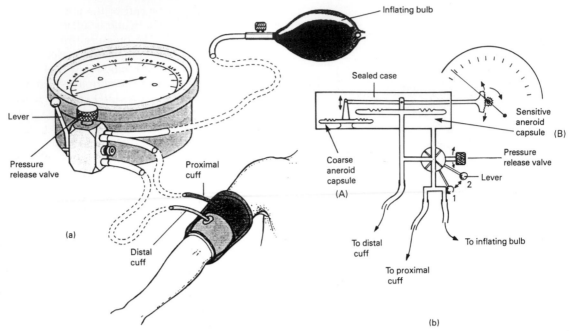

**Figure 16.9** The von Recklinghausen oscillotonometer (see text). Reproduced from Ponte, J and Green, D, (1986) *A New Short Textbook of Anaesthetics*. Edward Arnold.

accuracy at the systolic pressure. The actual blood pressure is indicated by releasing the lever back to position 1, at which time the scale indicates the cuff pressure.

It is now common practice to use electronic techniques, again relying on the oscillometric principle. Electronic oscillometric blood pressure monitors make use of a conventional pneumatic cuff surrounding, usually, the upper arm. Some manufacturers use a single tube to connect the cuff to the monitor whilst others use two tubes, separating the pump tube from that along which the pressure in the cuff is sensed. Figure 16.10 shows the principle of the technique. At the centre of the machine is a microprocessor which controls all the other components. The pump inflates the cuff to above the expected systolic pressure, which is measured by the pressure transducer. The air in the cuff is then allowed to leak slowly out via a solenoid valve, either smoothly or in a series of discrete steps. As the pressure in the cuff falls, the signal from the transducer varies, as shown in the graph. This signal is amplified in two ways: (1) After passing through a low-pass filter, it is amplified by a comparatively low-gain amplifier, the output of which is then proportional to the cuff pressure at that instant. (2) The signal is also passed through a high-pass filter, which effectively removes the electrical signal due to the slowly changing cuff pressure, and then through a high-gain amplifier so

that the comparatively high-frequency oscillations due to the oscillations of the arterial wall alone are amplified. It can be seen that these oscillations begin at the systolic pressure, are a maximum at the mean pressure, and finally disappear at the diastolic pressure. The signals from both these amplifiers are then passed through an analogue-to-digital converter (ADC) to the microprocessor. The microprocessor, apart from controlling the pump and the solenoid valve, calculates the systolic, diastolic and mean pressures and controls the display and alarms. The microprocessor also compares the results for systolic and diastolic pressures with what would be expected from the mean pressure. This is done because the most accurate measurement made by these machines is the mean pressure, as the maximum oscillations are much more easily detected than the points at which the oscillations *just* start and disappear.

It is possible that the values of blood pressure obtained with this technique do not exactly correspond to those obtained by direct intra-arterial measurement at the radial artery. This is often due to under-damping of the direct arterial pressure signal, but it has also been shown that pressure measured by the oscillometric technique is comparable to central aortic blood pressure. The heart rate is always displayed at the same time since it is so easy for the microprocessor to calculate this from the period between each oscillation.

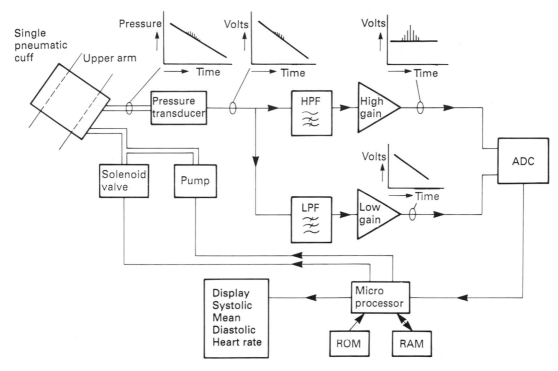

**Figure 16.10** Schematic diagram of the automatic non-invasive arterial blood pressure monitor using the oscillotonometric principle.

Oscillometric non-invasive blood pressure monitors may also have integral printers that record the blood pressure, heart rate and time at pre-set intervals.

The only major disadvantage of the conventional oscillometric blood pressure monitor is that it can make only discrete blood pressure measurements, at best, once every 2 minutes or so.

A recent development is a non-invasive blood pressure monitor using a very small pneumatically inflated cuff applied to a finger. The cuff also contains an infrared photo-plethysmograph. The technique is based on the concept that if an externally applied pressure is equal to the arterial wall pressure at all times, the artery will not change in size. If the arteries under the cuff are therefore kept at the same size, the blood volume contained within them will remain constant as will the absorption of the infrared light and therefore the photo-plethysmogram signal will remain constant. A microprocessor-controlled servo-system maintains the cuff pressure so that the light absorption remains constant. The pressure in the cuff is therefore instantaneously the same as that in the artery and a continuous blood pressure reading is therefore available.

# Temperature Measurement

The commonest method of measuring patient temperature is still by use of a mercury-in-glass clinical thermometer. However, remote-reading thermometry is much more convenient with the anaesthetized patient, using one of three electronic methods.

The resistance wire thermometer relies on the property of, usually, a platinum wire changing its electrical resistance linearly with temperature.

Thermistors are semiconductor temperature sensors that have the advantage that their change in resistance is greater with temperature than the resistance wire thermometer, but the change is not entirely linear and the calibration may drift with ageing. Thermistor temperature sensors may be extremely small — so small as to be able to be applied to the tympanic membrane.

Thermocouple thermometers rely on the Seebeck effect, in which a potential difference occurs at the junction between two dissimilar metals when they complete an electrical circuit. This voltage is very small and needs either amplification or a very sensitive galvanometer. The advantage of the thermocouple thermometer is that all couples made with the same materials will behave identically and therefore the calibration will not change should the couple be replaced.

# Assessment of the Neuromuscular Junction

A transcutaneous nerve stimulator may be used to assess blockade of the neuromuscular junction. This consists of a battery-powered pulse generator of sufficient output voltage to cause depolarization of a nerve passing subcutaneously when the electrodes are applied to the skin surface. The output must be low enough that no damage is caused and that skeletal muscle is not caused to contract directly, other than due to depolarization of the nerve supplying it. It is possible to select between a single pulse, a train of four, or tetanic stimulus. The effect of neuromuscular blockade is routinely assessed by observing the muscle twitches initiated by the stimulator. However, it is possible to measure the contractions more quantitively either by arranging a strain gauge force sensor to measure the force of the contraction, or by detecting and recording the electromyogram signal generated by the muscle.

This device should not be confused with the therapeutic TENS (transcutaneous electrical nerve stimulation) machine used for pain relief.

# 17 Atmospheric Pollution

## Introduction

There have been many epidemiological studies on the alleged adverse effect of chronic exposure to trace concentrations of anaesthetic gases and vapours in operating theatres and recovery rooms. The evidence is somewhat conflicting and/or inconclusive. Commonly quoted references suggest that:

- There is a common tendency to increased incidence of spontaneous abortion in female anaesthetists, anaesthetic nurses, and also the wives of men working in theatres.
- There is an increased incidence of minor congenital abnormalities amongst children of anaesthetic personnel.
- There appears to be an abnormal sex ratio among children born to anaesthetists, with a higher incidence of female children being born.
- There is an increased incidence of subjective complaints (headaches, fatigue, sleep loss, nervousness, pruritis).
- There is a higher rate of cancer (leukaemia and lymphoma) amongst exposed females.
- There is a higher incidence of liver disease in anaesthetists.
- There is an increased incidence of renal disease in exposed females.
- Dentists exposed to chronically high levels of nitrous oxide have developed neurological symptoms suggestive of a vitamin $B_{12}$ deficiency. This finding has been confirmed in rats chronically exposed to nitrous oxide.
- Animal studies (in rats) also show that chronic exposure to nitrous oxide has resulted in litters that are reduced in number and size compared with control animals.

It must be stressed, however, that some epidemiological studies did not confirm some of these claims.

It would seem prudent, however, to reduce levels of anaesthetic agents in the operating theatre environment, especially with the recent introduction (October 1989) in the UK of a government-approved code of practice 'Control of substances hazardous to health' (COSHH). This code of practice has been drawn up under the auspices of the Health and Safety Commission's (HSC) Advisory Committee on Toxic Substances and has been approved by the HSC under section 16 of the Health and Safety at Work Act (1974) for the purpose of providing practical guidance on the control of substances hazardous to health in the workplace.

This code came into force on 1 October 1989 and covers a wide variety of substances including anaesthetic gases and vapours. COSHH regulations require an employer to protect employees by:

1. assessment of risk;
2. prevention or control of exposure;
3. installation of control measures and maintenance of them as well as regular examination and testing of the control measures;
4. monitoring of exposure at the workplace;
5. provision of health surveillance;
6. provision of information and training.

Under item 2, COSHH recommends that 'Exposure should be controlled to a level to which nearly all the population can be exposed day after day without adverse effect on health'. However, there are no exposure standards for anaesthetic agents in the UK, with the exception of trichloroethylene (Trilene); the upper acceptable limit for this agent is an average of 100 ppm in any 8-h period of potential exposure. This reference exposure is usually expressed as an 8-h TWA (time-weighted average). The COSHH recommendation for other agents is that their concentration should be reduced as far as reasonably practicable.

Recommended exposure limits for anaesthetic gases and vapours in the United States are those set out by the National Institute for Occupational Safety and Health (NIOSH), which are as follows:

*Enflurane* 75 ppm (575 mg/m$^3$)
*Halothane* 50 ppm (400 mg/m$^3$)
*Nitrous Oxide* 50 ppm (91 mg/m$^3$)

The exposure limits are also based on the 8-h TWA.

Recent surveys have shown that when no steps are taken to avoid pollution, these limits are exceeded. For instance, two studies reported in the published code (COSHH) showed from a twenty-hospital survey that the levels of halothane varied between 0.1 and 60 ppm and for nitrous oxide between 200 and 300 ppm when no steps were taken. A twenty-seven-hospital survey showed the mean time-weighted average exposures to halothane were 1.7 ppm and to nitrous oxide 94 ppm.

# The Extent of Pollution

This depends on five factors:

- the amount of anaesthetic vapours employed;
- the size and layout of the operating theatre and any other place where anaesthetic vapours are used;
- the efficiency of the scavenging system;
- the efficiency of the air-conditioning and ventilating systems;
- the amount of leakage from the anaesthetic equipment.

## The amount of anaesthetic vapours employed

This may vary considerably. At one extreme is the non-rebreathing system used commonly in the UK, where there is a fresh gas flow of about 8 litres/min, of which 70% may be nitrous oxide, and to which the vapour of halothane or other agents may be added. Many anaesthetists in the UK feel that the employment of high flow rates contributes to simplicity and safety, and are not deterred from using them on economic grounds as yet, since they do not, personally, have to defray the cost of drugs used in the National Health Service. However, this attitude may well change in the near future.

At the other end of the scale are those who employ local and regional analgesia and total intravenous anaesthesia, or low-flow and closed systems. Discussion of the relative merits of these techniques as they affect the patient is not within the scope of this book.

## The size of the premises

'Dental chair' anaesthetics for extractions are fre-quently administered in small rooms. This, in itself, is probably of little importance, since the anaesthesia is of only short duration and most dentists employ general anaesthetics only occasionally, so exposure of the personnel (except the travelling anaesthetist!) is limited. However, the advent of inhalational methods for relative analgesia and sedation has resulted in much more prolonged exposure. In these techniques high flow rates of nitrous oxide may be used. This is discussed in greater detail in Chapter 11.

## The efficiency of the air-conditioning system

The frequency of air changes is often quoted. A figure of 20 per hour is usually considered satisfactory. However, the circulation of air throughout the theatre is often uneven, and frequently the recovery area, where the patient exhales anaesthetic agents, is poorly ventilated and there may be no arrangements for scavenging. The nurse attending the patient is often in direct line with the exhaled gases. There are two further considerations. The first is that some air-conditioning systems are wholly or partially recirculating, and may result in the vapours from one location polluting another. The second is that thought must be given to the siting of the external outlet of the extract system, which again may pollute other areas in which people work.

## Leakage

However efficient a scavenging system may be, its purposes will be defeated if gases and vapours are permitted to escape from the apparatus. Overt leaks from the high-pressure and regulated-pressure parts of the anaesthetic machine may be easily detected. Leaks from the breathing attachment may be less obvious, however, and may even be due to diffusion through the rubber or neoprene parts. The latter often absorb significant quantities of some of the volatile agents during the administration of one anaesthetic — only to release them during the next. For this reason new and unused breathing attachments should be used for the administration of an anaesthetic to a patient who exhibits sensitivity to a particular anaesthetic agent, for instance in the case of malignant hyperpyrexia.

Leakage may also result from carelessness when vaporizers are refilled.

# Control of Pollution

The control of pollution should be tackled along the

guidelines recommended in COSHH in the UK and NIOSH in the USA, namely:

1. Instilling an awareness in personnel working in the potentially affected environment.
2. Installation of effective scavenging equipment (see below).
3. Ensuring good working practices by
   (a) Always using the devices provided.
   (b) Daily inspection of these devices to establish that they are functioning.
   (c) Considering the use of low-flow systems where appropriate.
   (d) Checking for leaks in the breathing system.
   (e) Flushing out the breathing system (including the reservoir bag) through the scavenging device provided, at the end of an anaesthetic.
   (f) Considering capping off the breathing system at the end of an anaesthetic so as to prevent anaesthetic vapours that have impregnated the breathing hoses from polluting the environment.
   (g) The filling of anaesthetic vaporizers in a fume cupboard that includes a spill tray.
4. Efficient room air-conditioning so as to remove any pollutant that may have inadvertently escaped. (A minimum of 15 changes per hour with a balanced supply and extraction process.)
5. Regular monitoring of the theatre environment.

What constitutes regular monitoring appears to many anaesthetists to be the most difficult issue to resolve. Monthly or fortnightly checks might miss a week in which the levels could, due to a fault, contravene COSHH guidelines. An employer (the hospital) if sued by an employee could well find the case difficult to defend.

The extent of pollution in the theatre environment is now continuously quantifiable with the recent introduction of low-cost, non-dispersive infrared analysers that measure trace quantities of anaesthetic agents. A single analyser (e.g. the Ullair Gas Handling Unit) can be set to measure 12–24 sampling lines and record the extent of pollution at the sites on a continuous basis, logging the results on a chart recorder and producing an alarm when excessive levels are recorded.

# Scavenging Systems

A scavenging system is designed to transport waste gases and vapours from a ventilator or breathing system and to discharge them at some safe remote location. The various items that have been de-veloped to meet these needs include a *collecting system*, which conveys waste gases from the breathing system via *transfer tubing* to the *receiving system*. The receiving system behaves as a reservoir to store surges in the flow of waste gas. From here these gases have to pass via a *disposal tubing* to the *disposal system*. Two or more of these items may be embodied in a single item of equipment.

Waste gas may pass passively through the receiving and disposal system, using only the power generated in exhalation by the elastic recoil of a patient's lungs (passive scavenging), or it may be assisted through some form of gas or electrically powered apparatus which generates a sub-atmospheric pressure (active scavenging). Only systems that employ active scavenging are able to deal with the wide range of expiratory flow rates (30–120 litres/min) seen in anaesthetic practice, especially when certain ventilator systems are used. These systems (as opposed to passive systems) are, therefore, the only ones that can be recommended. And this is provided that they meet the specification and performance criteria approved by those countries in which they are in use (e.g. BS 6384:1987 UK).

## The disposal system

### Active systems

The subatmospheric pressure, required to power the disposal system, is usually provided by an exhauster unit, see Fig. 17.1 (although other devices are mentioned below). This works in a similar fashion to a fan and requires a low level of maintenance and no lubrication. The size of the unit depends on the number of scavenging sites to be supplied. Large exhauster units can provide waste gas flow rates of up to 2400 litres/min, servicing 20 sites. Large sites often have a 'Duty' and a 'Standby' unit which are linked. The 'Standby unit' is designed to operate automatically if the 'Duty' unit fails, as well as during periods of high demand. Although the exhauster unit is sited outside the operating theatre suite (sometimes a considerable distance away), the operating control switch is sited at a convenient location within the theatre suite.

Waste gas is fed into the disposal system via a terminal unit, sited on a wall or flexible pendant, both in the anaesthetic room and in the operating theatre. The unit contains a sealed female Schrader type socket which opens when the male probe from the receiving unit is connected.

Pressure fluctuations within the disposal system are controlled within precise limits by a vacuum/

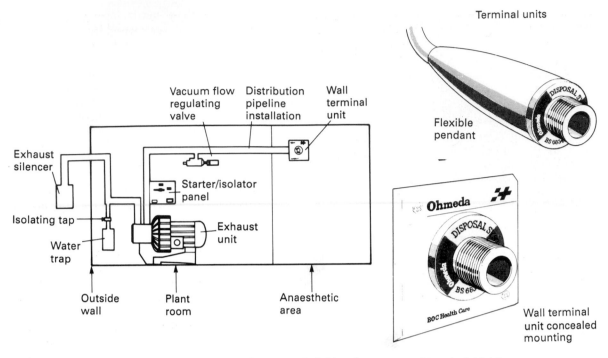

**Figure 17.1** A disposal system showing the exhauster unit (left) and two types of terminal (right).

flow regulating valve. It consists of an adjustable spring loaded plate covering the valve aperture and behaves as an air-entrainment valve should the vacuum exceed a predetermined level. This level is set, by adjusting the spring tension during commissioning of the system, to provide the correct flow rates. A number of valves may be fitted to large scavenging systems so as to protect and control specific areas.

The exhauster unit discharges the waste gas to a suitable outside wall via rigid pipework. A water trap, with an isolating tap, is included in this pathway to drain any accumulated condensation.

The use of an existing hospital piped vacuum system has often been advocated in the past. However these systems cannot be recommended as they may be unsatisfactory in design and may well be dangerous as:

- Scavenging requires a high flow system with a small pressure gradient between the terminal unit and the exhaust unit, whereas the piped vacuum in a hospital utilizes a lower flow with a larger pressure gradient between the vacuum pump and the terminal unit.
- The extra demand upon the medical vacuum for this purpose may result in other users being deprived of an adequate medical vacuum in an emergency.

- The displacement (flow rate) of the vacuum line may be inadequate to cope with the high flow rate and the pulsating nature of the output of some ventilators.
- The outlet of the vacuum system may be so located that the expired gases would pollute areas where other personnel are working.
- More importantly, as vacuum lines do not contain safety valves (vacuum/flow regulating valves, see above), there is a danger that an excessive 'vacuum' may be applied to a patient.

Other methods of providing active gas scavenging have been employed. These include:

- A venturi system, powered by compressed air, which may be used in place of the exhauster unit described above.
- A system such as the ejector flowmeter which is attached to each anaesthetic machine (see Fig. 17.7).

## Passive systems

In passive systems a wide-bore tube passes through one of the walls or the roof of the building and terminates in a ventile (Fig. 17.2). A ventile is a device which depends on the wind to entrain the exhaust gases or air. Unfortunately, the passive system can be relied upon to operate satisfactorily

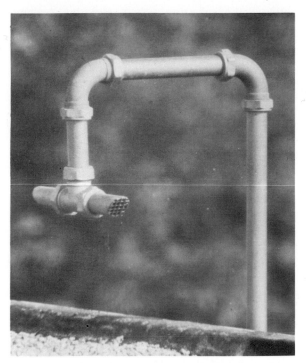

Figure 17.2  A ventile for passive waste gas disposal.

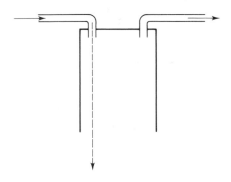

Figure 17.3  A receiving system constructed in such a way that a bolus of gas may pass straight out through the open end.

only when the outlet is installed in a suitable position and when the wind is blowing from the desired quarter. It may be affected by the proximity of other buildings. Under adverse conditions the flow may be in the opposite direction, and, because it would be possible for the scavenged gases from one operating theatre to be expelled into another, each point must have its individual ventile. Branching of the pipework is unsatisfactory. Usually the system terminates on the roof. As the waste gases pass to the cooler areas above the ceiling of the operating theatre, they become denser, thus tending to slow their flow, and water vapour may condense and run back down to the theatre, possibly carrying infection. A water trap is therefore essential.

## The receiving system

The exhaled gases emerge intermittently from the breathing system, their volume and flow pattern varying according to the type of apparatus in use. For example, with spontaneous respiration there may be a fresh gas flow of, say, 8 litres/min, and therefore that is the volume of gases to be scavenged per minute; however, the peak flow rate, during the period when the APL valve is open, may be much higher (up to 45 litres/min). Furthermore some 'bag in bottle' ventilators discharge driving gas as well as

exhaled gas into the scavenging system. This may well produce flow rates of in excess of 100 litres/min. It is important therefore to match the performance of the receiving system to that of the anaesthetic equipment.

It would be difficult to design a disposal system that could cope with these great fluctuations. Therefore the receiving system contains a reservoir for the expired and driving gases, from which they are passed more evenly to the disposal system. The container may be either a reservoir bag or an open-ended vessel of rigid material. There may be problems with the latter — for instance, if it is constructed as shown in Fig. 17.3, the gases emerging from some of the breathing systems and ventilators may flow with such a velocity that they pass as a 'bolus' straight out of the open end. If, however, the arrangement is as shown in Fig. 17.4, the bolus enters the disposal tubing directly.

If the reservoir is in the form of a closed bag, it is necessary to install two safety valves: one that opens to allow the escape of gases if the pressure within the system rises above a predetermined level, say, 10 cmH$_2$O (~ 1 kPa), to guard against accidents in which a part of the tubing could be obstructed; and the other that opens at a subatmospheric pressure of 0.5 cmH$_2$O (50 Pa), to admit atmospheric air if the

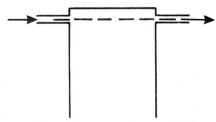

Figure 17.4  A receiving system constructed in such a way that a bolus of gas tends to pass straight into the transfer tubing.

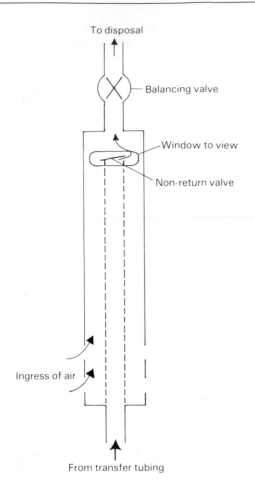

To disposal

Balancing valve

Window to view

Non-return valve

Ingress of air

From transfer tubing

**Figure 17.5**   An air-break, which allows for the ingress of air to satisfy any excess demand by the disposal system. It performs the functions of both the receiving system and the disposal tubing.

demand of the disposal system becomes excessive. This is also known as the 'patient safety protection system' or 'interface system'. In one instance the absence of this provision led to a situation where the closure of the APL valve during inspiration was prevented and the reservoir bag of the breathing system promptly emptied!

As an alternative, an 'air-break' (Fig. 17.5) may be installed, as a fixture on the wall or pendant. This performs the function of the receiver, over- and under-pressure relief valves and the disposal tubing. The transfer tube is all that is required. If a single disposal system serves more than one air-break, a balancing valve in each air-break is necessary.

The receiving system may be mounted on the anaesthetic machine, fixed to the wall of the operating theatre or placed in some intermediate position. Whichever is the case, the transfer tubing

between the collecting system and the receiving system should be fitted with 30-mm tapered connections. The disposal tubing, if detachable, should have fittings *other than* 30-mm, or 22-mm tapers in order to prevent interchangeability with any other part of the anaesthetic apparatus.

## The collecting system

The collecting system collects the gases leaving the anaesthetic equipment. It may consist of a shroud (Banjo fitting) that surrounds the APL (Heidbrink/ expiratory) valve as shown in Fig. 17.6a. When this is installed at the patient end of a breathing system (Magill/circle system), it may prove to be very heavy in use, dragging on the facemask or endotracheal tube. To prevent this, breathing systems such as the Bain and the two versions of the Lack and Humphrey (i.e. parallel and coaxial) were developed in which the APL valves were resited at the machine end. Figure 17.6b shows the shrouded APL valve on the Penlon version of the Bain.

Because an APL valve must inevitably present some resistance to expiration and also because the attachment of the collecting system to it may present mechanical difficulties, varies 'valveless' breathing systems have been described. One such system is described below.

(a)

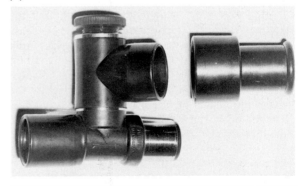

(b)

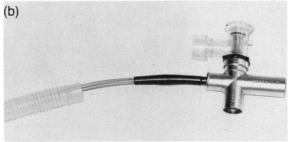

**Figure 17.6**   APL valves with shrouds (Banjo fitting) for connection to a gas scavenging system.

## The Hafnia breathing systems*

In the Hafnia breathing systems, which are modifications of the Mapleson A, B, C and D and circle systems, the APL valve is replaced by a relatively narrow tube through which excess gases are evacuated by an ejector flowmeter. The advantages claimed for the Hafnia are that scavenging is efficient and that owing to the constant active evacuation of excess gases, the pressure within the breathing attachment is kept at ambient and there is minimal resistance to expiration. If one considers the modification of the Mapleson A system (see Fig. 9.22), one finds that whereas during spontaneous breathing with the traditional form the fresh gas flow (FGF) may be reduced to less than the patient's minute volume without rebreathing, in the Hafnia modification, the FGF rate to prevent an increase of $PCO_2$, has to be 135% of the patient's minute volume. This is because in the former, the APL valve opens only at intervals to permit the escape of expired gases, while in the latter, evacuation is continuous and at times during the cycle *fresh* gases are withdrawn.

### The ejector flowmeter

The ejector flowmeter (Fig. 17.7) assists the removal of waste anaesthetic gases from the breathing attachment. It consists of an ejector (venturi) powered by compressed air or oxygen at a pressure of at least 100 kPa (15 psi). The entrained gases pass through a flowmeter, their rate being controlled by a flow control valve. By careful adjustment of this valve the rate of withdrawal of gases from the breathing attachment can be equated to that of the FGF, thus maintaining a status quo within the breathing attachment, with neither under- nor over-pressure. The resistance to expiration is reduced virtually to zero. Since this is an active system, a passive disposal system may be used. There may be condensation of water vapour, and therefore a water trap is fitted, which may be filled with silica gel.

To give some idea of the performance of the ejector flowmeter, 2.4 litres/min of driving gas at a pressure of 100 kPa ($\sim$ 15 psi) would be required to remove 7.5 litres/min of waste gases.

An ejector flowmeter is of use not only to equate the evacuation of waste gases with the FGF, but also to verify that the ejector is functioning correctly. In one investigation concerning over 100 ejectors

without flowmeters, it was found about half were failing to achieve the expected performance, and one was actually blowing 4.5 litres of air plus the waste gases into the atmosphere of the theatre!

The significance of atmospheric pollution and the general principles of methods by which it may be reduced having been discussed, some examples of the equipment available will now be described.

Collecting systems for scavenging in paediatric breathing systems are discussed in Chapter 14.

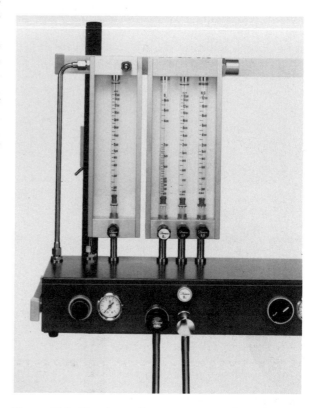

**Figure 17.7** The ejector flowmeter mounted on the back bar.

# Examples of Scavenging Systems

## The Penlon system

In the Penlon system there are a number of components from which those that are necessary to meet the local requirements may be chosen. They may be used in conjunction with an active or passive disposal system.

The collecting system consists of either a special APL valve or a direct connection to an expiratory port, for example of a ventilator.

---

* *Hafnia*, an old Latin word meaning Haven, was the Roman name for Copenhagen.

*Transfer tubing.* The inlet connector of the transfer tubing has a 30-mm female taper and may incorporate a positive pressure relief valve which opens at a pressure of 10 cmH$_2$O. The tubing itself is 22-mm plastic hose, and the outlet has a 30-mm male taper.

There are three different devices for the reception of waste gases and their disposal.

## 1. The Papworth block (Fig. 17.8)

This is a receiving system with a 2-litre reservoir bag, two inlets with a 30-mm female taper, and an outlet for a push-on 32-mm hose. There is an overpressure relief valve which opens at 10 cmH$_2$O (1 kPa) pressure and an underpressure relief valve (air entrainment valve) which opens at 0.5 cmH$_2$O

(50 Pa) subatmospheric. A V-plate bracket enables the Papworth block to be mounted either on an anaesthetic machine or on the wall. There is also a bung to occlude the second inlet if only one transfer tube is in use. It is noteworthy that the reservoir bag is labelled 'Do not squeeze bag'.

## 2. The Penlon integrated receiving and disposal unit

This unit (Fig. 17.9) is intended to be attached to an anaesthetic machine and to replace the Papworth safety block. It is similar to the above, except that it has the addition of a venturi flow inducer and therefore fulfils the role of an active disposal system. The venturi requires 3–4 litres/min of driving gas, at a pressure of 400 kPa ($\sim$60 psi). It can handle up to

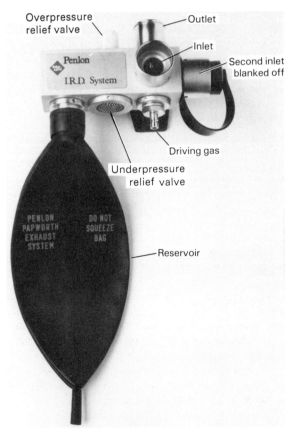

**Figure 17.8** The Papworth block. This is a receiving system that is usually mounted on the anaesthetic machine but may also be mounted on the wall. There are two inlets, the second of which may be blanked off when not in use. The outlet is connected via the disposal tubing to the disposal system. Note that there is an overpressure relief valve and an underpressure (air entrainment) valve.

**Figure 17.9** The Penlon integrated receiving and disposal system. This may be mounted on the anaesthetic machine itself. The model illustrated here contains a venturi driven by compressed gas which expels the waste anaesthetic gases via an otherwise passive disposal system. There is another version in which the waste gases are removed by the piped medical vacuum plant. Note that there are two inlets and that if only one is in use the other is blanked off by a specially provided plug.

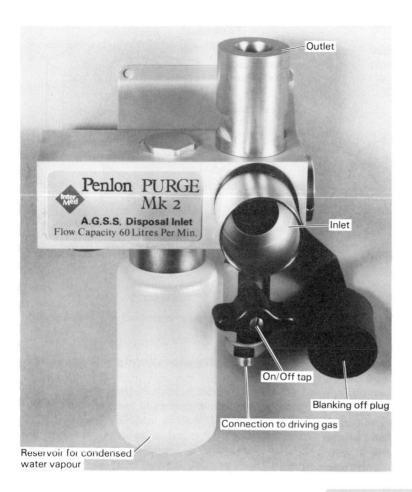

Outlet

Penlon PURGE
Mk 2

**A.G.S.S. Disposal Inlet**
Flow Capacity 60 Litres Per Min.

Inlet

On/Off tap

Blanking off plug

Connection to driving gas

Reservoir for condensed
water vapour

**Figure 17.10** The Penlon purge. This is a wall-mounted system which contains a venturi that entrains waste anaesthetic gases and expels them via an otherwise passive disposal system. The requirements for the driving gas are 4 litres/min at a pressure of 400 kPa (~ 60 psi) to dispose of up to 60 litres/min of waste gases. There is a reservoir to accommodate condensed water vapour which might run back from a passive disposal system.

60 litres/min of waste gases without imposing any positive pressure upon the transfer system.

### 3. The Penlon purge

This unit (Fig. 17.10) consists of a wall-mounted venturi, again using 3–4 litres/min of driving gas, at 400 kPa (~60 psi). It is connected to the Papworth receiving block by a 32-mm corrugated hose, and the outlet is a 35 mm parallel tube for fitting to the copper pipe of the passive system.

### The Penlon grille attachment (Fig. 17.11)

This is an attachment that can be screwed to the extract grille of the ventilating system. It may have a protruding or a flush 35-mm parallel connection. It is common practice to lead the gases through a short length of 35-mm pipe from the grille attachment to a position further within the ventilating duct, thus assuring that there is efficient scavenging.

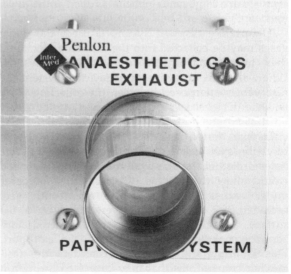

Penlon
**ANAESTHETIC GAS
EXHAUST**

PAP       YSTEM

**Figure 17.11** The Penlon grille attachment. This is attached to an existing extract grille of the ventilating system by screws or toggle bolts. There is a 30-mm female taper connection to accept the disposal tubing.

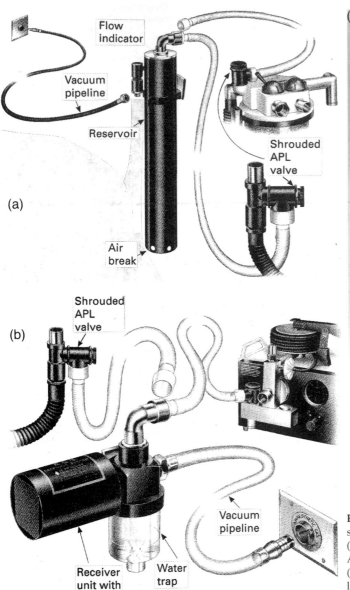

(a)

(b)

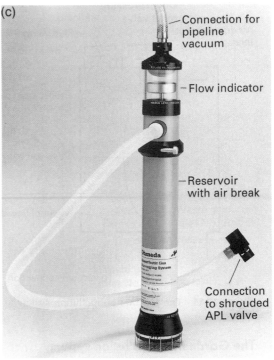

(c)

**Figure 17.17** The Ohmeda active gas scavenging systems (AGSS). (a) AGSS active 40 litres/min. (b) AGSS system specifically for use with Ohmeda AGSS extraction outlets rated at 110–130 litres/min. (c) Current version of Ohmeda AGSS rated at 120 litres/min.

## The Berner valve (Dameca)

The Berner valve (Fig. 17.18) can be used with spontaneous, assisted or controlled ventilation. Its mode of operation can perhaps be best understood if its components are considered one at a time. The two ports P and P′ (Fig. 17.18b) are connected within the breathing system. In this instance P is connected to the patient and P′ to a reservoir bag and the fresh gas flow. The head of the valve is mounted on a screw thread and thus may be screwed up and down. Let us start with it screwed fully up. At rest, the valve disc D, which is mounted on a guide G, is kept in contact with the lower

seating $S_1$ by the light spring L (Fig. 17.18c (1)). When the pressure in the breathing system reaches 1.5 cmH$_2$O, D is lifted to a midway position (Fig. 17.18c (2)), allowing excess gases to escape. During spontaneous inspiration the valve remains closed by the action of L, so preventing the admission of atmospheric air.

If the breathing bag is compressed sharply, so as to cause an increase of pressure within the system in excess of 3 cmH$_2$O, D rises so far that it engages upon the upper seating $S_2$, again closing the valve and thus permitting controlled or assisted ventilation (Fig. 17.18c (3)).

A problem arises, however, in that if the pressure

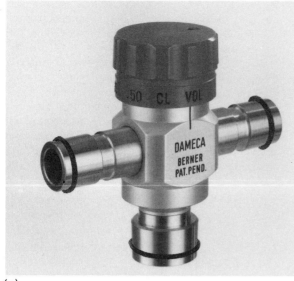

(a)

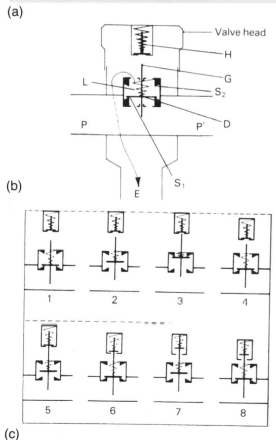

(b)

(c)

**Figure 17.18**  (a) The Berner valve. (b) and (c) Working principles (see text).

within the system were to be *maintained* at over 3 cmH₂O (as could happen during controlled ventilation, or during spontaneous ventilation as a result of the patient coughing), the escape of gas from the system would be prevented, because D would be kept permanently seated on $S_2$. To prevent this there is a second spring, H, of higher tension, attached to the valve head. When the valve head is screwed down from its uppermost position (marked 'VOL'), H and its plate impinge upon G and oppose the upward movement of D towards $S_2$ (Fig. 17.18c (5)). The pressure is progressively increased as the head is screwed further and when it is completely down to the 'CL' position (Fig. 17.18c (8)) pressure on the guide is such that D is kept permanently seated on $S_1$ and the valve is completely closed. By screwing the head down only as far as 'SP' (Fig. 17.18c (4)), the permanent closure of D on $S_2$ is prevented.

Since the pressure in the patient's air passages, and in the breathing system, varies with the degree of inflation of the lungs, the tidal volume may be selected by adjusting the valve head (and thereby the tension in H) so that the valve opens at the appropriate pressure, allowing excess gases to escape (Fig. 17.18c (6) and (7)). Under these circumstances the tidal volume at any particular setting will be constant, provided that the patient's compliance does not alter. The valve head is calibrated for pressures of 5, 20, 35 and 50 cmH₂O.

The expired gases are taken away through a port E, to which a length of corrugated hose may be attached to act as a reservoir. The vacuum hose used to achieve scavenging may be introduced either into the downstream end of the corrugated hose or to a small side-branch, which is fitted to the back of the valve body in some models.

## Absorption systems

Alternative methods may be employed for the removal of the vapours of volatile anaesthetic agents from waste gases. Activated charcoal, in canisters of 1 kg, absorbs volatile anaesthetic vapour efficiently. It has a low resistance and may be incorporated in the expiratory limb of a breathing system (Fig. 17.19). The canister increases in weight as the vapour is absorbed, and this may be monitored by a spring balance on which it is mounted. When the weight reaches the level stated, it should be discarded. Care must be taken to ensure that it is disposed of in a safe location, where it will not permit the vapour to be released and pollute the atmosphere breathed by other people. Used canisters should not be allowed to fall into the hands of drug

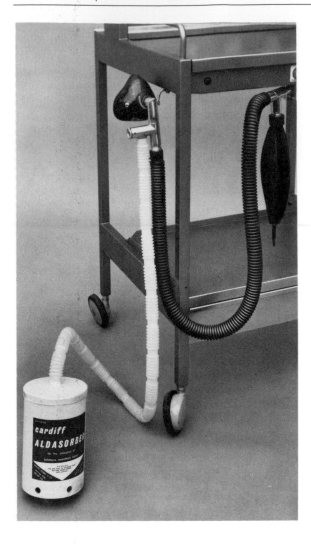

addicts, who have been known to heat them in order to gain the release of vapour. Indeed, the use of heat to release this has been employed in one type of canister, which being made of suitable metal, may be placed in the autoclave in order to discharge it. If this system is employed, one must again ensure that the discharge of vapour-laden steam from the autoclave is to a safe location.

Unfortunately, recent research incriminating nitrous oxide rather than the volatile anaesthetic agents, has rendered the employment of the relatively simple Aldasorber less appropriate.

**Figure 17.19**   The Aldasorber.

# 18 Infusion Equipment

## Basic Components of Infusion Equipment

The majority of intravenous infusions are administered by gravity from flexible plastic bags and plastic bottles using pre-sterilized, disposable giving (administration) sets. These giving sets are of several types:

- simple fluid administration — no filter, approximately 15 drops/ml;
- blood and fluid administration — with clot filter, approximately 15 drops/ml;
- fluid administration with micro dropper — no filter, approximately 60 drops/ml;
- burette, 100–150 ml in volume, with or without micro dropper;
- platelet giving sets.

Simple fluid administration sets must not be used to administer blood without a filter.

The rate of infusion depends upon:

- the height of the fluid container above the infusion site;
- the resistance to flow due to the giving set;
- occlusion of the tubing by a rate-controlling device;
- the physical properties of the fluid to be administered;
- the bore of the administration cannula;
- the back pressure in the veins of the patient.

The manufacturers of giving sets quote the size of drops, which may be 15–20 drops/ml, but it must be realized that the actual volume of the drops depends upon the physical properties of the fluid being administered. For more accurate control of fluid administration such as is required in paediatric practice, giving sets with micro-droppers may be used. Most micro-droppers when using normal clear fluids have a drop rate of 60 drops/ml. With a burette, increased safety is ensured as only volume for 1 h can be administered. Platelet transfusions require special platelet giving sets to reduce the risk of platelet aggregation occurring in the giving set, as would occur with conventional blood giving sets.

### Rapid infusion

When rapid infusion of blood or other fluids is required, the rate of administration may be increased by the use of a Martin's pump (Fig. 18.1), which is used when the infusion solution comes from a rigid bottle, or by a pressure infusing device (Fig. 18.2) when it is in a plastic bag. This may consist of an inflatable pressure bag, which may even be contained in a rigid box to increase the speed at which pressure may be applied.

Whenever fluids are administered intravenously at a rapid rate, provision should be made for warming them to body temperature, otherwise serious cooling of the body may ensue (Fig. 18.3).

### Accurate infusion control

It is often necessary in anaesthesia, in intensive care and in the management of pain, to be able to infuse drugs accurately and safely at a continuous rate over

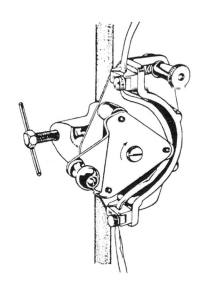

**Figure 18.1** A Martin's infusion pump.

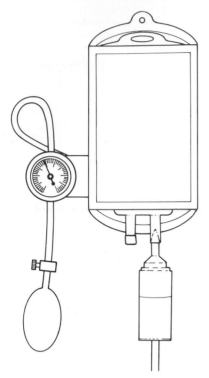

**Figure 18.2**    Pressure infusion device.

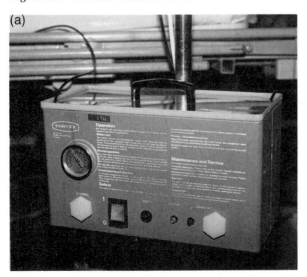

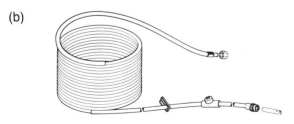

**Figure 18.3**    (a) Hot water blood warming system. (b) Coil through which the blood passes.

long periods of time. Large-volume infusions may be administered accurately by using an infusion 'pump', whereas infusions at very slow rates may be given using a syringe pump or driver.

A classification of so-called infusion pumps is shown in Fig. 18.4.

### Electronic drop counters

Electronic drop counters do not control the rate of infusion, but they accurately inform the user of the rate of infusion. A small beam of light, which may be infrared and thus invisible, is passed through the drop chamber of the giving set and interruptions of this beam are detected by a photoelectric cell. From a measure of the time between drops, the rate of infusion is electronically calculated and displayed. These devices are only as accurate as a knowledge of the size of individual drops, and this size must be programmed into the device each time it is used. Obviously the rate of infusion may not remain constant between estimations with these devices.

### Principles of infusion pumps

Most of the so-called infusion pumps are similar in appearance but may be very different in principle and in the accuracy of infusion rate. Some do not actually *pump* the liquid but use gravity as the source of energy. It is therefore necessary when using infusion pumps to ascertain the mechanism by which they work.

*Infusion controllers.* The infusion controller (Fig 18.4) usually uses a photoelectric drop counting system in conjunction with some form of adjustable occlusion of the infusion tubing controlled by a microprocessor. The infusion is by no power other than gravity, but is controlled by the microprocessor, which adjusts the clamp mechanism to compensate for changes in resistance to flow in the cannula or the patient's vein. This method of infusion is more accurate than by simple manually controlled giving sets and always includes alarms which are activated if the infusion rate cannot be maintained.

*The stepper motor.* The driving force in the majority of infusion pumps and electronic syringe drivers is an electrical machine called a stepper motor. The stepper motor may be directly controlled from a digital microprocessor system. The speed of a conventional electric motor driven from either an a.c. supply or a d.c. supply may vary with voltage, mechanical load or the frequency of the supply. It is difficult without electronic feedback to control such

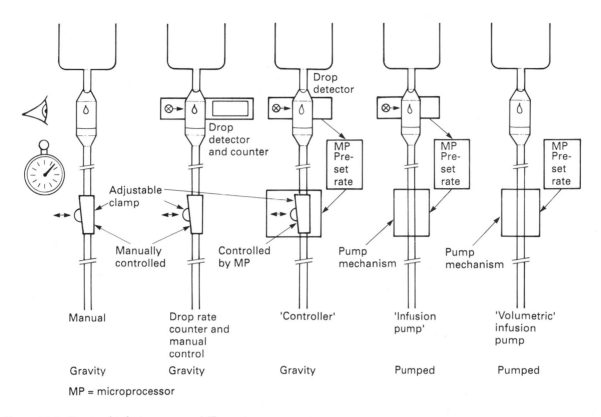

**Figure 18.4**   Types of infusion pumps. MP = microprocessor.

a motor accurately. The stepper motor is designed so that a series of pulses applied to the stator windings of the motor cause the shaft to rotate by a fixed amount for each pulse, typically 1.8°, 2.5°, 3.75° or 7.5°, irrespectively of the load, within certain limits. Infusion systems may be designed so that a pulse generator, whose frequency may be varied, can produce accurate control of an infusion and the frequency adjustment may be calibrated directly in millilitres per hour.

## Infusion pumps

Pumped infusion systems overcome the variation in infusion rate caused by back pressure, tubing resistance and the vertical height of the reservoir container or bag above the patient.

The driving mechanism of infusion pumps may be a peristaltic arrangement or may use a small syringe with associated valve in the manner of a conventional piston-pump.

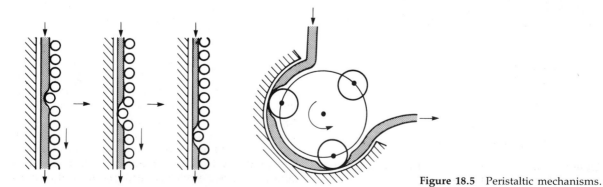

**Figure 18.5**   Peristaltic mechanisms.

The principle of the peristaltic infusion pump is shown in Fig. 18.5. The tubing of a giving set is rhythmically compressed by a series of rotating rollers or by a ripple with a series of mechanical 'fingers' as shown. The stepper motor driving either of these two mechanisms is controlled by a microprocessor.

Figure 18.6 shows a typical syringe-type infusion pump mechanism. This is also driven by a stepper motor controlled directly by a microprocessor. The volume of the syringe is usually about 5 ml. The syringe 'cassette' is supplied sterile and disposable. Fluid is drawn in rapidly from the reservoir bag into the syringe in less than 1 s. The valve is then actuated so that the syringe contents are expelled at the required rate into the patient, and then the process is repeated. Although, in theory, this produces an intermittent flow, it also produces a very accurate overall infusion rate with only 1-s interruptions infrequently.

The low-budget infusion systems rely upon drop counting to control the infusion rate. The required

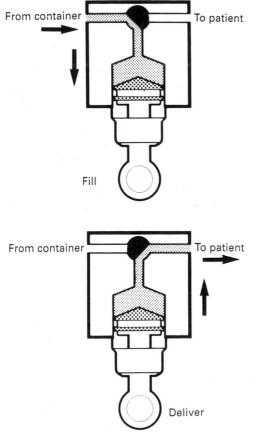

**Figure 18.6**   Principle of a syringe-type volumetric infusion pump.

infusion rate is dialled-in on the control panel and the 'dedicated' microprocessor in the pump compares the required rate with the rate of drops passing the photodetector, and thus maintains the stepper motor at the desired speed. The rate of infusion is once again dependent upon the drop size and the rate selector will have been calibrated for a specific giving set and for a specific fluid. The size of the drops will be dependent upon the physical properties of the fluid being infused and its temperature.

## Volumetric infusion pumps

The most accurate infusion pumps are the so-called volumetric pumps. With the volumetric pump the rate of infusion is determined by the precision of the pumping mechanism, be it a syringe system or high-quality silicon tubing in a peristaltic pump (Fig. 18.7). A drop counter is no longer required but may be provided as a means of detecting an empty reservoir bag. As a drop counter is not used for the actual flow measurement, variation in drop size does not effect the infusion rate. Volumetric systems are more expensive and the giving set or cassette *must* be that supplied by the pump manufacturer.

## Syringe drivers

The simplest mechanical syringe driver is driven by a clockwork mechanism. However, these are only obtainable at a single fixed rate of infusion and therefore find little use in anaesthesia and intensive care. Clockwork syringe drivers are mainly used for narcotic infusions for pain control in terminal care or occasionally for heparin infusions. There is a range of small battery-operated syringe drivers (see Fig. 18.8). These pumps are mainly used for insulin infusion and the relief of cancer pain with narcotic infusions. They may have a variable rate that is adjusted with a small screwdriver. The driving mechanism is a miniature d.c. motor that is switched on and off intermittently and drives a screw-threaded rod (or a screw) which is linked to the syringe plunger, causing its advancement. These syringe pumps are small and light enough to be worn in a holster by an ambulant patient.

Syringe drivers used in intensive care and anaesthesia usually make use of stepper motors, again connected to the syringe plunger by a lead screw. Thus each pulse applied to the stepper motor causes the advancement of the syringe plunger by a known amount. The pulse generator driving the stepper motor may be calibrated from 0.1 ml/h to 99.9 ml/h in steps of 0.1 ml/h. It is important that only

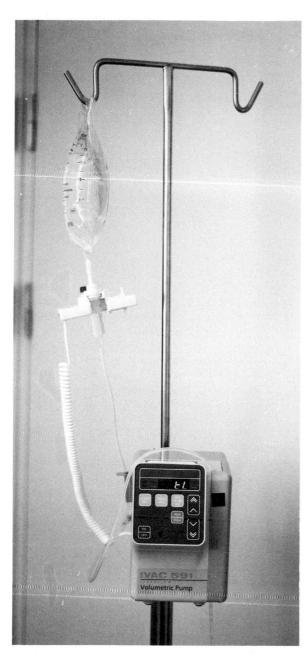

**Figure 18.7**  Volumetric infusion pump.

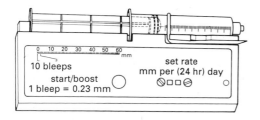

**Figure 18.8**  Graseby syringe driver.

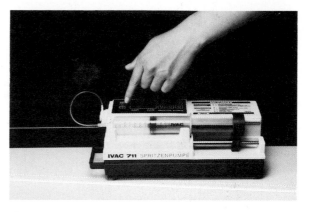

**Figure 18.9**  A syringe driver.

syringes recommended by the manufacturer are used, otherwise the calibration will be adversely affected. These syringe drivers (Fig. 18.9) may be free-standing or pole-mounted, and are mains driven, but may have a rechargeable battery option for the transport of patients. Electronic syringe drivers have alarms for occlusion and empty syringe.

# Patient-controlled Analgesia

Improved control of postoperative analgesia may be obtained by the use of patient-controlled analgesia systems. These consist of a syringe driver with an override facility that is controlled by pressing a button that the patient has in his or her hand. The rate of the background infusion and the size and maximum frequency of the patient-controlled boluses may be pre-set by the anaesthetist. Most of these devices record the times at which the patient has demanded and received the extra boluses.

# Filtration

Intravenous fluids should be filtered to protect the patient from microscopic foreign material. Blood for transfusion that is more than 24 h 'old' should be filtered (Fig. 18.10) to remove micro-aggregates that form from the breakdown products of the cellular components and platelets. Blood filters are of two basic types. *Screen filters* function as 'sieves' and are usually constructed from a woven mesh. They have a regular pore size, often of 40 μm. The efficiency of a screen-type filter at removing foreign matter increases progressively with each unit of blood passed as the pore-size tends to decrease progres-

Figure 18.10 A blood filter.

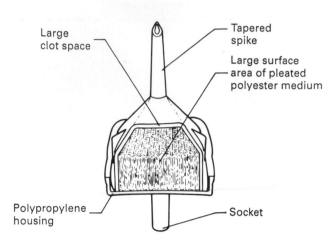

Large clot space

Tapered spike

Large surface area of pleated polyester medium

Polypropylene housing

Socket

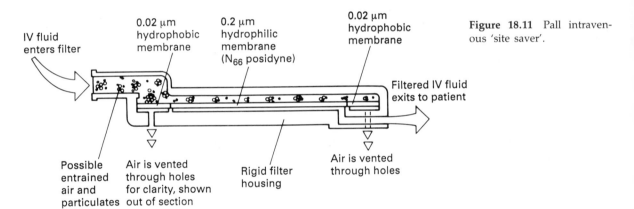

Figure 18.11 Pall intravenous 'site saver'.

IV fluid enters filter

0.02 μm hydrophobic membrane

0.2 μm hydrophilic membrane (N$_{66}$ posidyne)

0.02 μm hydrophobic membrane

Filtered IV fluid exits to patient

Possible entrained air and particulates

Air is vented through holes for clarity, shown out of section

Rigid filter housing

Air is vented through holes

sively down to 20 μm. Screen-type filters are said to be less damaging to the red cells than are depth filters. *Depth filters* consist of a pack of synthetic fibre, often Dacron, not formed into a mesh. The mechanism of 'filtration' is actually by adsorption of unwanted material, down to a size of about 10 μm, onto the surface of the fibres. This adsorption is probably due to electrical charge differences between the particles and the fibres. With the depth filter the efficiency at removal of unwanted material decreases with each unit of blood, probably due to channelling in the pack of fibres.

Intravenous crystalloids may be filtered with much finer sieve-type filters to remove foreign particulate matter including bacteria. The Pall 'intravenous site saver' extends the life of the giving set, which should normally be replaced every 24 h, to up to 96 h. The construction of the 'site saver' is

shown in Fig. 18.11. All particulate matter larger than 0.2-μm is removed by a 0.2 μm filter membrane. Air is also continuously vented through a hydrophobic membrane which has 0.02 μm pores, thus protecting the patient from air embolism. Use of the 'site saver' also protects against microbiological contamination.

## Autotransfusion

When a large blood loss may be expected during surgery, it may be possible to re-use the patient's own blood, provided that is uncontaminated and free from clots. Uncontaminated blood is aspirated by the machine, anticoagulant is added and it is stored temporarily in a reservoir. It may then be transfused back into the patient via a filter.

# 19 Medical Suction Apparatus

## Introduction

Suction apparatus is vital to the safe practice of anaesthesia and intensive care, and is probably the single most important piece of resuscitation equipment. It is used for clearance of mucus, blood and debris from the pharynx, trachea and main bronchi and during surgery for providing a clear field for the surgeon. Special suction apparatus is used for other purposes, for example gastrointestinal drainage, wound drainage and pleural drainage.

The three essential components of medical suction apparatus are:

- source of the vacuum;
- the reservoir or collection vessel;
- suction tubing.

Other refinements that modify the performance are discussed later.

Suction apparatus may be operated from a vacuum or gas pipeline; or it may be transportable, usually powered by mains electricity and supported on castor wheels; or truly portable, powered by a battery or cylinder of gas or by human energy (hand- or foot-operated).

The efficiency of the suction apparatus depends upon:

- the displacement, i.e. the volume of air at atmospheric pressure that the pump is able to move per unit time;
- the degree of negative (subatmospheric) pressure that can be produced by the pump, with particular regard to the time taken to achieve it;
- the internal resistance of the suction apparatus and the length and diameter of the suction tubing;
- the viscosity of the matter to be aspirated.

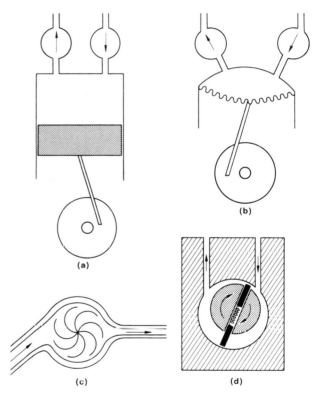

**Figure 19.1** Vacuum pumps. (a) Piston pump.
(b) Diaphragm pump. (c) Rotary vane 'vacuum cleaner' pump. (d) High-pressure rotary vane pump.

## Source of Vacuum

An electric motor or other source of rotational energy may be used to drive a mechanical pump, various forms of which are shown in Fig. 19.1.

Figure 19.1a shows a piston pump, which is capable of creating a high vacuum but, in transportable models, has a comparatively low displacement. Figure 19.1b shows a diaphragm pump,

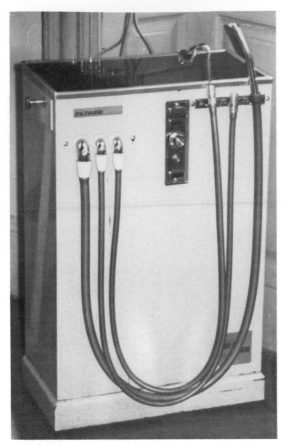

**Figure 19.2** A high-volume aspirator, which is used particularly in the dental operatory.

which is a variation of the piston pump; it is mechanically much simpler but often has the disadvantage of being much noisier than the conventional piston pump. Figure 19.1c shows a rotary pump, which may be designed to produce a very high displacement as would be required in the high-volume aspirator (Fig. 19.2) used in the dental surgery. It works in the same way as the suction source in a vacuum cleaner, and does not produce a very high degree of vacuum. It is also comparatively noisy. Figure 19.1d shows a form of rotary pump that can produce a high vacuum.

Note that the pumps shown in Fig. 19.1a and d usually require a special hydraulic oil, the level of which should be periodically checked, and topped up if required.

A bellows may be used (Fig. 19.3) as the vacuum source as in the foot-operated suction apparatus shown in Fig. 19.4.

Pneumatically driven pumps usually work on the injector (Fig. 19.5) or venturi principle. They may be driven by compressed air, oxygen, steam or water. A high vacuum or a high displacement may be achieved, depending on the design of the injector. When driven from an oxygen cylinder, these pumps are very wasteful of oxygen, but they have the virtue of being portable.

A piped vacuum source may be installed using a high-capacity pump connected to a large reservoir in a central position. The patient end of the pipeline is fitted with a self-closing non-interchangeable valve similar to that on the oxygen and nitrous oxide pipelines, to which the collection vessel and suction tubing may be attached. A vacuum regulator may also be fitted at this point to adjust the force of vacuum applied to the patient. The central pump, which operates intermittently to maintain the vacuum in the central reservoir, is controlled by a pressure switch. It is common practice to install two pumps so that one may be in use while the other is undergoing maintenance.

Traps should be installed in the various branches of a large piped system to intercept any liquid or solid accidently aspirated into it. The output of the vacuum pump should either be discharged to the exterior of the building or be fitted with a filter to prevent the spread of infection.

## The Collection Vessel

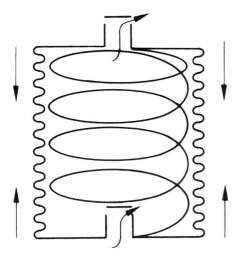

**Figure 19.3** The bellows-and-spring pump. The bellows is closed by the pressure of the foot and reopened by the recoil of the spring.

Whatever the source of the vacuum, the size of the collection vessel is important. Sufficient capacity should be allowed for all the matter to be aspirated.

(a)

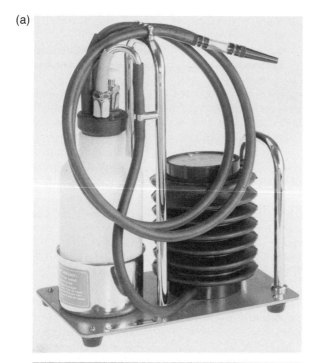

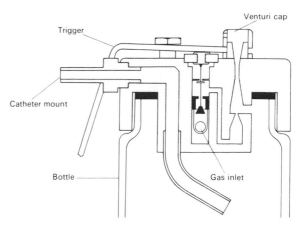

**Figure 19.5** An injector suction unit.

(b)

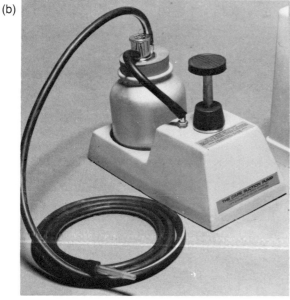

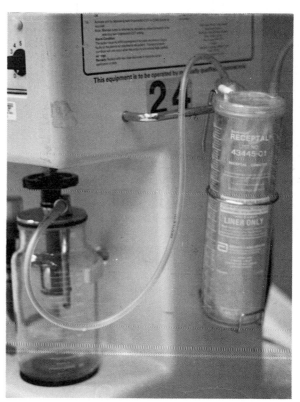

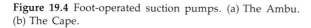

**Figure 19.4** Foot-operated suction pumps. (a) The Ambu. (b) The Cape.

**Figure 19.6** Receptal disposable collection vessel system.

Too big a capacity, however, will not only be cumbersome but will also increase the time taken for the vacuum to build up in it, even if the inlet from the patient is completely occluded. The interface between the collection vessel and the rest of the apparatus should be kept clean and free from damage and the sealing washer should be kept in

good order. A common cause of failure in suction apparatus is a leak at this point. The vessel should be graduated so that the volume of an aspirate such as blood can be estimated. The neck of the collection vessel should be large enough to allow adequate cleaning (Fig. 19.6).

With the increased danger of infection from

aspirates, as with AIDS and other serious infections, there is an increasing trend towards the use of collection vessels with disposable liners so that staff never have to come into contact with the aspirate when cleaning.

# The Suction Tubing

The internal diameter and length of the suction tubing should allow the greatest possible amount of suction at the patient end. The behaviour of fluids, as discussed in Chapter 1, shows that the resistance of the delivery tube is reduced by keeping it as short and as wide as possible. Whereas a tube of 6-mm bore may present little resistance to air, it will considerably impede the passage of blood, mucus and vomit.

The flow of air alone through the tubing may be laminar, but when it is mixed with liquids or solid matter it is likely to become turbulent, increasing the resistance. The wall of the suction tubing must be of sufficient firmness and thickness to prevent collapse under the vacuum or kinking.

### The suction nozzle or catheter

It may be necessary to use a long, narrow catheter, as, for example, in bronchial suction, but otherwise excessive length should be avoided. Suction 'ends' should taper to the nozzle so that as much of the length as possible may be of the wide diameter. The shape of the tip should be smooth so as to prevent damage to delicate surfaces, and it is sometimes

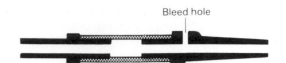

**Figure 19.7** The bleed hole in a suction nozzle, which can be occluded by the operator's finger. Note that there may be a transparent window to allow the operator to observe the material that is being aspirated.

desirable to have two or more holes, so that if one is blocked, possibly by mucous membrane being sucked into it, the other will continue the suction. This type of blockage is more common when the vacuum is too high, in which case provision may be made to admit air into the delivery tube or collection vessel by means of a bleed valve or hole. If there is a hole in the proximal end of the suction catheter or Yankauer handpiece, it may be occluded when required by a finger (Fig. 19.7). This is particularly useful when performing endobronchial suction. The advantage of placing the bleed valve or finger-hole at this point is that it does not reduce the flow along the suction tubing.

# Refinements of Medical Suction Apparatus

The following refinements may be added to a suction apparatus, in the positions indicated in Fig. 19.8. This is a diagram of a transportable suction apparatus, as opposed to a pipeline or manually operated machine whose components are different.

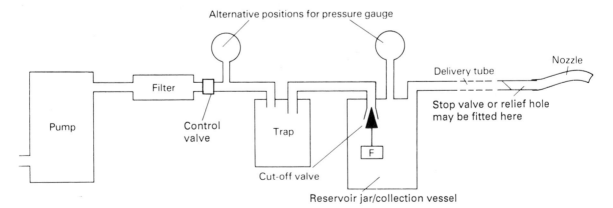

**Figure 19.8** The components of a transportable suction apparatus. The pump may be protected from infected material, which could be drawn from the reservoir jar, by a trap or filter. There is a cut-off valve within the reservoir jar that operates when the level of fluid in the jar is sufficiently high to raise the float F, so as to prevent any foreign material being aspirated into the pump. There are alternative positions for the pressure gauge. A trigger valve may be fitted close to the nozzle in order to maintain a constant standby vacuum in the reservoir jar.

*Cut-off valve.* This is fitted inside the collection vessel, and usually consists of a float which, being lifted by the rising level of aspirate, operates a valve to shut off the connection with the vacuum source. Its purpose is to prevent liquid from a full collection vessel entering the pump mechanism and causing failure, or entering the pipes of a pipeline system.

Occasionally, a cut-off valve, having been closed, is held closed by the vacuum acting upon it. It is then necessary, after emptying the reservoir, either to stop the vacuum source or to pull the float down again and so reopen the valve. The cut-off valve has to be designed so that its operation will not be upset by particulate matter in the aspirate.

*Bacterial filter.* This may (in fact, should) be fitted to prevent air that has been contaminated during its passage through the apparatus from infecting the atmosphere when it is blown out of the pump. It is best placed between the collection vessel and the pump so as to protect the latter. A container packed with wool wadding makes a fairly efficient filter — providing that it is dry. If it becomes wet, it will become ineffective and may also obstruct the airflow. Filters should be changed at regular intervals, depending on their size, lest they themselves become a source of infection. If there is no filter, a small quantity of disinfectant solution may be added to the reservoir, but this is not very effective.

*Vacuum control valve or regulator.* This may be fitted between the pump and the collection vessel. A vacuum control valve is a bleed valve, which when opened, admits air, thereby reducing the degree of vacuum. A vacuum regulator operates on a similar principle to a pressure regulator and so no energy is wasted by allowing air into the system. It is usual to use a vacuum regulator to control the degree of vacuum in a pipeline system terminal unit.

*Vacuum gauge.* These gauges, which are normally marked in mmHg or kPa, are fitted to the tubing between the vacuum control valve and the collection vessel, or immediately above the collection vessel itself. Note that modern vacuum gauges operate so that the needle goes anticlockwise as the vacuum increases. However, there are still many in use that work clockwise with increasing vacuum.

*Foam prevention.* Foam may be a problem in the collection vessel, since it causes closure of the cut-off valve when the vessel is far from full. It may even pass the valve and contaminate the filter or the pump, causing failure. Foam may be suppressed by the addition of methylated spirits (highly flammable), or

more effectively, by silicone-based emulsions.

*Stop valve.* This valve may be used to occlude the delivery tubing to close the nozzle. It allows the build-up of a vacuum during a stand-by period and is particularly useful when the pump gives a low displacement.

*Two collection vessels.* There are two ways in which two vessels rather than one might be used. In one arrangement a selector enables the second vessel to be used and the first one to be isolated when it is either full or leaking owing to a fault in a washer or chip in a jar. It is of particular importance when large volumes of fluid, as in ascites or major haemorrhage, are being aspirated.

In the second arrangement the jars are in series, so that if the first vessel is overfilled, the overflow goes harmlessly into the second without contaminating the pump or pipeline. This series arrangement may be the result of the addition of a disposable collection vessel system to a conventional single-vessel suction apparatus. Unfortunately the mechanical principles, though simple, are not always appreciated by the theatre staff, and misconnections are common.

## Pipeline Vacuum Units

Piped vacuum systems are now installed in most major hospitals. The 'behind the wall' equipment and terminal outlets are described in Chapter 4.

There are two types of local vacuum unit.

- Free-standing floor units, often with two large collection vessels, used for surgical purposes in the operating theatre.
- Those that are wall mounted and often plug straight into the pipeline outlet, as shown in Fig. 19.9, and have a single collection vessel. There are several types of these controllers available for specific purposes. The most common type is the so-called high-suction, which can be adjusted to provide up to the full vacuum pressure available from the wall outlet. Low-suction controllers are especially limited to provide safe suction for intrapleural drainage or nasogastric suction.

## Choice of Suction Apparatus

When selecting a suction apparatus for a particular purpose, the following points should be considered.

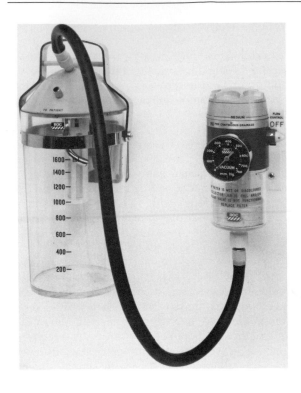

**Figure 19.9** A pipeline vacuum unit. On the right is the controller, which is plugged directly into a flush-fitting outlet (obscured in this picture). On the left is the reservoir jar.

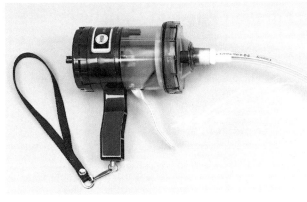

**Figure 19.10** Vitalograph hand-operated suction apparatus with applicator.

- Must it be portable? If so, should it be manually operated (Fig. 19.10) or powered by a gas cylinder, using an injector? If not, should it be powered by electric motor or pipeline?
- Is a high displacement needed?
- Is a high vacuum needed?
- What size should the collection vessel be?

It is also important to ascertain, for an electrically driven suction machine, whether it is rated for continuous or intermittent use, as some are intended for intermittent use only and prolonged periods of operation could lead to the motor overheating and failing. Such units are labelled appropriately.

High-volume aspirators, which use a pump similar to a vacuum cleaner, usually have three suction tubes of different diameters or with different nozzles (Fig. 19.2). Under no circumstances should those nozzles that are not in use be obstructed, since the free air passing through them is used to cool the motor, which may otherwise overheat. These suction machines are most commonly found in the dental surgery, especially where a jet or spray of water is used for cooling the operation of the high-speed turbine drill.

# Standards and Testing

As with all other medical equipment there are published Standards for design and manufacture. These Standards include descriptions of tests for the safety and efficacy of suction apparatus. The relevant Standards are listed in Appendix 3. Some of these tests are too complex to be performed routinely in the hospital setting.

A simple test to prove the efficiency of a high-vacuum suction apparatus may be performed as follows. A litre or so of water, so hot that the hand can only just be immersed in it, is placed in the collection vessel, which is then placed in its operating position. The vacuum source is then applied and the patient end of the delivery tube is occluded. By the time the vacuum has built up to its maximum, the water should be boiling.

# 20 Cleaning and Sterilization

## Introduction

The last few years have seen a major increase in the availability of single-use items of anaesthetic equipment such as endotracheal tubes, airways, breathing systems, reservoir bags, soda-lime canisters and even APL valves. Together with the advent of low-resistance bacterial and viral breathing system filters (see later) to protect ventilators and non-disposable breathing systems, a major reappraisal of the facilities required to carry out many of the recommended cleaning and sterilization procedures may well be required in many hospitals. However, in less-fortunate countries where the above facilities are unavailable, this chapter is still highly relevant.

Although it is generally agreed that all items, such as endotracheal tubes and airways, that come into direct contact with the patient should be sterilized, there remains a considerable divergence of opinion as to the degree of sterility required for anaesthetic machines and ventilators. Whereas in some hospitals anaesthetic ventilators and the breathing attachments of anaesthetic machines are regularly sterilized, in others this is seldom done. The fact that there is little evidence of cross-infection of patients, when sterilization is neglected, in general anaesthetic practice should not be allowed to condone such negligence. There are certain circumstances in which thorough cleansing and sterilization are universally accepted as necessary. Such occasions are when a patient with a virulent infection or tuberculosis has been anaesthetized, or when a patient with a respiratory infection has been maintained on a ventilator in an intensive care ward. In such cases, special precautions may be taken, and these are discussed later. It can be argued that any patient who is ventilated over a prolonged period becomes infected, and so does the ventilator. In practice a compromise is drawn between complete sterilization after each case and what may be regarded as the minimum required. Most instances of cross-infection from ventilators that have been reported are from intensive care wards where patients are on prolonged treatment, rather than from the operating theatre. Undoubtedly the risk of cross-infection is increased where little time elapses between cases.

At this juncture we should distinguish between decontamination, disinfection and sterilization. *Decontamination* consists of the physical removal of infected matter and can be achieved by a thorough washing or scrubbing. It renders an object both bacteriologically and ethically more acceptable and does not necessarily require high temperatures or chemical agents. Modern decontamination devices include the automatic washing machine and the ultrasonic washer. Some detergents are particularly useful; for example, it is claimed that Neodex 'gets under and lifts off contaminating material'. Certainly, if dirty airways and endotracheal tubes are dropped into a solution of 'Neodex' (20 ml/5 litres of water) immediately after use, they appear very clean when they are removed at the end of the day's work. *Disinfection* implies the removal or killing of most or all infective organisms, with the exception of the most resistant ones such as spores. This is regarded as adequate for many purposes and may be done by cold chemical methods or by pasteurization, which is particularly suitable for materials that do not well withstand the higher temperatures of autoclaving. *Sterilization* implies the killing of all organisms, including spores, but the methods employed require either expensive and sophisticated equipment (irradiation) or the employment of temperatures that may damage the article being sterilized.

Note that not all methods of sterilization or disinfection remove such things as chemical contamination. The term 'decontamination' has often been used erroneously where 'disinfection' was more appropriate, since no attempt at the removal of the contaminant was included in the attempts at destruction of the contaminating organisms.

The stages in the process are therefore:

- general cleaning and decontamination, and then, if required;
- disinfection;
- sterilization.

# Decontamination

A system for the decontamination of the corrugated hose, reservoir bags, facepieces, airways and endotrachael tubes, as well as other small items of anaesthetic equipment, is available in the form of the Scotts' SL40 anaesthetic apparatus decontaminator (Fig. 20.1). This machine resembles a dishwasher and cleans the equipment and then pasteurizes it by raising the temperature to 80°C and holding it at that level for 10 min. The pasteurization combines the process of decontamination with disinfection. An earlier model employed stabilized gluteraldehyde but this proved to be uneconomical.

Of particular use for small pieces of equipment, and for equipment of intricate shape, is the ultrasonic washer. This consists of a bath of water in which the objects are immersed and in which they are subjected to ultrasonic vibration. The water contains detergent, and for specialized purposes, as in the dental operatory, other chemicals such as ammonia may be used to break up the resins and alginates that are common contaminants.

If no further treatment in the way of disinfection or sterilization is required, articles such as facemasks may then be thoroughly washed and rinsed in hot water and then hung up to dry.

It should be noted that decontamination is a very important part of the process. If articles are not sufficiently decontaminated, then some of the methods described below may not be totally successful. For example, cases of cross-infection have been documented from equipment that was insufficiently cleaned and which was subsequently sterilized using ethylene oxide.

# Disinfection

One of the most suitable methods for the disinfection of anaesthetic equipment is pasteurization. This consists of heating the article to a temperature of 70°C for 20 min or 80°C for 10 min. It is most conveniently done in a water bath, but may also be done in the low-pressure autoclave. It is not so efficient as boiling, but does kill most infective agents and is usually considered adequate for perishable articles and where absolute sterility is not necessarily required. Whereas plastic and rubber articles may soon lose their shape and antistatic properties as a result of repeated boiling, they are less damaged by pasteurization. The antistatic properties may be restored, where this is still required, by the weekly application of a suitable spray.

One of the problems arising in the use of the water bath is that rigid discipline is required to ensure that it continues for the necessary length of time. Not only must the temperature be maintained but one must also prevent the addition of extra items while the process is continuing, thus recontaminating those already being treated.

## Boiling

Relatively small articles, including facemasks, may be boiled in water for 5 min. This is a fairly efficient method of disinfection, provided that one maintains the discipline mentioned above for pasteurization. Boiling is satisfactory for any article made entirely of metal and also for those made of

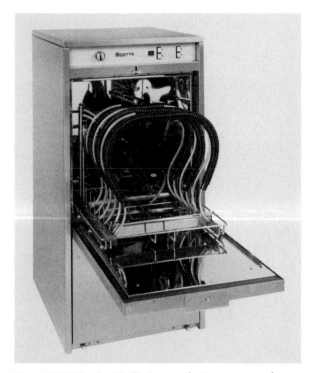

**Figure 20.1** The Scott's SL40 anaesthetic apparatus decontaminator. Note that different trays may be used in the same machine to wash and disinfect other equipment, including surgical instruments.

rubber or neoprene. The process should be timed from the point when the water returns to the boiling point after the introduction of the last item to be treated. Large, cold articles may lower the temperature significantly!

### Chemical methods of disinfection

A number of organic agents possess the ability to kill bacteria and viruses. The efficacy of these compounds depends on their concentration, the length of time in contact with the article to be treated and their individual potency. Most are in the form of liquids, into which the various objects to be treated are immersed. The liquid may also be impregnated onto a cloth, which is then used for wiping down smooth surfaces. The agent (if suitable) may be employed as a nebulized mist or fog (see below). Some agents may exist as a gas or vapour at room temperature, and can be blown through equipment or even whole rooms (fumigation).

*Liquids.* Alcohol, in the form of 70% ethyl or 70% isopropyl alcohol in water, is a fairly efficient disinfectant. (Pure alcohol is not as effective as the aqueous form.) It is used mainly to wipe down hard surfaces such as anaesthetic machines.

Chlorhexidine may be used in various concentrations. It is a non-detergent chemical disinfectant. Facemasks may be soaked for half an hour in a 0.05% solution in water. Quicker disinfection (2 minutes) may be attained by using a 0.5% solution in 70% alcohol. This solution is also useful for swabbing down equipment such as anaesthetic machines. Detergent chemicals should be avoided since they may cause damage to the rubber parts of anaesthetic apparatus.

Chloroxylenol has frequently been used, particularly for facemasks. A dilute solution should be used and the facemasks rinsed in clear water for 2 hours after immersion. However, there is a danger that the patient may develop facial skin rashes as a result of sensitivity to chloroxylenol, which is absorbed into the rubber of the facemask; so this agent is best avoided.

Hypochlorite solutions have recently been shown to be highly effective in decontaminating and disinfecting material infected with the human immunodeficiency virus (HIV).

Several agents have been used to disinfect ventilators. These include 70% alcohol in water, hydrogen peroxide, various aldehyde preparations and a proprietary mixture of dimethyl phenols in an alcoholic/detergent base. Alcohol should not be used to disinfect a ventilator which is electrically powered, where a risk of explosion exists. The ventilators should then be run for several hours in fresh air, to clear the disinfectant from the tubing and the internal parts of the breathing systems.

As shown in Fig. 20.6 the use of bacterial filters may also provide a very high degree of protection against the contamination of those ventilators of which the breathing systems cannot be separately sterilized.

*Mists and fogs.* Mists or fogs of disinfectants may be used for equipment such as older types of ventilators with non-detachable and non-autoclavable patient gas pathways. They may even be used for an entire room full of equipment. In the case of ventilators, the agents are best nebulized in an ultrasonic nebulizer (see Fig. 13.7). Care must be taken to make sure that the nebulizer does not run dry, since some types may be damaged if this happens. Larger fogging machines (Fig. 20.2) are available that are capable of treating a whole operating theatre. Recently doubt has been expressed about the efficiency of fogging a whole theatre. Also, evidence has been reported of damage to electrical apparatus by corrosion. However it is described here since the principle is satisfactory and it is the nature of the disinfectants themselves that presents problems. The advent of new agents may bring fogging back into vogue.

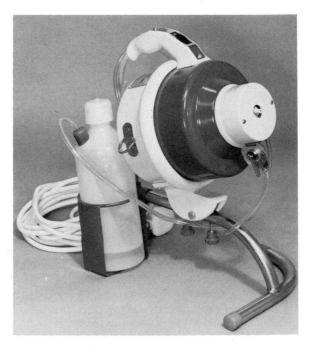

**Figure 20.2** A fogging machine.

*Vapours.* Formaldehyde vapour (H.CHO) is only moderately efficient as a disinfectant and requires the presence of water vapour. It is essential therefore that there is sufficient generation and circulation of the vapour. It is commonly produced from paraformaldehyde tablets, which contain 95% formaldehyde in a polymerized form. The vapour formation depends on sublimation, which takes many hours to complete and may be inefficient. The nebulization of a formalin solution (which contains at least 38% w/w of formaldehyde) is a more efficient means of generating sufficient vapour. A high vapour concentration is required to ensure satisfactory disinfection.

*Chemical compounds which may disinfect and sterilize.* Gluteraldehyde solutions have become very popular as disinfectants, providing, in suitable concentration, a wide spectrum of activity against bacteria, viruses and fungi. Prolonged exposure to these agents kills bacterial spores and so they can also be classified as sterilizing agents. The concentrations of agent and the exposure times required to sterilize equipment may vary with the agent and can be found on the product labelling. These solutions are non corrosive to equipment, however there is a high degree of skin and mucous membrane irritation due to contact with the liquid as well as inhalation of the fumes. Developed allergy to these agents is well known. Preparations using stabilized gluteraldehyde are thought to sensitize personnel less readily and are suitable alternatives. Such reactions mentioned above would be drastically reduced if these agents were regularly handled in a fume extraction cabinet.

Fogging and fumigation have become largely historical treatments, as modern ventilators have detachable and autoclavable gas pathways (see below.)

# Sterilization

## Autoclaving

In autoclaving, the most effective method of sterilization, the articles to be treated are placed in a chamber with a gas tight door. Steam is admitted not only to the chamber, but also to the jacket surrounding it, in order to raise the temperature within. The various stages of the process are usually controlled automatically, and finish with a vacuum stage in which the remaining moisture is removed. Small portable autoclaves generate their own steam by electricity and are independent of the boiler house.

The steam is at a temperature considerably above the boiling point of water and therefore at a high pressure. The time required depends on both the pressure and temperature developed, as shown below:

| Time | Pressure | | Temperature |
|------|------|------|------|
| 30 min | 15 psi | 101.3 kPa | 122°C |
| 10 min | 20 psi | 135 kPa | 126°C |
| 3 min | 30 psi | 202.6 kPa | 134°C |

Articles such as facemasks, which consist of canvas covered by rubber, are liable to be damaged, but red rubber endotracheal tubes may be autoclaved perhaps 10 or 20 times. Many plastic items are likely to be damaged. Articles may be prepacked in envelopes or boxes of suitable material before autoclaving, and chemical 'tellers', in the form of Browne's tubes (which contain a liquid that changes colour after the appropriate temperature treatment) or Thermalog strips (which act in the same manner), may be included in the pack to demonstrate that the heat process has been adequate and that sterilization is complete. Alternatively, the pack may be sealed with a special adhesive tape that shows, by colour changes, that the heat process has been adequate.

Autoclaving is the most efficient, quickest, simplest and probably the most cost-efficient means of sterilization for use in the hospital. Other methods of sterilization mentioned below are appropriate only when autoclaving is contraindicated.

Although high temperature and pressure autoclaving is a most efficient method of sterilizing (as opposed to mere decontamination), there are many items which would be irreparably damaged by this process.

There are two systems which lend themselves particularly to anaesthetic equipment, as in each case an anaesthetic machines can be wheeled bodily into them, always, of course, according to makers' instructions.

## 1. Low pressure, low temperature steam (LTS)

This is performed in a chamber somewhat similar to the high temperature autoclave. However, the pressure within is about 37 kPa (5.5 psi) *absolute* (in other words subatmospheric) in order to maintain the steam as a vapour at approximately 74°C. This is efficient at disinfection in that it kills most vegetative organisms, but not spores.

The addition of the vapour of formaldehyde to

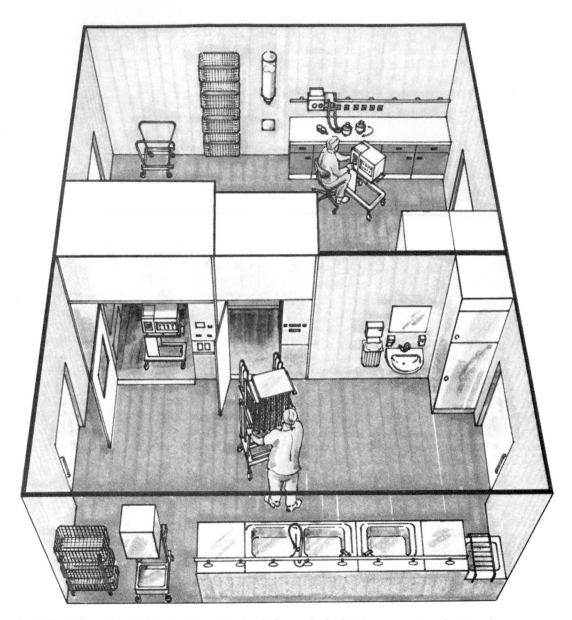

**Figure 20.3**   The Dräger 'Aseptor' fumigation cabinet, which may be built into an operating theatre suite.

this, called *low pressure steam and formaldehyde (LTSF)* renders this process very much more efficient, and kills many if not all spores. It does, however require very careful programming, including vacuum extraction, and 'pulsing' of the steam and formaldehyde. This is a process in which the latter are pumped in and out of the chamber, so that the changes in pressure assure that the vapours penetrate completely all the articles being treated.

Relatively small LTSF chambers of about 4 ft³ may be used to sterilize fibrescopes, whereas others, with doors at both ends may be so large that articles

such as anaesthetic machines or even beds may be wheeled in. The development of LTSF would seem to be at a stage when there are still difficulties in assuring their reliability, but some authorities consider that they may well replace ethylene oxide for many purposes.

## 2. Formaldehyde cabinets

*The Dräger 'Aseptor'.* This is an entire system (Fig. 20.3) in which a 'dirty' and a 'clean' room may be separated by the cabinet into which large items of equipment may be wheeled, or in which small items may be attached to the nozzles through which formaldehyde vapour is introduced. In earlier models the formaldehyde was then neutralized with ammonia, but in later ones this is no longer necessary, since the formaldehyde does not adhere to surfaces. This is because the temperature and humidity are controlled at suitable levels: approx. 45°C and 90% r.h.

It would seem that with the use of formaldehyde alone, the incidence of damage to even domestic electronic equipment, such as television sets, is very rare.

### Dry heating

Some articles are suitable for sterilization by dry heat. They may be wrapped in special craft paper and then placed in a thermostatically controlled hot air oven at 150–170°C for 20–30 min. This method is not suitable for plastics or rubber. All-glass syringes may be sterilized by dry heat, provided that the temperature is raised and lowered slowly to prevent breakage by uneven expansion. Most lubricants deteriorate and should not be used on syringes. Metal plungers should be removed from the barrel of the syringe before heating, or the barrel will be fractured. Dry heat is the method of choice for some ophthalmic instruments.

### Ethylene oxide or propylene oxide

*Ethylene oxide or propylene oxide* gas may be used for sterilizing equipment and in particular those articles that are damaged by other methods. The difficulty is that a special sterilizer is required. This consists of a chamber resembling an autoclave, in which both humidity and temperature are controlled. The process is expensive and takes several hours. Ethylene oxide is very flammable, and is used in a 5–10% mixture with a gas such as carbon dioxide or 'Arcton 12' (dichlorodifluromethane) to prevent explosion risk. Heat and water vapour are also required. The expense and mechanical difficulties of this method usually limit it to use in specialist departments and for perishable items.

Provided that it is properly used, ethylene oxide is an efficient sterilizing agent, but makeshift arrangements such as enclosing large items of equipment in plastic bags, may prove unsatisfactory.

After sterilization in ethylene oxide, a period of 5–7 days must elapse before the gas is entirely eliminated from rubber and plastic. This period of 'elution' may be speeded by the use of an aeration chamber.

Ethylene oxide cannot be used to sterilize polystyrene, since it has an adverse effect on this material.

### Gamma irradiation

The use of γ-rays requires a large, expensive and sophisticated plant, which is appropriate to the sterilization of large quantities of disposable goods, rather than the resterilization of individual pieces of equipment in repeated use. This method is quite inappropriate for any but the largest of hospital groups and will not therefore be described here.

## Routine Disinfection and Sterilization of Anaesthetic Equipment

### Anaesthetic machines

At the end of every day's work, the external surfaces of the anaesthetic machine should be thoroughly cleaned with a solution containing soap or 70% alcohol or with a suitable disinfectant solution, such as 0.5% chlorhexidine (Hibitane) in 70% alcohol. The breathing attachments should be removed and the corrugated hose, reservoir bags, expiratory valves, elbows and catheter mounts thoroughly washed in hot soapy water, rinsed and hung up to dry. The immersion of these parts in some types of detergent solution is ill-advised, since the surface of the rubber parts may be damaged. They may safety be soaked in a solution of 0.1% chlorhexidine in water for 1 hour. If the anaesthetic machine is not to be used immediately, it is better to cover it after cleansing.

At intervals any reuseable breathing systems, tubing, fittings, etc. should be autoclaved. This is by far the most satisfactory method of sterilization, but its too frequent use may result in softening of the rubber parts and a reduction of their antistatic properties. Rubber breathing bags may be damaged by autoclaving. Increasing use is being made of neoprene, a synthetic substance, and silicone rubber that stand up better to heat treatment.

### Circle absorbers

Some circle absorbers are constructed of materials that would be damaged by heat sterilization, in which case the following is advised. The reservoir bag and corrugated hose should be treated as above. The glass domes on the unidirectional valves may be unscrewed and the valve discs carefully removed and cleaned, and the dome wiped out with a spiritous solution, such as 70% alcohol, or a 0.5% chlorhexidine solution. When refitting the dome one should make sure that the sealing washer is in place. From time to time the soda lime canister should be emptied and thoroughly cleaned. This is partly in the interest of sterility, and partly to remove small particles of soda lime from the thread of the canister, which otherwise would cause corrosion and wear and might prevent an airtight fit.

The contamination of circle absorbers may be reduced if, during use, the hoses are allowed to fall in a deep U-loop. This tends to cause droplets of moisture containing infection to 'fall out' before they reach the absorber. Bacterial filters, as described in Chapter 12, may be used to protect the absorber from infection.

Many modern circle absorbers may be autoclaved, and this is obviously more satisfactory.

### Elbows, APL (expiratory) valves, catheter mounts and small fittings that are made partly of rubber

These may be soaked in chlorhexidine solution or boiled. Autoclaving may cause the rubber to deteriorate rapidly in some makes, whilst in others the manufacturers recommend it. They may be pasteurized in the decontaminator shown in Fig. 20.1.

### Ventilators

The tubing and reservoir bag should be removed and treated in the same manner as the anaesthetic machines. The exterior of the ventilator should be swabbed down in an antiseptic solution, such as alcohol or chlorhexidine, and carefully dried. It should be remembered that there are three parts of a ventilator requiring separate consideration, namely (a) the air or gas passages, a distinction between the inspiratory and expiratory sides being sometimes possible (Fig. 20.6), (b) the exterior of the cabinet, and (c) the space within the cabinet but outside the respirator pathways, which may become contaminated by expiratory gases. In respect of the above it should be remembered that the infection that contaminates a ventilator during one operation may be distributed around the theatre during the next — therefore contamination of the ventilator is to be avoided.

### Facemasks

Immediately after use facemasks may be immersed in a suitable soap solution. A suitable concentration is 5–10 ml of spirit soap per litre of water. At the end of every day's work the facemasks should be taken out, thoroughly washed in a hot soapy solution, rinsed in hot water and hung up to dry. They should not be cleaned with detergents or with substances such as trichloroethylene, since these tend to damage the surface and make them sticky. (This damage is particularly likely in the case of facemasks made of rubber with a silicone rubber finish.) Facemasks should not be autoclaved, since with many types not only may the rubber perish but also structural damage may occur.

### Reuseable endotracheal tubes (red rubber) and airways

Endotracheal tubes and airways should also be dropped into the bucket of soap solution immediately after use. They should later be cleaned out with a long narrow brush specially made for the purpose (Fig. 20.4), thoroughly rinsed and then either autoclaved or boiled for 3 minutes. Autoclaving is undoubtedly the most efficient method of sterilization, but endotracheal tubes tend to become soft with repeated treatment in this manner and do not usually stand up to many more than 10 or 20 treatments. Undoubtedly, this is justifiable, even

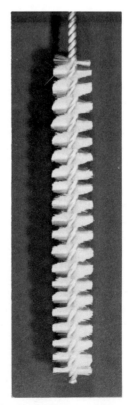

**Figure 20.4** A brush for cleaning endotracheal tubes, etc.

though this reduces the lifespan of the tube. Connectors are best removed from the tubes before heat treatment, so as to prevent permanent stretching. The cuff should be tested at some time during the process to ensure that there are no leaks.

Airways and endotracheal tubes made of latex rubber and thermoplastic materials require careful handling during autoclaving or boiling. Plastic articles, in particular, are liable to lose their shape when heated, and until perfectly cold again should not be distorted in any way. Armoured endotracheal tubes should be handled with especial care, since if they are crushed with forceps, the armour will be distorted and the lumen of the tube diminished.

Silicone rubber armoured tubes often have a self-sealing attachment on the cuff inflation tube. In this case it should be confirmed that no water or air remains in the cuff, or the self-sealing end should be maintained open by a dummy syringe without a plunger, otherwise during autoclaving the cuff may become overdistended and rupture (see Fig. 9.48).

### Perspex articles

Perspex articles, such as transparent soda-lime canisters, should not be heat treated, but after washing may be wiped out with a 70% alcohol (not chloroform, which dissolves Perspex) or 0.9% chlorhexidine solution.

## Special Precautions for Infected Cases

Where a patient is known to have an active respiratory infection (including tuberculosis) or to be a source of transmission of hepatitis B (serum hepatitis) or HIV (human immunodeficiency virus), special precautions should be taken. If an appropriate Mapleson system is to be used, the reservoir bag, bag mount, corrugated tubing, APL valve, elbow and facepiece should be removed from the anaesthetic machine immediately after the operation and placed in a specially labelled (biohazard) plastic bag. To this are added other items that have been in contact with the patient, such as the head harness and retaining ring and the airway and endotracheal tube (if these are not of the disposable type). These items should all be thoroughly washed and then if possible autoclaved; failing this, they should be boiled or soaked in a chemical sterilizing solution, such as one of those mentioned above. If a low-flow system is required, a Waters' canister may be used. After use, all the

metal parts may be autoclaved and the rubber or plastic parts treated in the same way as above. The laryngoscope handle should be swabbed with alcohol or chlorhexidine solution and the blade either autoclaved or soaked in 0.5% chlorhexidine in 70% alcohol solution for at least 3 minutes. The anaesthetic machine and any other surfaces that may have been contaminated should be swabbed down with alcohol or chlorhexidine solution.

The use of bacterial and viral filters such as that shown in Figs 20.5 and 20.6 may reduce the contamination of breathing attachments and may therefore be deemed desirable in such cases.

## Storage of Sterile Objects

Facemasks and other parts of breathing systems should be hung up to dry and then stored in a dust-free cupboard or drawer. Reuseable airways and endotracheal tubes, following decontamination and rinsing, should be dried and individually packaged before autoclaving.

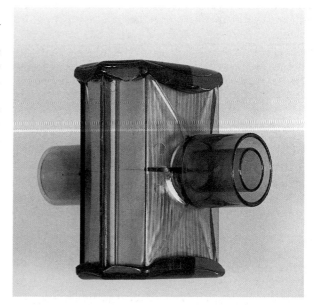

**Figure 20.5** A bacterial filter.

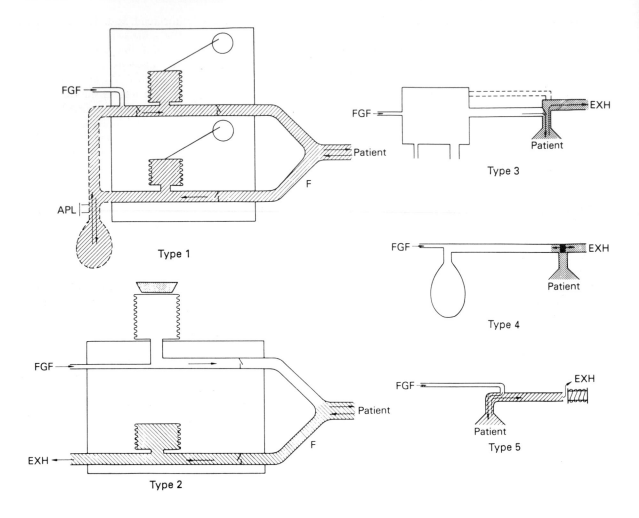

**Figure 20.6**   To show the extent of contamination of a ventilator according to the type of breathing system employed, and the need for sterilization. FGF = Fresh gas flow. EXH = Exhaust (to scavenging system if required). Type 1—Engine-driven closed-circuit anaesthetic ventilators, such as the Cape Waine. Since the expired gases are stored in a reservoir and then returned to the inspiratory side, the whole of the breathing system becomes contaminated and requires sterilization. The filter shown in Fig. 20.5 may be fitted at F to prevent such contamination. If the reservoir bag is removed and there is no rebreathing, then only the expiratory side becomes contaminated. Type 2—Gas-driven ventilators, such as the Manley MN2 or MP2. Only the expiratory side becomes contaminated. In the case of the MP3, this may be detached for sterilization. Type 3—Gas-driven ventilators, such as the Bird Mark 7. Only the expiratory valve becomes contaminated and may easily be sterilized. Type 4—Minute volume dividers, such as the East–Freeman automatic vent. Only the valve itself and the expiratory limb become contaminated. Type 5—The mechanical thumb. The whole attachment except for the fresh gas delivery tube becomes contaminated.

# 21 Instruments and Aids to Anaesthesia

## Laryngoscopes

Visualization of the vocal cords for intubation was popularized by Sir Robert Macintosh and Sir Ivan Magill in the early 1940s. It was during the insertion of a Boyle–Davis gag that Sir Robert conceived the idea of his laryngoscope, which is still the most popular design in use today and has spawned a wide variety of modifications. It consists of a blade that elevates the lower jaw and tongue, a light source near the tip of this blade to illuminate the larynx and a handle to apply suitable leverage to the blade. The handle also contains the power supply (battery) for the light source. This blade is so hinged on the handle that, when it is opened to the right-angle position, the light comes on automatically.

### Blades

Macintosh designed a slightly curved blade (Fig. 21.1) with a small bulbous tip that was to be inserted anterior to the base of the epiglottis in an adult. The child and infant blades were not designed by him and he condemned them as being anatomically wrong and unnecessary. Blades for infants and children tend to be either straight or with a shallow curve at the tip only. Figure 21.2 shows the wide variety of blades currently available and the choice of blade for routine use is probably

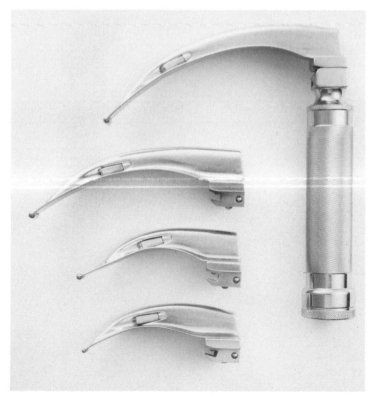

**Figure 21.1** The Macintosh laryngoscope with four sizes of hook-on blade.

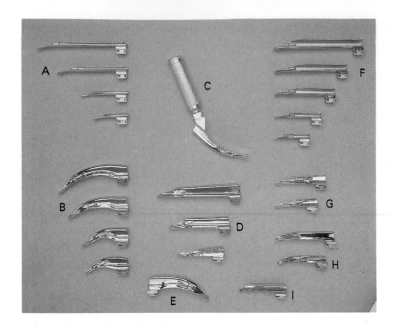

**Figure 21.2** Laryngoscope blades. **A**, Miller pattern: 3, large; 2, adult; 1, infant; 0, premature. **B**, Macintosh pattern: 4, large; 3, adult; 2, child; 1, baby. **C**, Macintosh polio blade. **D**, Soper pattern: adult; child; baby. **E**, Macintosh pattern left-handed version. **F**, Wisconsin: large, adult, child, baby, infant. **G**, Robertshaw's: infant and neonatal. **H**, Seward: child and baby. **I**, Oxford: infant.

largely a matter of personal preference. Most blades are detachable from the handle for ease of cleaning and change of blade size where appropriate. The 'hook on' connection which allows easy detachment is very convenient and was developed by Welch Alleyn Ltd in the early 1950s.

The extended blade normally forms a right angle with the handle. However this may prove difficult to insert in patients with abnormal anatomy, e.g. limited neck extension or large breasts, or who are in unusual situations (e.g. in a cabinet ventilator). Various alternative angles for blades have been produced by modifying the 'hook on' angle (e.g. the polio blade, Fig. 21.3) or by producing a handle with multiple locking positions, (the Patil–Syracuse handle, Fig. 21.4).

The electrical system of the laryngoscope has been greatly improved in recent years, but some points are still worthy of note. The bulb unscrews from the light carrier. On most bulbs the central contact is a 'blob' of solder, but there still remain others in which it is a small wire coil, which may need bending and adjusting so that it will reach the contact in the light carrier but not short circuit on to the side (Fig. 21.5).

The light carriers, if detachable, for different blades are not interchangeable and should be removed and cold sterilized when the blade is autoclaved. The electrical contacts between the handle and the mount of the blade may need cleaning from time to time with some fine abrasive

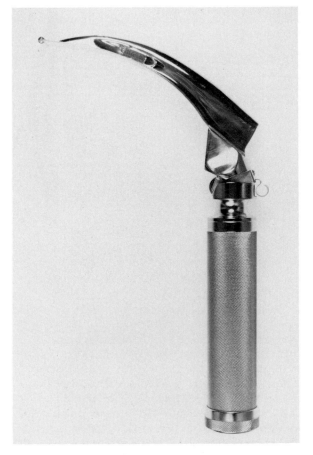

**Figure 21.3** The Polio laryngoscope.

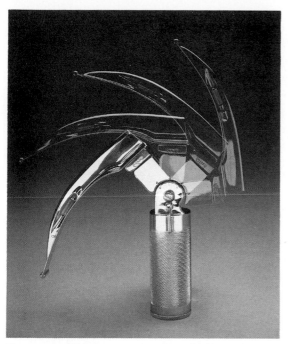

**Figure 21.4** Patil–Syracuse handle, which allows multiple locking positions of the attached laryngoscope blade.

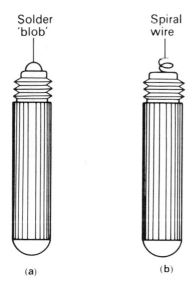

**Figure 21.5** Laryngoscope bulbs. Notice the solder 'blob' contact on (a) and the wire spiral on (b).

material or a smooth file. In some cases the handle may be removed by loosening the retaining screw a couple of turns and then, while pressing the knurled head inwards, slipping the blade off the handle.

When replacing the batteries in the handle, it should be ensured that the spiral spring is still in the base of the battery compartment; leak-proof batteries should be used. (It is most aggravating to find, in an emergency, that not only are the batteries exhausted but they have also corroded within the handle, making replacement impossible.)

The laryngoscope blade may be cleaned between cases with soap and water, applied using a scrubbing brush, followed by spirit or chlorhexidine swabbing, and should be autoclaved, without the light carrier, as often as circumstances permit.

## Left-handed laryngoscopes

At least one company (Penlon) manufactures a Macintosh laryngoscope the blade of which is the mirror image of that to which we are accustomed. The left-handed laryngoscope is not, as sometimes imagined, for use by an anaesthetist who is left-handed, but for patients in whom the nature of the teeth or maxilla make it undesirable to exert pressure upon a particular area. This may be due to complicated dental restorations, loose or ill positioned teeth, or the presence of cysts or tumours of the maxilla, to which damage could be caused by pressure of the laryngoscope. A left-handed laryngoscope should be carefully marked and kept in an appropriate place. Those with no experience will be amused to find how difficult it is to use it to begin with. It would be wise to obtain some practice with it so that when a difficult case does arise the user will be familiar with it.

## Bronchoscopes

There are simple emergency bronchoscopes which work on the same principles as laryngoscopes. The proportions are different, however, and a smaller bulb is employed.

It is an advantage to obtain blades that fit the same universal handle as the laryngoscope. They are made in various sizes, a set of three diameters, viz. 11 mm, 8.5 mm and 3.5 mm, being convenient.

Figure 21.6 shows three blades for the Magill emergency bronchoscope, which incorporates a side tube through which oxygen may be blown. By occluding the open end with the finger, the patient's lungs may be inflated with what becomes a type of T-piece system. Although this may be less convenient for the operator than a jetting device (Chapter 12), it is pointed out that this is an *emergency* bronchoscope to be used at times when the latter may not be available. Metal suction tubes or plastic suction catheters may be used for aspiration.

Figure 21.6 Magill emergency bronchoscope blades.

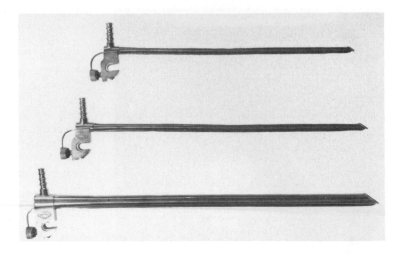

# Recent Advances in Laryngoscope Design

## Light source

Many currently produced laryngoscopes are produced with the light source now sited within the handle and with the light projected to the tip of the blade via a fibre-optic bundle (see below). This bundle may be manufactured as an integral part of the blade (Fig. 21.7), making the blade very easy to clean and sterilize. The siting of the light source within the handle also increases the reliability of this design over traditional light sources sited on the blade. Rechargeable nickel–cadmium batteries are gaining popularity as the power source for these laryngoscopes.

## Flexible fibreoptics

The object of the flexible fibreoptic system is to transmit light from a powerful external light source through an instrument that, being flexible, can be passed through a series of curvatures, and return to an eyepiece or camera an image of the area being illuminated. It may be used for endoscopy by various routes: for example, laryngoscopy, bronchoscopy, oesophagoscopy and colonoscopy. The pathways through which the illumination and the image pass consist of bundles of thousands of very fine glass fibres. Typically these fibres have a diameter of the order of 20 μm. Each consists of a central glass core surrounded by a thin cladding of another type of glass having a refractive index different from that of the core. As will be seen in Fig. 21.8, the light ray passing down the fibre is

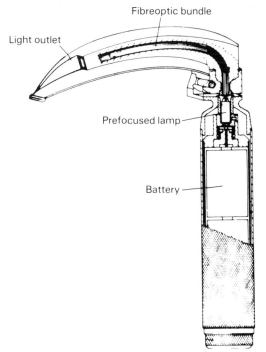

Figure 21.7 The Heine fibreoptic laryngoscope. Note that the lamp is within the handle, thus avoiding unreliable electrical contacts between the handle and the blade.

repeatedly internally reflected from the interface between these two elements of the fibre. A bundle of these fibres is called a guide. In the case of a light guide the fibres are arranged in a random fashion, whereas with the image guide the ends of the fibres at each end of the bundle must be precisely located relative to each other. Each fibre carries the light from one small portion of the image in the same way that many small dots make up the printed representation in a book or newspaper of an

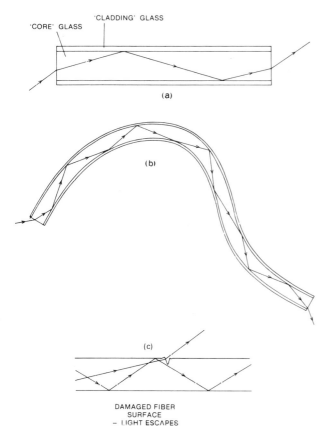

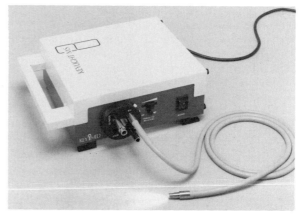

**Figure 21.9** A light source and guide.

**Figure 21.8** (a) A single optical fibre. Note that the light ray is repeatedly internally reflected from the interface between the core and cladding glass. (b) If the fibre is curved, the ray is still internally reflected within it. (c) If the surface of the fibre is damaged, the light ray may not be totally internally reflected and some light may escape from the bundle.

original photograph. The fibres are so fine that they are easily flexible and they are lubricated so that they can move relative to each other. The whole bundle may therefore be flexed.

The light source of a fibrescope (Fig. 21.9) is usually powered by the mains electricity supply and contains a lamp very much brighter than that seen at the distal end of a laryngoscope. It provides sufficient illumination not only for visualization, but also for the taking of colour photographs with a suitably adapted camera.

The trunk of the instrument may carry all of the following: an optical bundle (image guide), one or two light guides, a channel for suction or air insufflation, and another channel for the passage of instruments such as biopsy forceps. At the distal end of the optical bundle there is a suitable lens to focus the image on the ends of the fibres; at the proximal end there is an eyepiece that may be focused. The eyepiece mount also carries a connection for the vacuum/insufflation channel and a valve to make a seal for the instrument channel. A fibreoptic bronchoscope is shown in Fig. 21.10.

The care of the fibrescope and of light cables in general is of great importance. The optical bundles in particular are extremely expensive to manufacture and are easily damaged. Although they can be flexed into acute angles of relatively small radii, they are easily damaged if they are pinched or knocked, as for example by a towel forceps on the operating table, or by being shut in the lid of the case in which they are transported. The covering over the distal 6 cm or so of the instrument is very delicate, and it is at this point that the greatest flexion takes place. It may well have to be replaced at about yearly intervals; the whole instrument being serviced every 6 months, according to the maker's instructions.

After use, the instrument may be cleaned by wiping it with a solution of aqueous chlorhexidine and then rinsed in water. It can be disinfected between cases with a glutaraldehyde based solution, but it is essential that in older models the eyepiece and head of the instrument are not immersed in the

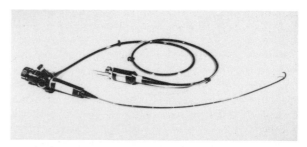

**Figure 21.10** A fibreoptic laryngoscope.

solution, otherwise water may track down between the fibres and damage the lubricant between them. If the trunk is immersed in the sterilizing solution, it should not be hung vertically, since the pressure at the lower end may be sufficient to drive water inside the cable and damage the lubricant as mentioned above. There are specially designed dishes into which the instrument is laid horizontally, with the head supported well above water level. Currently marketed models are now totally immersible and these restrictions do not apply. Disinfectant solution may be sucked through the channels, and there is also a small brush which may be used to clean the instrument. Although the instrument may be better protected by returning it to its carrying case after sterilization, it is, in fact, better to hang it vertically in a cupboard with the eyepiece at the top, so that any moisture contained may evaporate.

### Fibreoptic laryngoscopes

These instruments are invaluable as an aid to difficult intubation either by the oral or nasotracheal route. A number of techniques involving their use have been advocated, but all of them require regular practice on routine cases before they can be of benefit in an emergency or difficult situation.

# Sprays

Nebulizing sprays are used for the topical (surface) application of local analgesic solutions, such as 4% lignocaine, to the larynx and trachea, and sometimes of vasoconstrictors to the nose. The general principle is the same in all of them: a jet of air is blown through a venturi and 'sucks up' and nebulizes a solution of the agent to be used. Figures 21.11 and 21.12 show two popular types.

All of these sprays tend to block up if they are not cleaned shortly after use, because the solution remaining at the nozzle dries out, leaving crystals that block the small orifice. This may be avoided by rinsing them out with distilled water or spirit after use.

The spray may be cleaned after use by any cold sterilizing solution, but a scrub with a brush and soapy water followed by soaking it in 70% alcohol for 3 minutes is considered adequate. In the air inlet to the bulb there is a ball or flap valve. The analgesic solution has a tendency to run back into this and cause corrosion. In the case of the Swerdlow spray (Fig. 21.12) the ball may be removed for cleaning by unscrewing the knurled nut, care being taken to avoid losing the small retaining spring.

The two other common problems encountered with the Swerdlow spray are that the washer that seals the joint within the container is often damaged by over-tightening, and that the small length of tubing with the sinker often falls off. The tubing

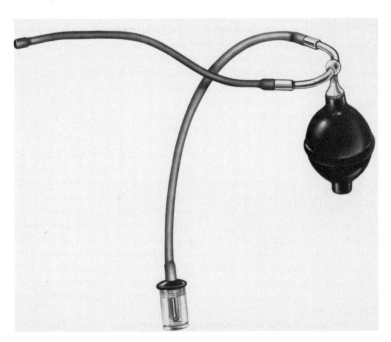

**Figure 21.11** The Macintosh spray.

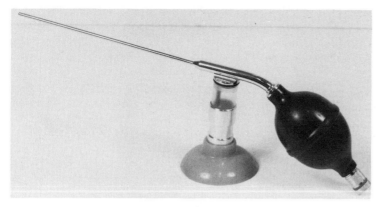

Figure 21.12 **Figure 21.12** (a) The Swerdlow spray. (b) Working principles. Note that the diameters of the tubes leading to the nozzles are very small and if analgesic solution is allowed to collect and crystallize out in this area the spray will be blocked. (c) The one-way valve.

(a)

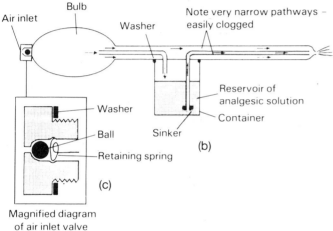

Air inlet

Bulb

Washer

Note very narrow pathways – easily clogged

Washer

Ball

Retaining spring

Sinker

Reservoir of analgesic solution

Container

(b)

(c)

Magnified diagram of air inlet valve

may be replaced by a piece cut from the pilot tube of an old red rubber cuffed endotracheal tube.

The maintenance in good working order or otherwise of the sprays may be taken as an index of the efficiency of the theatre technician!

# Bougies and Stylets

Occasionally at laryngoscopy the larynx may be only partially visualized or hidden behind the epiglottis and beyond reach with the normal curvature of an endotracheal tube. Intubation may possibly be then accomplished by either (a) altering the curvature of the endotracheal tube using a malleable plastic-coated metal stylet or (b) initially inserting a long, thin gum-elastic bougie and using this as a guide over which the tube may be passed ('rail-roaded') into the trachea. A bougie and stylet are illustrated in Fig. 21.13.

Malleable metal stylets should be plastic-coated so that, in the event of a metal fracture (from repeated

bending), part of the stylet will not detach and disappear into the bronchial tree. Most are designated as single-use only to prevent potential fracture occurring.

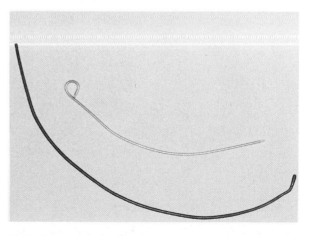

**Figure 21.13** A bougie and a stylet.

# Berman Intubating/Pharyngeal Airway

This airway has a circular cross-section with a complete longitudinal split down one side (Fig. 21.14). It may be used either as a pharyngeal airway or a guide to intubation. In the latter mode, when the airway is inserted in the mid-line and the tip reaches the patient's vallecula, a small endotracheal tube may be passed through the airway and into the larynx. The airway is also extremely useful as a guide in fibreoptic oral intubation. The large internal bore of this airway holds the pharyngeal structures out of the way and also protects the fibrescope tip from pharyngeal secretions. The longitudinal split in the airway facilitates its easy separation from the fibrescope and allows subsequent railroading of the endotracheal tube into the larynx.

The following schedules are included as a guide for the benefit of those who are required to equip a new anaesthetic department.

# Schedule 1: The Standard Anaesthetic Unit

*Boyle's anaesthetic machine*, complete with the following:

- Rotameter (flowmeter) unit for $N_2O$, $O_2$, $CO_2$ and (if required) air;
- Boyle's vaporizing bottle, where still used;
- temperature-compensated vaporizers;
- Cardiff swivel outlet;
- Mapleson breathing system;
- circle absorber unit;
- emergency oxygen flush control;
- provision for $CO_2$ cylinder;
- provision for medical suction;
- monitoring equipment;
- shelves — steel;
- top shelf;
- drawer unit;
- pipeline attachment;
- cylinder labels (Fig. 21.16);
- pressure relief valve;
- oxygen warning device.

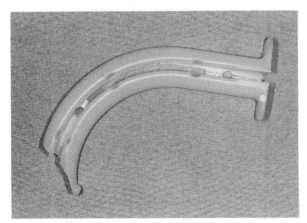

**Figure 21.14** Berman intubating/pharyngeal airway.

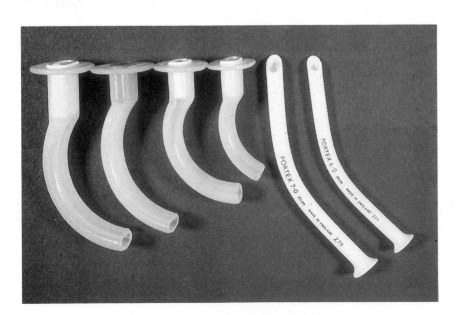

**Figure 21.15** Artificial airways. (Left) Guedel oropharyngeal airways. (Right) Nasopharyngeal airways.

*Other extras*:

- facemasks, various (M & IE, BOC, etc.);
- cylinder keys (Fig. 21.17);
- spares (reservoir bag, corrugated hose, expiratory valve, etc.);
- airways, various (Fig. 21.15)
    Guedel oropharyngeal airway
    Nasopharyngeal airway;
- endotracheal connectors;
- endotracheal tubes;
- laryngoscopes, adult and paediatric;
- laryngeal sprays;
- Magill's endotracheal introducing forceps (Fig. 21.18);
- syringe and Spencer Wells' forceps for inflating endotracheal cuffs;
- Spencer Wells' forceps (Fig. 21.19a);
- Guy's tongue forceps (Fig. 21.20);
- Mayo's tongue and towel forceps (Fig. 21.21) or Thompson's tongue forceps (Fig. 21.22);
- large Kocher's forceps (Fig. 21.19b);
- scissors;
- mouth gags (Figs 21.23–21.25);
- mouth wedge and prop (Fig. 21.26);
- suction end (Yankauer's or other);
- stethoscope;
- Ayre's T-pieces;
- Magill emergency bronchoscope, combined with various sized blades;
- suction catheters;
- kidney dishes and gallipots;
- Clausen's, Connell's or other head harnesses (Fig. 21.27);
- Hudson's head harness (Fig. 21.28);
- catheter mounts (Fig. 9.78);
- plastic buckets;
- armboards;
- ampoule holder block;
- 9-drawer cabinet(s);
- bandages, adhesive plaster, etc.;
- analgesic ointment and lubricating jelly;
- drip stands;
- intravenous infusion equipment.

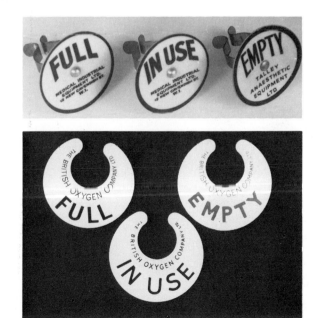

**Figure 21.16** Various cylinder labels.

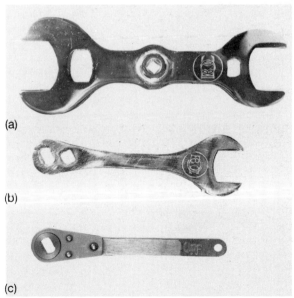

**Figure 21.17** Cylinder keys. (a) For bull-nosed cylinders. (b) For pin index cylinders. (c) A ratchet type for pin index cylinders.

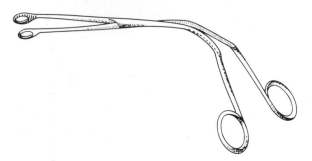

Figure 21.18 Magill's endotracheal introducing forceps.

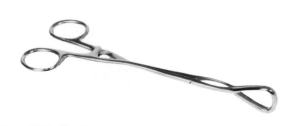

Figure 21.20 Guy's tongue forceps.

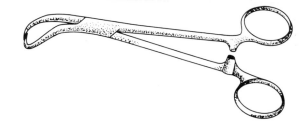

Figure 21.21 Mayo's tongue and towel forceps.

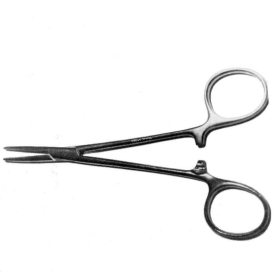

(a)

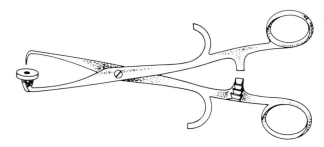

Figure 21.22 Thompson's tongue forceps.

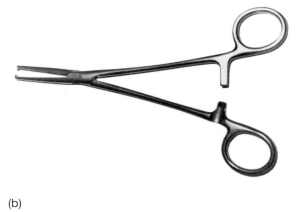

(b)

Figure 21.19 Artery forceps. (a) Spencer Wells'.
(b) Kocher's.

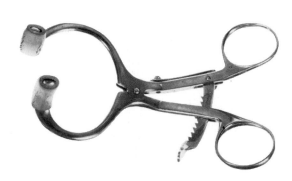

Figure 21.23 Sydenham's modification of Doyen's mouth gag.

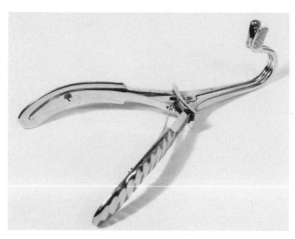

**Figure 21.24** Ferguson's mouth gag.

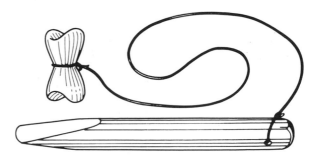

**Figure 21.26** Wooden mouth wedge and prop.

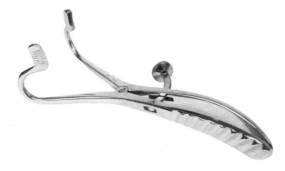

**Figure 21.25** Mason's mouth gag.

(a)

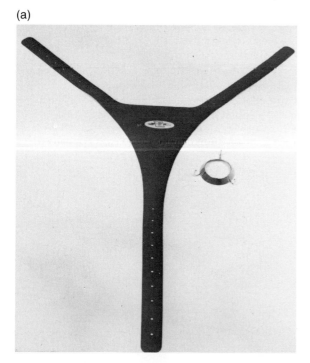

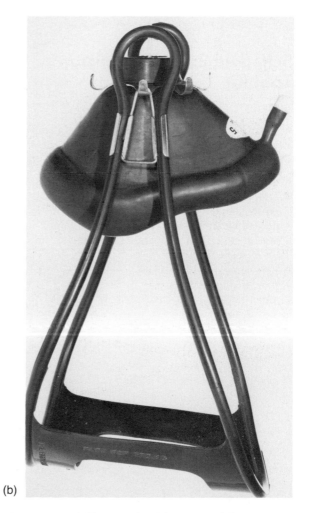

(b)

**Figure 21.27** (a) Clausen's head harness and ring.
(b) Connell's head harness.

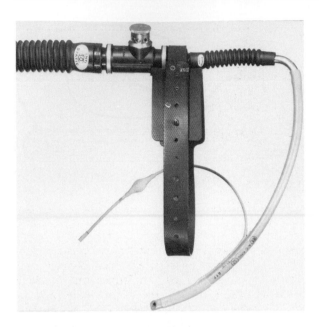

**Figure 21.28** Hudson's head harness.

# Schedule 2: The Technician's Tool Kit

A set of tools for the technician who has completed a training scheme organized by a manufacturer should include:

- various screwdrivers, including Phillips;
- a set of spanners up to ½-in Whitworth and equivalent metric sizes;
- adjustable spanners, one small, one large;
- set of hexagonal wrenches (Allen keys), imperial and metric sizes;
- pair of combination pliers;
- pair of diagonal cutters;
- small hacksaw and spare blades;
- set of files;

- ball-pein hammer;
- wooden mallet;
- sharpening stone;
- oil can;
- vice mounted on the bench;
- crimping tool and spare ferrules — *available only to a suitably qualified engineer*;
- spare bulbs for laryngoscope and bronchoscope;
- spare batteries;
- spare washers, including those for cylinder yokes, soda-lime canisters, sprays, etc.;
- torch;
- direct-current electric test meter;
- grease and other specified lubricants;
- manufacturers' instruction manuals for machines and ventilators;
- pressure gauges of various types.

# 22 Electrical Hazards and their Prevention

## The Mains Electric Supply

Since many items of anaesthetic apparatus and monitors are powered by electricity, it is important to understand some of the principles involved. The 'mains' electric supply is not *direct current*, flowing uninterruptedly in the same direction, as is produced by a battery; for good engineering reasons it provides an *alternating current*, in which the flow is constantly changing from one direction to the other in a rapid and regular manner. The number of complete cycles of this change of direction, or its *frequency*, is 50 per second in the UK and 60 per second in some other countries, for example the USA. The two conductors in a cable therefore cannot be said to be *positive* and *negative*, as would be the case with direct current; but since one is at, or at about, the same potential as earth (because it is connected to earth at the transformer), this is said to be *neutral* or *return*, and the other conductor to be *live*. Because of this earthing of the neutral conductor, any person (or object) who is connected to earth would complete the electric circuit by touching the live conductor, even if no contact were made with the neutral one. Figure 22.1 shows how under certain conditions the circuit may be completed by, say, an earthed diathermy plate, resulting in fatal electrocution. (In most modern diathermy machines the plate is 'earth-free'.) Stringent precautions should be taken to ensure that the polarities are correctly identified and connected for all mains electrical apparatus. Furthermore, the interruption of the neutral conductor alone could result in

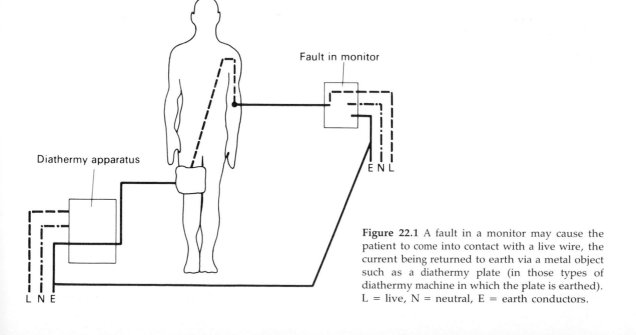

**Figure 22.1** A fault in a monitor may cause the patient to come into contact with a live wire, the current being returned to earth via a metal object such as a diathermy plate (in those types of diathermy machine in which the plate is earthed). L = live, N = neutral, E = earth conductors.

apparatus being at a live potential and yet not operating. Any contact with apparatus in this condition could, if it has not been disconnected from the mains supply, lead to electrocution. It cannot be overemphasized that if a fault exists, the services of a competent technician should be sought.

The inclusion in an electric supply cable of a third conductor that connects the metal chassis, frame and enclosure of the apparatus to the earthed point of the supply ensures that under faulty conditions, such as an internal short in the equipment, the chassis and enclosure would not be rendered live. This wire is said to be the *earth* conductor.

*Fuses* interrupt the electric supply in the event that the current passing through them exceeds a predetermined level that might cause overheating or damage. They may be installed in the mains supply circuit, in the plug-top at the end of the lead to the apparatus, or in the apparatus itself. They usually consist of a fine-gauge wire, which melts if the current passing through it exceeds that against which it is intended to offer protection.

## Accidents associated with the mains electric supply

There are three ways in which the mains electric current, or equipment powered by it, may endanger the patient:

- electrocution;
- burns;
- ignition of flammable materials, leading to fire or explosion.

### Electrocution

Until recently the only concept of electrocution was one in which two remote parts of the body such as the hands were applied to the two poles of a 240-V mains electric supply.

Figure 22.2a shows how the current may pass through a wide segment of the body so that at any one point within the trunk, the actual 'current density' may be of low order.

The current flowing depends on several factors, including the electrical resistance of the skin at the point of contact. This is particularly influenced by moisture or dryness.

Let us consider the passage of current from one hand to the other, or from one hand to a foot. If the current exceeds 1 mA, a tingling sensation is felt (Fig. 22.2a). If the current is increased, the sensation becomes progressively painful. A current in excess of about 15 mA produces a tonic contraction of the muscles, as a result of which the patient is unable to release his grip upon the electrode: this is known as the 'no let go' threshold (Fig. 22.2b). A current in excess of 75–100 mA can result in ventricular fibrillation (Fig. 22.2c).

A very high current, in excess of 5 A, produces a tonic contraction of the myocardium which could, if irreparable damage has not occurred, be followed, when it ceases, by a normal rhythm. Such a high current is unlikely to be encountered in clinical practice, other than during defibrillation.

Electrocution may cause death relatively slowly by the tonic contraction of the respiratory muscles, leading to asphyxia, or more rapidly by ventricular fibrillation. The onset of ventricular fibrillation may be somewhat delayed, being preceded by ventricular tachycardia, which causes circulatory failure, but which may revert to normal rhythm if stopped in time.

It will be remembered that the neutral pole of the mains electric supply is connected to earth at a point remote from the patient. Since all conductors have some resistance, however low, a loss known as *volts drop* occurs along these conductors, so that the neutral conductor is not *exactly* at earth potential at the patient end of the circuit. This difference in potential can cause 'stray voltage' and may lead to a 'stray current'.

Since earthed electrodes may be attached to more than one part of the patient, and from more than one piece of apparatus supplied by different mains sockets, it is recommended that the earth connections on all the socket outlets in a single clinical area be interconnected by a conductor of low resistance to minimize voltage differences between them. Similarly, all exposed metal objects such as radiators, water pipes, etc. are interconnected to a good earth.

Figure 22.2a, b and c shows the effect of a current passing between the extremities. When it passes across the patient's trunk only a small part of it passes through the heart. However, recent advances in medicine and surgery have led to the placement of electrodes on, within or close to the heart. Under these circumstances a very much smaller current, possibly as low as 100 μA, can result in ventricular fibrillation (Fig. 22.2d) since all the current passes through the heart. A very small potential, such as the stray voltage in the mains neutral lead, could be sufficient to produce electrocution in this way. This phenomenon is known as *microshock*.

There are two ways of preventing accidents caused by unwanted currents returning to earth. One is to install an isolating transformer, the output of which is carefully isolated from earth, and the second is to detect unwanted currents passing to

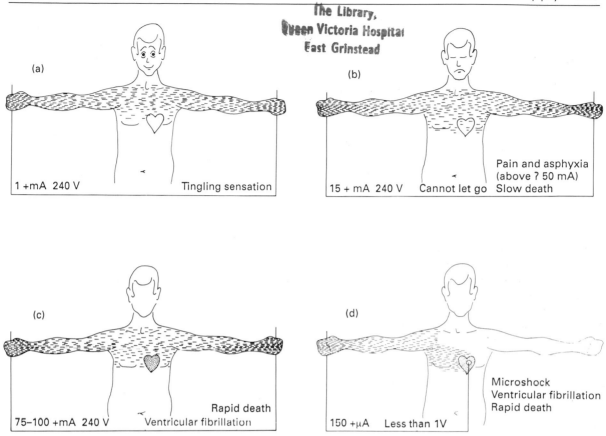

**Figure 22.2** (a) A current in excess of 1 mA passing through the body may produce a tingling sensation. (b) If the current exceeds about 15 mA, muscles are held in tonic spasm; the victim cannot let go and will eventually die of asphyxia. (c) When the current exceeds 100 mA, ventricular fibrillation and rapid death will occur. (d) If one electrode is applied to the right ventricle of the heart itself, a very small current can result in ventricular fibrillation.

earth by a device that may then *either* sound a warning *or* automatically switch off the supply. There are advantages and disadvantages of each of these and they will be discussed below.

Such a transformer may supply all the outlets for a whole operating room or theatre suite. This is referred to as *safe patient power* (Fig. 22.3). Apart from the expense, the problems are that if there are several appliances in use, and each of these has a small earth leakage current that is harmless in itself, the sum of all these currents may be sufficient to trip the relay and cut off the power to some piece of vital life-support equipment. Similarly, a fault in one piece of equipment may cause the cessation of power to another. If the relay operates a warning device rather than a circuit breaker, it may be observed too late or be unheeded by staff who do not appreciate its importance. Isolating transformers

may be used in another and, in the author's opinion, more satisfactory manner. They may be included in the circuitry of each individual item of mains-operated electromedical equipment that can be connected to a patient. The patient circuit is earth-free and said to be *fully floating*. The enclosure of the equipment may be earthed, or completely insulated.

The second method of improving safety is to install a current-operated earth-leakage circuit breaker (COELCB, also known as an 'earth trip' or residual current circuit breaker) (Fig. 22.4). This may be installed in the electric supply to a whole operating room or theatre suite, or may be installed in each item of equipment. The live and neutral conductors each take a couple of turns or so (both exactly the same) around the core of a toroidal transformer. A third winding is connected directly

**Figure 22.3** Safe patient power. The output of the isolating transformer is free from earth. Should earth leakage occur above a prearranged level, the relay will either disconnect the supply to the input of the transformer or sound a warning device. L = live, N = neutral, E = earth connectors.

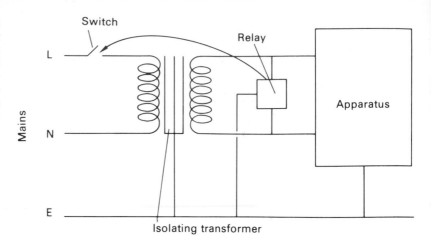

to the coil of the relay that operates the circuit breaker. If the current in the live and neutral conductors is the same, the magnetic fluxes cancel themselves out. If they differ, there is a resultant field which induces a current in the third winding and this causes the relay to operate and break the circuit. A difference of as little as 30 mA can trip the COELCB in as short a time as 0.03 s. It may be manually reset, and may also have a test button to check its operation.

A similar device may be used instead merely to give a warning of excess earth leakage, or it may perform both functions.

COELCBs may present problems similar to those of isolating transformers, except that they are less expensive. They operate so quickly, and as a result of such a low earth leakage current, that they very greatly reduce the possibility of serious electric shock.

In the UK electrical safety in clinical areas is achieved by a high standard of earthing of the fixed wiring, by good earthing of enclosures and by fully floating patient circuits where appropriate. Further safety may be achieved by using battery-operated equipment. In some cases the battery may be recharged between periods of use by 'plugging in' to the mains supply.

## Burns

Where an electric current passes through the skin, whether intentionally or not, electrical resistance leads to the generation of heat. Depending on the amount of heat produced, the area over which it is applied and the rate of cooling by the blood circulation, burns may result. This matter is discussed further below, in connection with diathermy.

## Fire

Sparks occurring at switches or from the interruption of the supply by the removal of a plug could ignite flammable vapours. They are prevented in the operating theatre by the installation of sparkproof switches (see Fig. 22.5), and electrical socket outlets that 'capture' the plug, preventing its withdrawal while the switch is turned on. All electrical apparatus in the operating theatre that does not comply with these precautions is kept outside the 'zone of risk', as described later in this chapter.

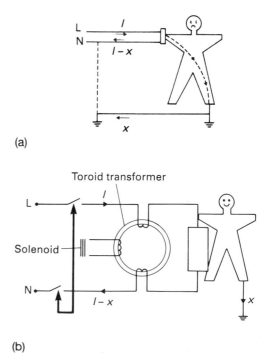

**Figure 22.4** (See facing page for caption.)

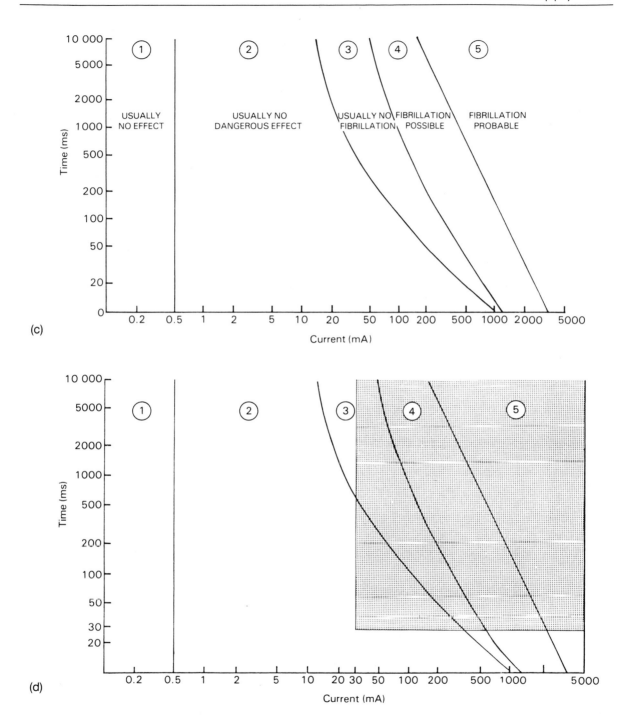

**Figure 22.4** (a) If a load is taking a current of $I$ amps from the live conductor L and $x$ amps is returning via the patient and earth, then the current in the neutral conductor N will be $(I - x)$ amps. (b) A current-operated earth-leakage circuit breaker (COELCB). The imbalance between the currents in the live L and neutral N conductors is sufficient to set up a field in the toroidal transformer sufficient to induce in the third winding a current that will trip the solenoid and therefore disconnect both the live and neutral supply. (c) The effects of a current passing through the human body (hand to hand or hand to foot). Zone 1, usually no effect; zone 2, usually no dangerous effect; zone 3, usually no danger of ventricular fibrillation; zone 4, ventricular fibrillation possible; zone 5, ventricular fibrillation probable. (d) The shaded area denotes the protection given by a COELCB.

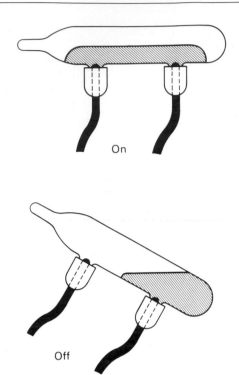

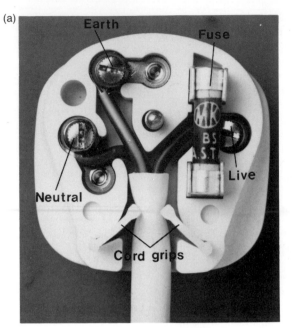

(a) Earth    Fuse

Neutral    Live

Cord grips

Figure 22.5 The contact of a sparkless mercury tip switch.

Note that this 'zone of risk' no longer includes the whole operating theatre.

The correct wiring of electrical plugs is essential; this is shown in Fig. 22.6. Fatal mistakes have occurred when the wire intended to be earthed has been connected to the live terminal. Further, when new electrical apparatus is being commissioned, the voltage for which it is intended, and the setting on the voltage control panel (when one is installed), should match that of the mains supply.

# Fire and Explosion

For these to occur there are three prerequisites: combustible material, oxygen to support combustion, and a source of ignition.

The risks arise from two sources:

- the use of high-pressure oxygen and high concentrations of oxygen at atmospheric pressure;
- the use of flammable anaesthetic agents.

Burning consists of the chemical combination of a 'combustible' material with oxygen. Energy is liberated in the form of heat, and if it takes place in a confined space the pressure may be increased

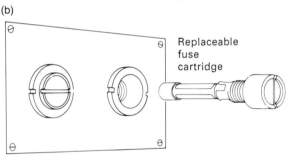

(b)    Replaceable fuse cartridge

(c)

|         | 'Old' British | 'New' International |
|---------|---------------|---------------------|
| Live    | Red           | Brown               |
| Neutral | Black         | Blue                |
| Earth   | Green         | Green/yellow        |

Figure 22.6 (a) The correct wiring of a ring main 13-A plug top. (b) A cartridge fuse as fitted in portable electrical equipment. (c) Colour coding for flexible electrical cables.

greatly. Rapid liberation of heat and the rise of pressure result in an explosion.

## High-pressure oxygen

When there is a rise in the pressure of a gas, heat is generated. If a flammable material such as oil or grease, in a confined area, is suddenly subjected to oxygen at the pressure of a full cylinder (~ 2000 psi

(140 000 kPa)), the heat generated is sufficient to ignite it and cause an explosion. This, incidentally, is the principle of the compression-ignition (diesel) engine.

Therefore, oil, grease or other flammable materials should be kept away from apparatus in which high-pressure oxygen is used.

Under some conditions nitrous oxide may dissociate, producing nitrogen and oxygen, and the latter gives rise to the risk of an explosion. Therefore nitrous oxide cylinders should be treated with similar care.

## Anaesthetic agents

Cyclopropane, most ethers and ethyl chloride are explosive in anaesthetic concentrations.

Carbon dioxide, halothane (Fluothane), methoxyflurane (Penthrane) and enflurane (Ethrane), are not flammable, nor is nitrous oxide at atmospheric pressure. However nitrous oxide *does* support combustion even more fiercely than oxygen. Trichloroethylene also is non-flammable under the conditions in which it is used by the anaesthetist.

Fire or explosion may be caused by the ignition of gases or vapours within the anaesthetic equipment, or escaping from it, or of the vapour of a flammable substance that has been accidentally spilled or used for purposes such as the cleansing of the patient's skin.

Ignition of flammable mixtures may be caused by sparks from static electricity, from faulty electrical apparatus, from the cautery and diathermy apparatus, from electric motors, or from an electric plug-top being pulled out of the socket when the switch is turned on and current is flowing. Naked flames are seldom employed in operating theatres now, but they may be encountered in ophthalmic or dental surgery.

## Static electricity

Static electrical discharges have probably been responsible for most of the explosions that have occurred.

Today, when nylon and Terylene clothes are so popular, the clicking from sparks as static electricity is discharged is commonplace. Similar static charges are developed on dressing trolleys, operating tables and anaesthetic machines.

Although the quantity of static electricity generated in the operating theatre is relatively small, there is sufficient energy in the spark, when it is rapidly discharged, to ignite flammable vapours such as cyclopropane and ether. Arrangements should therefore be made not only to prevent the generation of static electricity but also to discharge slowly to earth any that does occur.

There is therefore an upper and a lower limit to the permissible electrical resistance between any part of the antistatic floor and earth. The resistance between two electrodes set 2 ft (60 cm) apart should nowhere be less than 20 000 Ω or more than 5 000 000 Ω. All mobile equipment in the operating theatre and anaesthetic rooms should make electrical contact with the floor. Trolleys, anaesthetic machines, etc. have wheels, the tyres of which are constructed of antistatic (conducting) rubber. In the absence of such precautions a metal chain, one end of which is attached to the frame of the trolley, is allowed to dangle onto the floor in such a way that at least three links are in contact with the floor. Such chains may become damaged or detached, and are sometimes wound round the frame so that they do not reach the floor. They are therefore a poor substitute for conducting rubber wheels and should be used only where it is necessary to update old equipment.

All footwear worn by the staff should contain conducting material. Tests should be made periodically with an instrument such as a Megger resistance meter to confirm that the electrical conductivity of the above items remains within the prescribed limits.

The most important precaution, however, is the use of antistatic (conducting) rubber or neoprene in the construction of the components of breathing attachments and other flexible parts of anaesthetic machines. As recently as 1982 an explosion occurred with cyclopropane, where a coaxial breathing attachment, the outer tube of which was of a non-conducting material, was damaged. Fortunately it was not in use with a patient at the time. An aerosol spray such as Croxtine (BOC) may be applied at intervals to any parts of the breathing system, but particularly to rubber and neoprene, to render them antistatic. This should, however, be considered as an adjunct to, rather than a substitute for, the proper materials being used.

Sparks may also be caused by the striking of metal against stone, as occurs when the metal end adaptor of a corrugated hose is dropped on a terrazzo floor.

In 1956 a working party set up in the UK by the Ministry of Health reported on the risk and prevention of anaesthetic explosions. This followed a period of 7 years during which 36 explosions had been reported, some of them fatal.

The term *zone of risk* was used to denote the area in which explosive mixtures were deemed to be liable to exist during routine anaesthetic practice.

Within the 'zone of risk' the following precautions were advised.

- There should be no naked flames.
- All electric switches should be sparkproof and electric plugs should be 'captive' while the switch is turned on.
- All parts, especially rubber tubing, etc. of anaesthetic apparatus should be constructed of conductive (antistatic) rubber or other material, and the operating theatre floor should be antistatic. Antistatic rubber, containing carbon, has sufficient conductivity to leach away static electricity, and yet has sufficient resistance to prevent so fast a discharge that a spark occurs.

All trolleys, stools and other mobile equipment should have tyres or feet of a conducting material. These are painted yellow or have a yellow flash or label to indicate that they are antistatic.

The 1956 working party defined the 'zone of risk' as extending from floor level to a height of 4.5 feet ($\sim$ 1.4 m) and 4 feet ($\sim$ 1.2 m) laterally from any anaesthetic apparatus. Because the anaesthetic machine is mobile, this included the whole anaesthetic room and operating theatre.

Since 1956 there has been a dramatic decrease in the incidence of explosions. This must be due in part to the advent, a couple of years later, of halothane, which quickly replaced cyclopropane and ether to a very great extent.

In 1968 Professor Vickers of Cardiff enquired into the possibility that the expensive precautions taken were more stringent than was really necessary.

Following investigations described in a paper in 1970, the Association of Anaesthetists of Great Britain and Ireland has recommended that the zone of risk be reduced to 25 cm around any part of the gas pathways of the anaesthetic machine or its breathing attachment.

In the UK and other countries this smaller zone of risk has been accepted. It is considered safe to install switches and socket outlets that are not sparkproof in the operating theatre provided that they are permanently attached to the wall. It is also recommended that they be at a height of approximately 15 inches ($\sim$ 40 cm) above the floor. This reduces the risk of damage to flexible cables. All mobile electrical apparatus, and socket outlets on the operating table or floor, should comply with the criteria for sparkproof precautions, since they may be placed within the zone of risk.

The above regulations do not seem to take account of the fact that an anaesthetic machine may be pushed up against a wall at a place where an electric fitting is positioned.

It would seem that the most important precaution for the prevention of explosions where inflammable agents are employed is the use of antistatic materials in the breathing attachments. Certainly, explosions are more likely on a cold, winter Monday morning when the air is dry, the water vapour having been precipitated as frost, and the operating list has not been running long enough to generate sufficient steam or water vapour to humidify the air within the operating theatre suite.

The cost of antistatic floors and sparkproof electric switches alone is high. In one operating theatre and its suite of rooms, 43 sparkproof switches were counted. It would be pertinent to ask how soon it will be possible to replace all explosive anaesthetic agents with non-flammable ones and save much expense and trouble. Perhaps the only reason for maintaining the present precautions is that ether, being cheap, simple to use and relatively safe, is still widely used in some parts of the world. Nevertheless, in many more developed areas, both ether and cyclopropane have been abandoned and antistatic and sparkproof precautions are being relaxed.

## Surgical Diathermy

The anaesthetist and his assistants are usually responsible for the correct connection of the diathermy machine. Therefore they should know something of those aspects of the use of diathermy that will concern them.

Surgical diathermy employs the heating effect of an electric current, and may best be explained by analogy with a domestic electric heater (Fig. 22.7).

Provided that the wiring and plug are in perfect condition and present no electrical resistance, the only part of the circuit offering resistance is the heating element itself, and it is only here that heat is produced.

The amount of heat produced depends on the current (measured in amps) and the resistance (in ohms) of the heating element through which it passes. The power developed is in this case converted to heat and may be expressed as:

$$W = RI^2$$

where $W$ = power (in watts), $R$ = resistance (in ohms), and $I$ = current (in amps). If the power is liberated solely as heat, 1 W will give 0.24 cal/s.

In the case of surgical diathermy power in the region of 50–400 W is commonly used.

Returning to the domestic heater, if the prongs of

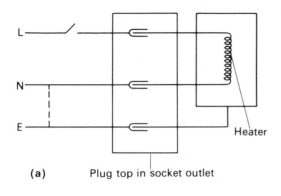

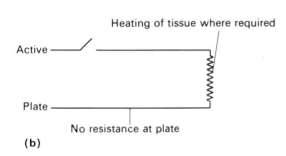

**Figure 22.7** Surgical diathermy. (a) An analogy with the circuit of an electric heater. L = live, N = neutral, E = earth conductors. (b) The circuit of surgical diathermy.

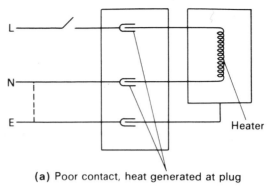

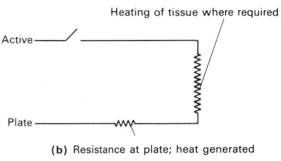

**Figure 22.8** (a) Poor contacts in the socket cause heat to be generated at the plug top. L = live, N = neutral, E = earth conductors. (b) An analogy with resistance at the indifferent plate in surgical diathermy, resulting in the generation of heat and the possibility of a burn.

the plug are dirty or a poor fit in the socket, there will be electrical resistance at this point too, and heat will be liberated there as well (Fig. 22.8).

This state of affairs is commonly found to exist when one pulls out the plug to extinguish an electric heater and the plug-top is hot enough almost to burn the hand!

To complete the analogy, the electric heating element represents the small piece of tissue grasped by the forceps, where it is designed to generate the heat. The plug and socket represent the indifferent electrode (plate) attached to the patient's leg. Should the contact between the plate and the patient present resistance, heat will be generated that may even be sufficient to burn the patient.

Excessive rises in temperature at the site of the plate may be prevented by:

- using a large plate so that any heat generated is spread over a wide area. A good contact may be assured if the plate is placed under the patient's buttocks, if this is possible;

- applying the plate to an area with good blood circulation, which will help to carry away the heat.

It is necessary to pass considerable currents through the human body to produce enough heat to have these effects. Under normal circumstances the accidental passage of an electric current through the body has a number of deleterious effects, including sudden death. However, it was found experimentally, many years ago, that although living tissues, especially conducting and contractile tissues, are very sensitive to direct current and low-frequency alternating current, this sensitivity markedly decreases as the frequency is increased beyond 10 kHz (see Fig. 22.9).

A sine waveform is used for cutting, and a damped waveform for coagulation (Fig. 22.10). The sine waveform may be produced by a valve oscillator, while a damped oscillation is best produced by the spark-gap generator. The more recent transistorized diathermy sets produce a satisfactory cutting current, but some users find that the interrupted waveform they produce for coagulation

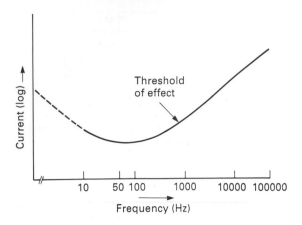

Figure 22.9 Variation of the threshold of pathophysiological effects of electric current with frequency.

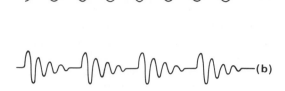

Figure 22.10 Waveforms for surgical diathermy. (a) A cutting current. (b) A damped waveform for coagulation.

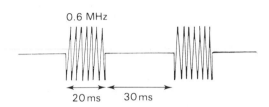

Figure 22.11 Pulsed waveform for coagulation from a transistorized diathermy set.

(Fig. 22.11) is not as satisfactory as that of the spark-gap.

The frequencies although not standardized, are in the region of 0.4 MHz in the spark-gap generator and 1–1.5 MHz in valve oscillators.

Modern apparatus is capable of producing modified waveforms that are intended for both cutting and coagulation.

The indifferent lead (i.e. the plate) is at earth potential in many diathermy sets and it is therefore important that it is connected to the correct terminal of the diathermy apparatus. If the plate were accidentally connected to the active terminal, the patient might be burned where his body was in contact with those parts of the operating table at earth potential, when the foot switch was depressed.

The above description is of a unipolar arrangement. However, some diathermy sets are capable of being used with a bipolar system in which the current passes from one blade of a pair of forceps to the other. The circuit is earth-free and the current does not pass through any part of the patient's body other than that grasped by the forceps (Fig. 22.12). The power required is small and it is electrically safer, but it is suitable only for the coagulation of small pieces of tissue or blood vessels. It is particularly suitable for ophthalmic and neurosurgical procedures.

## Accidents due to the use or misuse of the diathermy apparatus

These may be divided into two groups, first where the patient receives electrical burns, and second where fires or explosions are caused by the use of diathermy in the presence of flammable vapours.

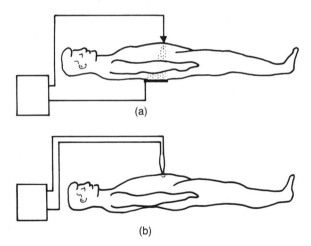

Figure 22.12 (a) Unipolar and (b) bipolar diathermy.

The second group of accidents may also be caused by hot wire cautery.

### Electrical burns

Electrical burns may be the result of:

- The accidental depression of the foot switch when the forceps or cutting electrode is in contact with some part of the patient that it was not intended to burn. This may be prevented by keeping the forceps in an insulated 'quiver' when not in use, and it is also minimized by the installation of a buzzer within the diathermy machine that sounds when the foot switch is depressed. The indicator light on the machine is useful as a confirmation that the apparatus is working, but is not usually heeded as a warning when it is accidentally operated.

- They may also result from poor contact between the plate and the patient, a burn occurring where it actually does touch.

  Some diathermy machines give an audible warning if the plate lead is not plugged in, or if the electrical continuity of the lead is broken. However, the fact that the warning is not given is not proof that the plate has been applied to the patient. Some transistorized sets have a fully floating output and the patient is unharmed if the indifferent electrode is neglected.

  Where the old-fashioned saline pad is used, it may have dried out, or too dilute a solution of saline may have been used. The plate may have been applied too loosely.

  The pad must completely envelop the plate and its terminal, otherwise metal parts might touch the patient's skin and cause burning or mechanical injury.

- Burns can also be caused by the electrical circuit being completed via the operating table and the floor, or other points through which the patient may be earthed, which may occur if the plate is not applied. It has been known for the tracheal mucous membranes to be severely damaged when the patient was earthed through the damp endotracheal tube and the anaesthetic machine.

- Another danger seldom appreciated is the risk of infarction when unipolar diathermy is used on an organ that has been temporarily raised on its vascular pedicle. The classical injury is that caused to the testis when raised from the scrotum on its vas. Figure 22.13 shows how the current density is greatly increased in the vas thus causing its destruction. If unipolar diathermy must be used, then the exposed testis must remain in contact with the rest of the body and its electrical conduction improved by the interspersion of a saline-soaked swab.

### Diathermy and pacemakers

The use of RF diathermy should be avoided in patients with internal or temporary external cardiac pacemakers as there is a risk of inhibition or even permanent damage. If diathermy must be used, the

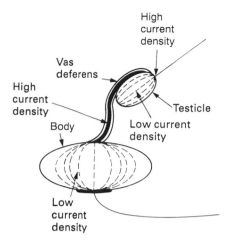

**Figure 22.13** The danger of high current density at other areas than that intended during surgical diathermy.

bipolar variety should be used and then only away from the anatomical site of the pacemaker and its wiring.

### Fires and explosions

Fires and explosions may be caused in the presence of any flammable vapour or liquid. It should be remembered that not only are some anaesthetic agents flammable, but so are ethyl and isopropyl alcohol, which are often used for cleaning the skin prior to operation. They may be soaked up by and remain in the drapes. This is particularly dangerous, since alcohol flames are barely visible where the part is strongly illuminated by the theatre lamp.

The cause of fire may be a spark at the active electrode itself, or a faulty mains lead, plug or foot switch.

Real safety lies in the abandoning of flammable vapours and liquids.

The external cases (enclosures) of most diathermy machines are made airtight, i.e. gasproof, but this state is difficult to maintain when the machine is to be wheeled about into rooms of varying temperature, so that pressures are developed across the gasproof seal. Also if, owing to over-use or electrical fault, the interior is heated and fumes are generated, a dangerous increase of pressure may occur, leading to rupture.

# 23 Lasers

## Introduction

Anaesthetists should be aware of the principles of lasers as they are finding increasing application in medicine and surgery and their employment gives rise to a number of dangers.

The term *laser* is an acronym derived from Light Amplification by Stimulated Emission of Radiation. The laser produces an intense beam of pure monochromatic light, that is light of a single wavelength or colour. The output beam may be of very small cross-sectional area and is virutally non-divergent. These properties mean that large amounts of energy may be delivered to very small areas of tissue with great accuracy. The wavelength of a laser is determined by the lasing medium used.

Although there are many more complex laser systems, the basic components of a laser are shown in Fig. 23.1. The lasing medium, which may be a gas, a liquid or a solid, is chosen from a study of the atomic electron energy levels upon which the laser depends. The atoms of the lasing medium are excited to high energy levels by a 'pumping' source, which may be a high-voltage discharge in the case of a gas or an intense flash of light from a flash-tube. Figure 23.2 shows the excitation and emission processes possible in a gaseous lasing medium. A photon of energy from the pumping source may be absorbed by a stable atom in its so called 'ground state' which then becomes an excited atom with an electron in a higher energy level. Spontaneous emission of a photon of energy occurs as the excited atom falls back to the ground energy level. If a further photon of pumping energy at the correct wavelength is applied to an atom in its excited state, then as it falls to the ground state two photons of energy will be emitted instead of one. This is known as *stimulated* emission. The emitted photons thus produced are in phase with, have the same polarization as, and travel in the same direction as the stimulating radiation. This mechanism is amplified by many of the escaping photons being reflected back into the lasing medium by the mirrors. Thus a chain reaction occurs, producing an intense source of light energy, some of which is allowed to escape through the partially reflecting mirror at the output end of the lasing medium. The output beam of the laser is usually directed to the tissues by a fibre-optic light guide.

The clinical use of lasers depends upon a compromise between (a) laser–tissue interaction, (b) absorp-

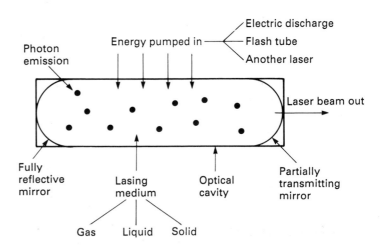

**Figure 23.1** Basic components of a laser.

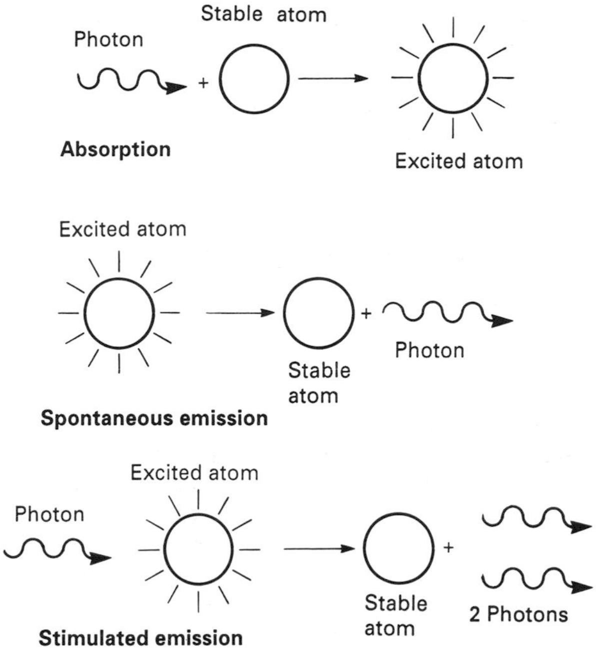

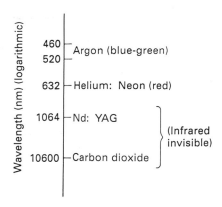

**Figure 23.2** Absorption, excitation and emission processes.

**Figure 23.3** The electromagnetic spectrum showing the wavelengths of emission of common medical lasers.

tion and penetration depth, (c) availability of a laser of the correct wavelength and power, and (d) availability of suitable fibres to transmit the desired wavelength to the tissues.

The spectrum in Fig. 23.3 includes the three most commonly used therapeutic lasers: carbon dioxide, argon and Nd : YAG.

The carbon dioxide laser energy is absorbed by water and thus the intracellular water is rapidly vaporized. The main use of the carbon dioxide laser is as a 'bloodless scalpel'. The blue-green argon laser beam is maximally absorbed by substances with the complementary colour, i.e. red. Thus the argon laser is used to coagulate blood in small vessels with very little effect on other more transparent tissues, for example the retina. The Nd : YAG (neodymium : yittrium–aluminium garnet) laser has a solid lasing medium and produces energy in the near infrared region of the spectrum that is absorbed deeply in the tissues. When invisible infrared lasers are used, it is common practice to make use of a low-powered visible-light laser such as a helium : neon laser at the same time, in order to aid in aiming the therapeutic laser accurately.

# Safety Aspects

Apart from the danger to the patient from the beam

of laser energy if it is misused, there is a risk to the operator and other persons in the operating environment. This is because of the long range of laser light due to the virtual non-divergence of the beam; thus increased distance from the source has little safety benefit. Even reflected laser light may be very dangerous to the eyes. Visible laser light transmitted to the retina of the eye may burn it irreparably, leaving a blind spot in the field of vision. A similar lesion over the optic nerve may result in total blindness of that eye. The cornea, lens and aqueous and vitreous humours partially or totally absorb far infrared laser radiation and therefore these tissues are more susceptable to damage than the retina. Laser radiation on the skin may be felt as a burning sensation, which is therefore self-protective provided that the victim is conscious and has not received an analgesic. There is an international classification for lasers which is shown in Table 23.1.

**Table 23.1** International classification of continuously working lasers

| | |
|---|---|
| Class I | Powers not to excede MPE* for the eye |
| Class II | Visible laser beams only<br>Powers up to 1 mW<br>Eye protected by blink-reflex time of 0.25 s |
| Class IIIa | Relaxation of Class II to 5 mW for radiation provided beam is expanded so that eye is still protected by blink reflex |
| Class IIIb | Powers up to 0.5 W<br>Direct viewing hazardous |
| Class IV | Powers over 0.5 W. Extremely hazardous |

* MPE = maximum permissible exposure.

## Protective Eyeware

Protective eyeware may be in the form of goggles or spectacles. Spectacles generally do not give as complete peripheral protection as goggles. It should be noted that different eyeware is required for different wavelengths of laser.

## Anaesthetic-related Risks

A further risk which is of special importance to the anaesthetist is the danger of fire due to oxygen enrichment of the local environment in which the laser is being used. This problem occurs not only during ENT surgery but also when the laser is inadvertently directed towards drapes under which high concentrations of oxygen and nitrous oxide may be present. The following precautions should be taken.

- No flammable anaesthetic agents or nitrous oxide should be used. (Nitrous oxide supports combustion as well as oxygen.)

- Non-reflective (matt black) instruments should be used, as the reflected laser beam is almost as powerful as the main beam.
- Inspired oxygen concentration should be no greater than 25% if possible.
- Non-flammable endotrachael tube, either using special materials or by covering a conventional tube with aluminium tape, should be used.
- Other tissues should be protected with wet swabs.

## Safety Codes

In the UK the Department of Health has published guidance on laser safety. This should form the basis of a set of local rules — a Safety Code — and the appointment of a Laser Protection Supervisor in every area in which a laser is in use. The Laser Protection Supervisor must not be the operator of the laser but should be observing the safety aspects during its use. The most important duty of the Laser Protection Supervisor is to make sure that all staff are wearing the correct eye protection throughout the laser session.

# 24 Hazards and the Psychology of Accidents

## Introduction

Operative mortality associated with anaesthesia has been variously quoted as between 1 : 1000 and 1 : 10 000 with approximately 1–3 deaths per 10 000 anaesthetics administered.

## The Changing Pattern of Accidents Associated with Anaesthetic Apparatus

Owing to the less frequent use of flammable and explosive anaesthetic agents and the institution of precautions to prevent explosions, particularly in connection with static electricity, accidents due to fire and explosion have been virtually eliminated. However, as flammable and explosive agents are now hardly ever used in the developed world, many new operating theatre suites are no longer protected against static electricity.

In recent years, deaths from electrocution have been reported, and following the elucidation of the concept of *microshock* one is left to wonder how many cases of ventricular fibrillation may have been caused in this way in the past.

Other factors that may influence the changing pattern of accidents are increasing complexity of equipment, disparagement of the mundane, and reliance upon assistance (nurse, technician or another anaesthetist).

The major causes for mortality and also of considerable morbidity are:

- insufficient oxygen supply to the brain;
- inadequate carbon dioxide removal;
- administration of excessive amounts of anaesthetic or other associated drugs;
- barotrauma to the lungs;
- obstruction of the airway.

Statistical evidence shows that about 70% of critical incidents can be attributed to human error and only about 13% due to genuine equipment failure. The scenarios leading to critical incidents are often multifactorial and it must remain the responsibility of designers and manufacturers of anaesthetic equipment, and the users, to minimize the possibility of their occurrence.

The administration and management of general anaesthesia may be depicted as a closed loop as shown in Fig. 14.1. The anaesthetist controls the anaesthetic machine and its accessories. These manipulations have a direct effect upon the patient and are, in turn, observed by the anaesthetist who then further adjusts the machine if necessary.

The anaesthetist's role is vital in that he or she composes the gas mixture, controls the ventilation (be it spontaneous or controlled), observes the response of the patient and must, if possible anticipate the surgeon and any changes in the patient's condition.

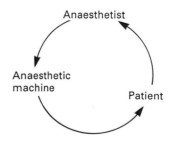

**Figure 24.1** Anaesthetic 'control loop'.

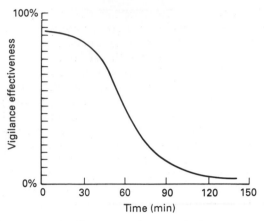

**Figure 24.2** An illustration of the kind of vigilance effect that can be expected in the performance of passive tasks with low signal rate. This shows a notable decline in performance after about 30 min. Reproduced from Hawkins, F.H. (1987), *Human Factors in Flight*. Gower Technical Press.

# Vigilance

Two important attributes of the anaesthetist must be considered for the safe conduct of anaesthetic practice: vigilance and decision-making ability. The level of arousal also affects the rate and the quality of both vigilance and the ability to make decisions correctly and rapidly.

Vigilance is defined in the dictionary as watchfulness or caution. Anaesthetic vigilance has been defined by Gravenstein (Editorial in *Journal of Clinical Monitoring* Vol. 2, no. 3, 1986) as a state of clinical awareness whereby dangerous conditions are anticipated. In 1943, research by the Royal Air Force showed that vigilance requiring continuous monitoring and detection of brief, low-intensity and infrequently occurring events over long periods is poor. This is illustrated in Fig. 24.2, which shows rapid fall-off in vigilance after a period as short as half an hour.

# Decision-making Ability

The *decision-making ability* of the anaesthetist is dependent upon training, experience and the feedback of information from the senses of the patient's condition, the anaesthetic machine, the monitoring equipment and the requirements of the surgeon.

Psychological research has shown that the human brain is able to make only a single decision at any one instant. The pathway for human information processing is depicted in a simplified form in Fig. 24.3.

Incoming physical stimuli are received by the sense organs and it is therefore necessary to make sure that stimuli are within the bandwidth of and are of sufficient amplitude for those organs. The brain will not necessarily perceive the same message from the stimuli on each occasion, as perception depends upon context and previous experience in handling similar stimuli. The information is *filtered* and these filters are controlled by feedback

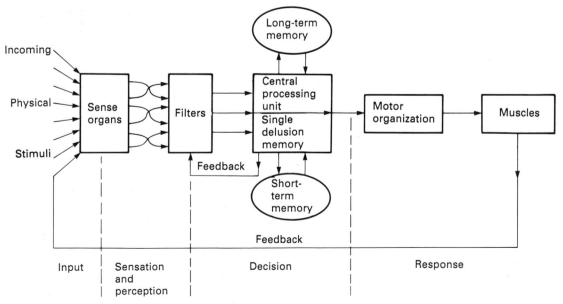

**Figure 24.3** Human information processing.

loops. At this stage, some of the information may be off-loaded into short-term memory and may be lost if other information bombards the senses simultaneously. The human brain has a single decision channel. All information to be processed must pass sequentially through this one channel. A person can attend only to one thing at a time, although he can change from one thing to another extremely rapidly; the danger of pre-occupation is obvious. Following a decision during which information from long-term memory may be used, a response is effected via the muscles. This is a grossly simplified description of an extremely complicated process.

## Arousal

Both vigilance and the ability to make decisions are affected by the anaesthetist's level of arousal. Arousal is the level of 'wakefulness' and is controlled by the reticular formation in the mid-brain. Arousal ranges from total stupor to hypomania. For any task there is a level of arousal at which one performs most efficiently, as shown in Fig. 24.4. Surprisingly, this optimal level decreases as the difficulty of the task increases, so that over-arousal is most likely to occur for difficult tasks. Over-arousal often occurs in emergency situations when difficult tasks may need to be carried out rapidly. Under-arousal for a particular task slows decision-making and makes it less accurate and also reduces vigilance. Under-arousal occurs with boredom and sleep-deprivation.

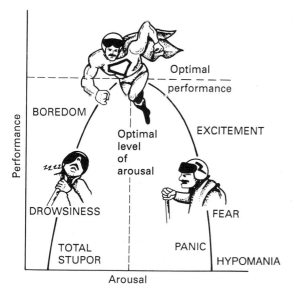

**Figure 24.4** The inverted 'U' curve.

Performance is also adversely affected by physical and mental ill health, hunger, environmental discomfort (temperature, humidity, noise), life-stresses (marriage, divorce, moving house, birth, illness or death in the family, legal problems, etc.).

Many of the factors mentioned may not be amenable to optimization but some are. The design of anaesthetic and monitoring equipment with safety and ergonomics in mind has now become a priority. Until recently the design of anaesthetic and associated equipment has been on a purely functional basis and typical arrangements 'just grew' as new developments occurred and, more probably, as money for purchase became available.

## Anaesthetist or Pilot?

Much of the aforementioned relates equally well to pilots and their aircraft. The reason is that there are many similarities between administration of anaesthesia and flying. Both skills are carried out by intelligent highly motivated professionals who have undergone many years of expensive training. Both have to carry out many routine but highly skilled procedures and remain vigilant for long periods of time, observing for one of many possible but hopefully rare, adverse occurrences that may be life threatening, after which skilled intervention has to be instituted rapidly. Both professions also have to work long and often unsocial hours in imperfect environments and yet have to maintain high standards that are imposed externally as well as self-imposed.

## Pre-anaesthetic Checklist

Many critical incidents could be avoided if another leaf was taken from the pilot's textbook — the pre-flight checklist. This is a *written* list of checks and measurements which must be made before every flight by every pilot, no matter how experienced or senior. The pre-anaesthetic checklist is now becoming more important with the increasing complexity of the equipment under the anaesthetist's control. A typical checklist is shown in Table 24.1. A more comprehensive checklist recommended by the Association of Anaesthetists of Great Britain and Ireland is to be found in Appendix IV.

**Table 24.1**   Pre-anaesthetic checklist

**At the beginning of the session**
1. Check all *controls 'off'*.
2. Check *gas supplies*, both cylinder and pipeline.
3. *Inspect* and check *function* of
   Oxygen supply failure alarm
   Oxygen/nitrous oxide ratio protection
   Oxygen flush
   Breathing system
   Mechanical ventilator and disconnect
   alarm
   Waste gas scavenging system.

**Before each case**
1. Check reserve oxygen supply.
2. Check function of breathing system.
3. Check vaporizer.
4. Check absorber, if in use.
5. Inspect equipment for
   Entotracheal intubation
   Intravenous infusion
   Resuscitation.
6. Check function of high-vacuum suction
   apparatus.
5. Apply and check monitoring systems.
6. Set appropriate alarm levels.

# A New Philosophy

Schreiber has elucidated the anatomy of the critical incident. The critical incident occurs when one or more of the components of the control loop (Fig. 24.1) behaves unpredictably, be it the machinery, the patient or the anaesthetist himself. The time course of a critical incident is shown in Fig. 24.5.

When an adverse condition begins, the danger of injury to the patient increases with time, as shown. There is a time delay before the problem is noticed by the anaesthetist and identified. Another delay occurs before the problem is corrected, after which there should be a recovery to safe conditions if the correction is made early enough. Excessive delay in noticing the problem or in its correction will lead to permanent injury.

As already described, the reliability of the human for constant vigilance over long periods of time is questionable and his ability to make decisions when bombarded with multiple sensory inputs is sorely put to the test. Monitoring during anaesthesia should not be limited to electronic surveillance of the patient's physiology but should also include monitoring of the equipment's performance and of the anaesthetist himself. Monitoring of the anaesthetist's performance may be done with automatic generation of the anaesthetic record chart, which may also form part of a *clinical audit*.

Research shows that alarm systems should be designed to make as long as possible the time available to correct a problem before injury begins. Examination of Fig. 24.5 shows that this may be accomplished by minimizing the pre-alarm period and making it as clear as possible to the anaesthetist what the problem is and its level of urgency.

Schreiber has also pointed out that the further along the system, from the gas and electricity supplies to the patient, a parameter is monitored, (Fig. 24.6) the greater the delay before the alarm is sounded and the greater the number of possible

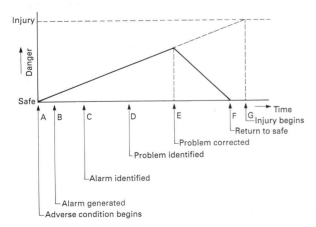

**Figure 24.5**   Diagram of Schreiber's time course of a critical incident as it would occur in anaesthetic practice.

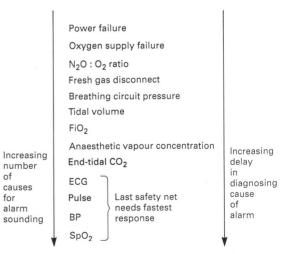

**Figure 24.6**   The further along the system, from supplies to the patient, that a parameter is monitored, the greater the delay before the problem is corrected.

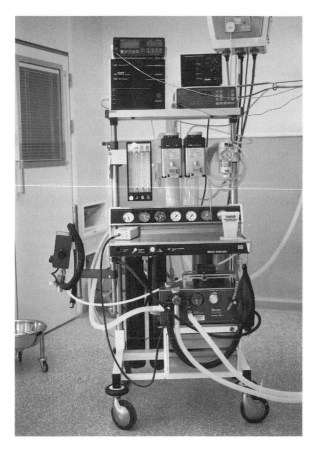

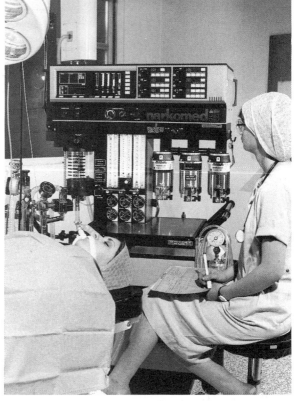

**Figure 24.7** Conventional anaesthetic machine with monitoring equipment. Note the wide and random distribution of the individual displays. Compare this with Fig. 24.8.

**Figure 24.8** Dräger Narcomed III anaesthetic machine with integrated monitoring and alarms.

causes of that particular problem. For example, if the oxygen supply fails, the oxygen supply alarm would sound immediately. Some seconds later, depending on the fresh gas flow into the breathing attachment, the inspired oxygen monitor alarm would become active. However, it may be more than a minute before the saturation as indicated by a pulse oximeter would fall below the critical level. Furthermore, the causes of a drop in $SpO_2$ are numerous compared to the causes of the sounding of the oxygen supply pressure alarm.

*Alarms* do not necessarily refer to emergencies but may indicate abnormal situations that may or may not have the potential to become emergencies. The ideal monitoring system should differentiate between *advisory*, requiring awareness, *caution*, requiring a prompt response, and *warning*, requiring immediate response. Ideally an audible warning differentiating between these three levels should draw the anaesthetist's attention to a visual indication of what the problem is. Figure 24.7 shows a

conventional anaesthetic machine with monitoring equipment mounted on it. Regularly, during an anaesthetic, the anaesthetist must scan all the visual displays indicated and when a crisis occurs, he or she must not only differentiate the alarm sounds but must then locate the apropriate display before making a decision as to the cause and then correcting it. The anaesthetic machine shown in Fig. 24.8 was developed to minimize the delay between the onset of an adverse condition and its detection and correction. Extensive use of 'human factors engineering' has lead to a machine with a structured alarm system with centralized displays for alarms and data, a centralized control panel for functions which apply to the entire system, a centralized connection panel for the physiological monitoring and a centralized power supply with automatic battery back-up in case of power failure.

The advantage of this integrated system (Fig. 24.9) is that information from each of the monitoring systems may be prioritized by a computer before

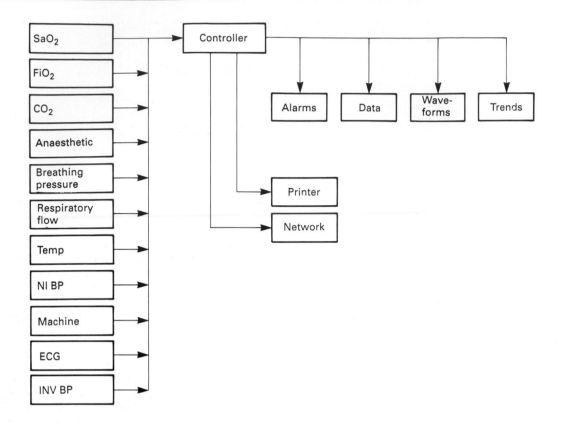

**Figure 24.9**   Integrated system architecture.

any alarm is sounded. The data may be displayed in the most convenient fashion for easy and quick assimilation and may also be printed to provide a permanent record.

# 'Standards' in Anaesthesia

In anaesthesia, the word Standards may refer to standards as written by BSI, ISO, CEN, CENELEC, ASTM, ANSI, etc. which refer to the minimum safety requirements for equipment design, or the standards that have been promulgated by professional bodies regarding the safe conduct of anaesthesia.

A condensation of the recommendations of the internationally recognized professional bodies includes:

**Essential**

1. Continuous presence of appropriately qualified anaesthetist (providing continuous clinical observation).
2. Oxygen supply failure alarm.
3. Continuous monitoring of cardiac output.
4. Observation of reservoir bag and chest excursion.
5. Ventilator disconnect alarm.
6. Oxygen analyser of inspired gas.
7. Electrocardiogram.
8. Non-invasive arterial blood pressure.

**Strongly recommended**

 9. Spirometry.
10. Pulse-oximetry.
11. Temperature.
12. End-tidal carbon dioxide.
13. Monitoring of neuromuscular blockade.

# 25 The Anaesthetic Room and Recovery Area

## Introduction

There is much debate as to whether anaesthetic rooms (in hospitals where they are still used) have a place in modern anaesthesia. Proponents claim that anaesthetic rooms:

- provide a more tranquil environment than the operating theatre for patients (especially children);
- provide ready access to a wide variety of equipment and drugs;
- provide a better teaching environment for junior staff, free from the stress of impatient surgeons waiting to operate!
- speed up the throughput of patients (the theatre may be cleared from the debris of the preceding case while the next patient is anaesthetized).

Those against anaesthetic rooms claim that:

- they are unnecessarily expensive, requiring a doubling up of expensive anaesthetic machines and monitors;
- they are potentially dangerous, as moving the patient (including transfer on to the operating table) increases the chances of disconnection of the breathing system and misplacement of intravenous access;
- there may well be a period of inadequate monitoring during transfer to the operating table.

It is the authors' belief that the anaesthetic room is an essential part of the building, in which not only will the patient experience a tranquil atmosphere but the anaesthetist can set about the induction of anaesthesia (possibly the most hazardous part of his work) undisturbed.

As anaesthetic rooms are still commonly used, information in this chapter is relevant.

The size and position of the anaesthetic and recovery rooms are too often dictated by factors outside the control of the anaesthetist. The following points, however, should be born in mind when the anaesthetist is in a position to influence design.

## Layout of the Anaesthetic Room

(1) The anaesthetic room, although requiring access to both the operating theatre and the theatre corridor, should not be used as a route for personnel passing between them. The layout should be such that the intrusions by surgeons and theatre staff are reduced to a minimum.

(2) The floor area should be sufficient to permit both of the patient's arms to be abducted and placed on armboards and there should be sufficient room at each end of the trolley to allow staff to pass from one side to another even with the doors open. The doors should be open in the direction in which the patient trolley passes.

(3) In a multiple theatre suite, the anaesthetic rooms should be similar, though they may need to be mirror images of each other. If the general layout permits, they should be close to each other and to an equipment store or parking area for bulky apparatus such as ventilators. Where each theatre technician is assigned to his own anaesthetic room, small departures from uniformity should be allowed to encourage his initiative and individuality.

## Contents of the Anaesthetic Room

### Furniture

Figure 25.1a and b shows a typical anaesthetic room. The cupboard space must be ample and should

(a)

(b)

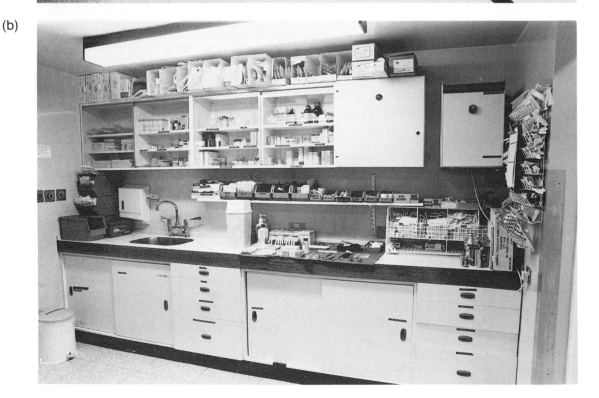

**Figure 25.1** The anaesthetic room. (a) The anaesthetic machine, mobile trolley, pedal bin (with plastic liner bag) for facemasks, a large refuse bin for paper and plastic waste, and the ceiling-mounted spotlight. (b) The sink, drug cupboard (including the DDA—dangerous drug administration cupboard), fridge, and rigid container for sharps disposal.

include a proportion of cupboards with glass doors, which may conveniently be at eye level above the worktop. Similar drugs (i.e. induction agents, etc.) should be grouped together, and the shelves suitably labelled. There should be a small, wall-mounted refrigerator with a visible temperature gauge for the stocking of drugs requiring cold storage (e.g. suxamethonium).

A double-locked cupboard should be available for the storage of controlled drugs and should be connected to an easily visible red warning light that is activated when the cupboard is opened.

A suitable colour-coded labelling system for syringes containing drugs should be available. It seems anachronous that ampoules containing the drugs are labelled, but when the drug is transferred to a syringe the syringe is not similarly labelled.

Below this cupboard space there should be a worktop of generous size at least 2.5 m × 0.5 m and which should incorporate a sink. The latter should have a surgical mixer tap, which should be high enough to fill a bucket but low enough not to splash the associated worktop. There should be a suitable liquid soap dispenser and a disposable paper towel rack available for an anaesthetist to wash his hands between cases.

Behind this worktop there should be a racking system to accommodate prepacked sterile articles such as needles and syringes. Below the worktop there should be sets of drawers to store stocks of appropriate endotracheal tubes, airways, intubation aids and spare equipment. Alternatively, these items may be stored on a mobile trolley that can be wheeled up to the patient when required. There should be a writing surface where the operating register and register for controlled drugs may be kept. A clock with a seconds hand should be placed in a position where the anaesthetist can see it during the induction.

The overall lighting intensity should be high, but not dazzling to the patient. There may be provision for an additional spot-light. Especially where infants are anaesthetized, a window or skylight is highly desirable to enable the patient's colour to be assessed by daylight. The promises by architects and builders to provide daylight by artificial means are not always fulfilled. Some fluorescent tubes give a close approximation to daylight. The colour rendering, that is the colour of the patient when illuminated, given by special 'daylight' tubes has been found to be the best, and this type should be used in all areas where patients are tended.

The anaesthetic room should also contain suitable disposal systems.

- Either a bucket two-thirds filled with suitable detergent soap solution or a pedal bin with a disposable plastic liner for placing soiled reuseable tubes, airways, facemasks, etc. prior to appropriate cleaning and sterilization.
- A suitable refuse sack and container for disposing of paper and plastic packaging of various items of anaesthetic equipment.
- A dedicated and puncture-proof 'sharps' container for the disposal of used needles and syringes.

The anaesthetic room should also contain a small stock of all the relevant equipment and solutions for intravenous infusion for both central and peripheral sites as well as suitable adhesive tapes and dressings for adequately securing these infusions.

## The anaesthetic machine

A small, lighter anaesthetic machine is commonly used in the anaesthetic room as it conserves space and is more mobile than its larger versions. It need not necessarily require a cascade-type double flow-meter since relatively high flows of anaesthetic gas are usually required during the induction of anaesthesia. For similar reasons, a circle system may also be unnecessary. Wall-mounted anaesthetic units are available that conserve space even further; however, they limit any alternative arrangement in patient position during induction.

Wall-mounted sockets for pipeline gas and vacuum supplies should be available (see below) with the suction unit machine-mounted so as to be readily available to the anaesthetist.

## Antistatic precautions

Traditionally, the floors of anaesthetic rooms and operating theatres have been constructed of antistatic material to reduce the possibility of static charge igniting flammable anaesthetics. As these agents have gradually been phased out, the insistence on antistatic precautions has been relaxed, although it may well be argued that for floors and instrument trolleys it should still be maintained because it reduces the static charge on trolleys that attracts dust that may well carry infection.

Until recently, all electrical fittings were required, by regulation, to be sparkproof; mercury tip-switches were usually employed. Subsequently, however, research has shown that ignition of anaesthetic vapours is not likely at a distance greater than 25 cm from the gaseous pathways of the anaesthetic machine.

There has been considerable relaxation of regulations (in the UK) with reference to electrical equipment mounted on walls and more recently on the anaesthetic machine. This has culminated in a report from a Working Party (Great Britain 1990) with the following recommendations.

1. *New buildings*. Antistatic precautions are no longer necessary unless the department of anaesthesia expressly wishes to use flammable agents.
2. *Existing buildings*. The department of anaesthesia should advice its Health Authority whether or not it wishes to continue to use flammable agents. The Health Authority must then decide whether to maintain or provide antistatic facilities.

If flammable agents are used, the recommendations set out in HTM 1 and HTM 2 (Great Britain) must be implemented. No electrically powered equipment should be used within the 'zone of risk' (as defined in Chapter 22) unless marked as suitable for use with these flammable agents. If any of these conditions cannot be satisfied, the use of flammable agents must be discontinued.

Assigned anaesthetic areas where antistatic facilities are not provided should be clearly marked with the sign indicating this (Fig. 25.2). If the decision is taken to abandon the use of flammable agents and consequently not to provide antistatic facilities, the Hospital Management should ensure that:

- all the relevant staff are informed of the decision;
- each anaesthetizing area has a warning sign;
- all anaesthesia equipment capable of delivering a flammable agent has been removed or suitably modified by an authorized person to prevent the administration of a flammable agent;
- departmental heads ensure that unsuitable equipment and flammable agents are not reintroduced.

When providing an electrical supply to an anaesthetic room, there should be at least four socket outlets for electrical plugs and two on each of the walls in the operating theatre. Fire-fighting instructions and apparatus should be placed in a position where they are available to the staff, but not where they frighten the patient.

The overall decor of the anaesthetic room should be reassuring and restful to the patient and should possibly include a picture or illustrated calendar and suitable cartoons when the patients are children.

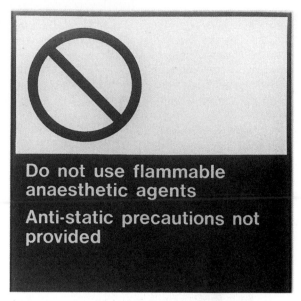

**Figure 25.2** Warning sign. Addition to the HTM 65 range of safety signs.

# Future Planning of Anaesthetic Services

When equipping a hospital from the start, it is convenient to make out a list of equipment for a 'standard anaesthetic room'. A copy of this list may then be taken and amended for each anaesthetic room according to the type of work to be done. A similar list may be made for the recovery area, and for anaesthetic apparatus required in theatre. Next a list can be compiled of equipment intended for general use in the theatre suite as a whole, specifying items such as ventilators, monitors, resuscitation equipment, etc. The anaesthetist may be asked also to order equipment for intensive-care and coronary-care units, for the accident department and for the treatment of cardiac arrests and other emergencies in the hospital. Typical lists are shown in Chapter 21.

# Pipeline Outlets

The pipeline outlets may be mounted on the wall, in the floor, in the ceiling or on a swinging boom (Fig. 25.3). Each arrangement has advantages and drawbacks. It is usually found more convenient to use wall-mounted outlets in the anaesthetic and recovery

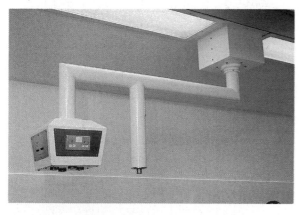

**Figure 25.3**   A swinging boom for medical piped gases.

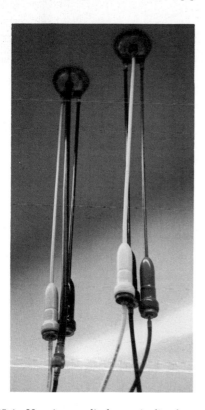

**Figure 25.4**   Hanging medical gas pipeline hoses.

The flexible tubing of a telescopic type is liable to damage and is not easily accessible for repairs and maintenance. A swinging boom is also liable to mechanical damage or failure and it is not always possible to prevent its traverse from coinciding with that of the operating light and other objects. A boom may also disperse dust in the operating theatre. Booms and rigid pendants may be fitted with electrical outlets, etc.

Piped gases and a vacuum may also be supplied through hanging hoses fitted with non-interchangeable connections (Fig. 25.4).

# Management of the Anaesthetic Room

Although the anaesthetic room is connected with both the operating theatre and the outside corridor, no member of staff should be allowed to use it simply as a passage between the two. It should be kept as the private domain of the anaesthetist, in which he is not disturbed during the induction of anaesthesia and the patient is not molested while still conscious. However, there may be times when minor procedures are best performed in the anaesthetic room rather than the operating theatre. Examples are endoscopies and operations for infected cases such as the simple incision of abscesses, etc. where the contamination and consequent re-cleaning of an operating theatre can be avoided. The atmosphere should be reassuring and quiet and the walls that the patient can see should not be covered with gloomy hazard notices and the like (Fig. 25.5).

There should be as much standardization as possible between all the anaesthetic rooms in one hospital, although obviously that attached to, say, an ENT theatre will require certain stock items that would not be found in one for orthopaedic surgery. For day-to-day management the care of each anaesthetic room should be assigned to one particular, named, technician who may identify himself with the efficient running of that particular area.

Care should be taken to avoid the contamination of unused equipment. For example, the worktop should be clean for the drawing up of drugs, etc. and all used equipment should be excluded. The anaesthetist should be discouraged from putting down on this surface used objects such as syringes and needles which are liable to be contaminated with the patient's blood, and laryngoscopes, airways and endotracheal tubes which, being contaminated with the patient's saliva, could well carry

rooms with a standard position above floor level (1.3 m for horizontally engaging probes; 1.6 m for vertically engaging probes) and suction units mounted on a special plate screwed on to the wall adjacent to them. In the operating theatre, a fixed pendant is usually the best arrangement. Although there is a possibility that the height at which it is fixed may be out of the reach of very short anaesthetists, there is less risk of mechanical failure.

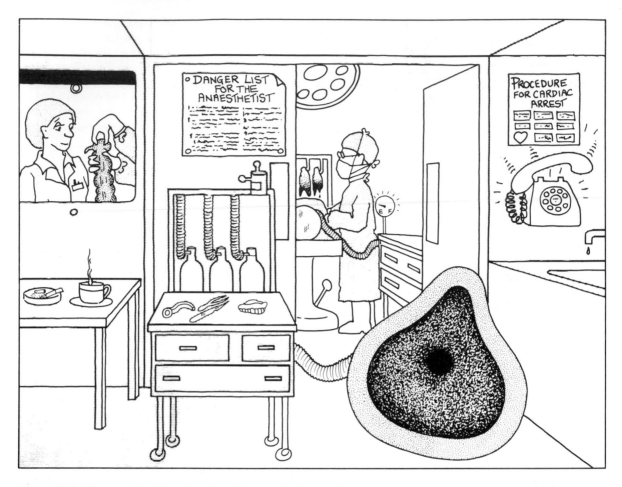

**Figure 25.5**   How a patient should *not* see the anaesthetic room!

infectious agents. Used endotracheal tubes, airways and laryngoscopes that are destined for re-sterilization should be kept in a container isolated from items such as syringes, needles and broken ampoules, in order to avoid the possibility of fragments getting into the items that will be re-used. For example, there have been cases where an endotracheal tube has been obstructed by the top of an ampoule that had got into it prior to resterilization.

Cleanliness is not only required to avoid the risks of cross-infection, but also to prevent too much contact with drugs, including antibiotics, to which an allergy may become established.

The anaesthetist may also be required to supervise the keeping of a register recording the details of operations and also to keep a record of controlled drugs used.

Nurses, technicians and anaesthetists should be aware of the location of drugs and equipment that may be needed in an emergency but only one of

which is kept in reserve in the whole operating theatre suite (e.g. fibreoptic laryngoscope and light source).

## Layout of the Recovery Area

It is equally important that there should be a satisfactory recovery area for the immediate postoperative period, up to the stage where the protective reflexes have returned and the patient is awake. Here again there are different practices. Some anaesthetists prefer to have a recovery area immediately adjacent to the theatre and anaesthetic room so that they may observe, through a suitable window, the supervision of patients as they recover from anaesthesia. In other situations one central recovery room may serve several theatres. The only disadvantage that this might have is that more

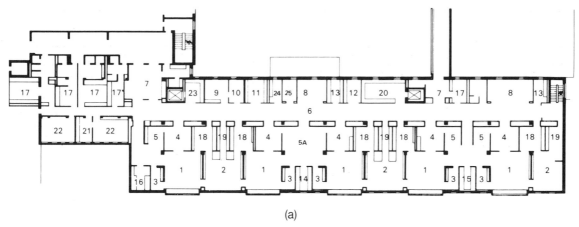

(a)

**Figure 25.6** (a) Plan of a multiple operating theatre suite. 1, Operating theatre; 2, sterilizing room; 3, scrub room; 4, anaesthetic room; 5, recovery area; 5A, larger recovery area; 6, clean corridor; 7, transfer bay; 8, trolley storage bay; 9, and 10, offices; 11, ventilator and anaesthetic equipment room; 12, superintendent's office; 13, general store; 14, special store; 15, Mobile x-ray storage; 16, anaesthetic department workshop/store; 17, changing rooms; 18, disposal and instrument cleaning room; 19, sterile pack store; 20, central sterile supply department (CSSD) and special instrument room (with lift direct to main CSSD); 21, kitchen; 22, sitting room; 23, dirty disposal room with decontaminating machine and lift to incinerator and CSSD dirty receiving room; 24, cleaner's room; 25, sister's office.
(b) Detailed plan of a single theatre unit. 1, Operating theatre; 2, sterilizing room; 3, scrub room; 4, anaesthetic room; 5, recovery area; 6, main theatre corridor. Note the direction in which the doors of the anaesthetic room open.

(b)

reliance is placed on a large number of skilled staff, since it is impossible for such a recovery room to be close to all theatres in a large suite. Referring to Fig. 25.6a it will be noticed that two recovery areas have been joined together by virtue of removing partitions to make one relatively large recovery room (5A) accommodating up to six patients. This type of system works satisfactorily, but it will be noted that the area is immediately adjacent to and visible from the neighbouring anaesthetic rooms and theatres.

Where the recovery area is not adjacent to the operating theatre suite, a suitable intercom system should be available so that the anaesthetist may be rapidly summoned to the recovery area if necessary.

Each recovery position should be equipped with:

- a regulated oxygen supply, preferably from the pipelines;

- suction apparatus with a selection of soft and rigid suckers;
- a selection of airways, syringes and needles;
- a bank of electrical sockets for connection on equipment;
- appropriate monitoring equipment, including ideally a blood pressure recorder, a pulse oximeter and an electrocardiogram;
- a suitable scavenging system.

For patient transport, patient trolleys should be equipped with an oxygen supply and medical suction.

### Anaesthetic related areas

*Cylinder store*. A cylinder storage area is required in an operating theatre or operating suite, even if there is a piped medical gas installation. Full cylinders may conveniently be stored on gently sloping shelves, those needed for use being drawn from the bottom of the slope and new ones being added at the top as the stock runs down hill. This ensures that the cylinders are used in rotation and none are held in stock for excessive periods of time.

*Fume cupboard.* A fume cupboard should be available in an operating suite (a) for the refilling of vaporizers and (b) for the cleaning and sterilization of equipment using aldehyde-based products so that the fumes do not induce a sensitivity reaction in theatre personnel.

*Administration office.* An administration office should be available for the designated person in charge of anaesthetic equipment (theatre sister or senior operating department assistant). The office should contain a filing system relating to the inventory of equipment and consumable stock, the names and addresses of relevant manufacturers, a system of recording the service history of the various items of equipment (log book) and a reporting system for equipment malfunction.

# 26 Administration, Supplies and Maintenance

## Introduction

The smooth running of an anaesthetic department requires that a designated person should be in charge who has developed a good liaison with the staff associated with supply, running and maintenance of the operating suite. These include the nursing staff, technicians, porters, EBME (electronic and biomedical engineers), pharmacist and supplies officer. The designated person in charge should collate an inventory of all equipment including:

- date of purchase;
- user manuals containing the serial numbers for spare parts;
- a record of the serial number and model number of the piece of equipment;
- guarantees for this equipment;
- the address and telephone numbers of the manufacturers and their representatives.

Each item on this inventory should have an individual file or have its own log book, which should show the model number and serial number, the anticipated scheduled service date, the date of completed servicing and by whom, and a section for reporting any faults.

This filing system should also have a section on hazard notices, cross-referenced to the equipment included in the inventory.

The anaesthetic department should have an area within the theatre suite for the storage of stock items (endotracheal tubes, breathing hoses, soda lime, etc.). These items should ideally be placed on shelving that is labelled for ease of recognition. A list of the stock carried should be regularly reviewed ('stocktaking'), so that there can be appropriate reduction or increase in the placing of orders. Failure to stocktake on a regular basis or to provide a well-ordered stock area often results in vast quantities of obsolete equipment that has no financial value. Stock ordering should be performed by the designated person who, in consultation with the department of anaesthesia, should decide the type of stock held. Expensive equipment (which might be used only occasionally) should only be ordered by a senior anaesthetist and not to satisfy some junior anaesthetist's passing whim.

The designated person in charge should also keep a 'faults book' for equipment. A laid-down procedure should be produced and displayed so that the personnel involved are aware of the channels for reporting faults on equipment. For example, an anaesthetic nurse or ODA (operating department assistant) discovering a fault prior to the anaesthetist performing his own pre-operative check would report this fault to the senior anaesthetist involved in that operating list. This anaesthetist would then decide whether the fault required the immediate decommissioning of the equipment and if so would make sure that the equipment was suitably labelled as faulty and not to be used. The fault (and date of discovery) would be entered into the fault book and the designated person in charge of equipment would be informed. This person would then contact the appropriate service contractor (either the manufacturer or local electronic and biomedical engineering department). If, on discussion with the senior anaesthetist, the fault is thought to be potentially dangerous, it should subsequently be reported to the local and/or national policing body. In the UK, this would be the Regional Scientific Officer based at the Regional Health Authority and the National Scientific Officer based at the Department of Health.

In the individual theatre, the anaesthetic nurse or operating department assistant should be responsible for each anaesthetic area in relation to stock and equipment. Again stock (drugs, endotracheal tubes, intravenous fluids, etc.) should be neatly displayed and organized and regularly topped up. It may be advisable for the designated person in charge of theatres to stipulate individual theatre stock levels. This person should also ensure that all anaesthetic equipment is clean, sterile (where appropriate) and in good working order. However, this does not absolve the anaesthetist from doing his own pre-anaesthetic checks (see Chapter 24) to ensure that the appropriate cylinders have been turned on, empty ones replaced, vaporizers replenished and the test carried out to ensure that pipeline hoses are correctly connected.

In addition to the above, the designated anaesthetist on an operating list should ensure that a register of the anaesthetics performed is completed, and that an operating list for that day is published and available with details of the patient, hospital number and operation planned.

It is also that person's responsibility to check the patient's identity and confirm the proposed operation, so that the planned anaesthetic is given to the right patient.

# Maintenance

The maintenance of anaesthetic machines falls into three categories.

- the day-to-day cleaning, replenishment of empty cylinders and vaporizers and general fettling;
- planned preventative maintenance (PPM);
- breakdown repairs.

In the case of essential apparatus, including life-support systems, the scale of equipment should be such that if any one particular item were to break down there would be sufficient reserves on which one could call to continue the service. In a large department it is preferable that there be one senior anaesthetist who has a particular interest in, and identifies himself with, the purchase and maintenance of equipment. All members of the department should be aware that no-one except an authorized person should be permitted to tamper with anaesthetic equipment. Items of anaesthetic equipment that are faulty should never be sent to the ordinary hospital engineer ('steam and drains' department), since although there are in these departments many mechanics who wish to be helpful and are only too pleased to render assistance when asked, they are often unfamiliar with the principles involved in anaesthetic equipment. Their well-meaning assistance or interference has only too often lead to accidents resulting from inappropriate repairs or alterations.

Maintenance should be carried out either by the manufacturer or by establishing within the hospital an electronic and biomedical engineering department (EBME) whose members may include both electronic and mechanical engineers. Many manufacturers provide suitable training courses for these personnel and approve them not only to carry out the supervisory duties mentioned above but also to make repairs and adjustments to equipment as required as well as routine servicing. However, the individual engineers must be aware of their own limitations.

## Planned preventative maintenance (PPM)

For many years, in the UK at least, it has been required that anaesthetic machines be routinely serviced four times a year and ventilators twice. Temperature compensated vaporizers are usually serviced as a separate item, and the recommendations vary from one type to another. Recently, however, the D.o.H. has changed the policy so that all anaesthetic equipment should be serviced 'according to the maker's recommendations'.

Records of PPM should be kept either in the equipment log books provided in the department or by collecting the service schedules supplied by the servicing engineer from the manufacturer. If the EBME department is responsible for maintenance, they should obtain comprehensive sets of diagrams, etc. of the equipment under their care and they should also keep a stock of spare parts sufficient to deal with the most common breakdowns. Such spares as reservoir bags, tubing, APL valves and catheter mounts should be kept within the anaesthetic department.

# Supply of Cylinders of Compressed Gases

In the UK these are normally ordered by the pharmacist and stock levels for each gas are agreed between him and the department of anaesthetics.

Some system should be employed to allow regular rotation of the stock of cylinders, so that those longest in store are used first. Labels such as those shown in Fig. 26.1 may be well intended, but in practice are of little use. A full cylinder is identified by the plastic dust cover around the outlet and an empty one by a suitable labelling system as is the custom of the particular hospital.

The administrative anaesthetist may also be responsible for contingency planning for a disaster

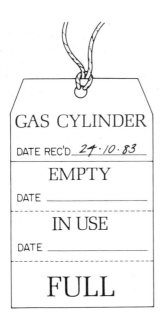

**Figure 26.1** A cylinder label.

(see Chapter 27). This means not only the provision of anaesthetic equipment to take to the scene of, for example, an air crash or industrial calamity within the area, but also the provision of equipment that can be used in the event of the failure of supplies within the hospital. There must, for example, be adequate reserve cylinders to provide a stand-by service, in the event of a failure of the piped medical gas system, until all patients being anaesthetized can be returned from the operating theatre with their operations completed.

All medical and nursing staff and technicians should know where this equipment is kept and the anaesthetist should be familiar with its operation. Portable anaesthetic equipment often differs markedly from that used in the theatre.

# Purchase of Equipment

Administrative arrangements for the purchase of equipment must obviously vary from one country to another. In the UK the proposed delegation of budgets to clinicians means that the yearly capital expenditure on equipment must be anticipated in order to bargain for a realistic equipment budget. It is here that the equipment inventory and stock utilization information is invaluable.

### Replacement of expensive items of equipment

A policy must be agreed between the anaesthetists as to the type of anaesthetic equipment to be ordered in this category so as to maintain a uniformity of standards and the standardization of equipment. This also permits the purchase of adequate spare parts and facilitates the emergency repair of equipment (where appropriate) by the EBME department. Having decided on the type of equipment, the department needs to calculate the cost price or the unit price of the item, the anticipated lifespan and the anticipated percentage increase in unit price at the end of the lifespan, and the number of items in each category to be purchased.

Some agreement should be arranged between the budget provider and the budget holder for the expenditure required to meet the introduction or new technology. The argument that the purchase of new equipment could reduce maintenance costs and reduce the expenditure on drugs, gases and materials is often a cogent one — as is the mention of legal problems that might occur if the equipment (or lack of it) failed to comply with that which could be deemed essential to prevent accidents.

### Stock orders and disposables

In the current financial climate, the department should agree the range and stock levels to be held within the department and an accurate record of useage should be kept.

### Non-stock ordering

Non-stock orders should be kept for items of equipment of low cost that are not regularly ordered and therefore not kept in stock. A contingency budget should be kept to cover items purchased in this category.

# 27 Provision of Anaesthesia in Difficult Situations and in the Developing World

## Introduction

There are certain situations in which it would be difficult or impracticable to provide sophisticated, heavy and bulky anaesthetic equipment on the scale to which we are accustomed in hospitals. Examples are domiciliary anaesthesia for a single patient and which may be for an emergency or planned minor surgery, and anaesthesia and resuscitation at the site of an accident or disaster. Also, in areas where under-development of transport and other facilities preclude the adequate supply of cylinders of nitrous oxide and oxygen and maintenance of anaesthetic equipment, special arrangements may have to be made.

## Domiciliary Anaesthesia

In a compact country such as the UK there is seldom any difficulty in providing a portable anaesthetic machine, complete, if necessary, with cylinders for the administration of a single anaesthetic. Minor surgery only would be undertaken. There are several satisfactory portable Boyle's machines, which function in the same manner as their larger counterparts, but very often only small cylinders are carried, and some form of rebreathing system, such as a circle absorber or Waters' canister, is appropriate. These portable anaesthetic machines may, if necessary, be used in conjunction with a manual resuscitator such as the Ambu, the Oxford bellows, or merely a reservoir bag to achieve artificial

ventilation if relaxants are used. Examples of these are shown in Chapter 12. Local, regional or intravenous anaesthesia are often the methods of choice at high altitudes, since the reduced atmospheric pressure may make it difficult to achieve adequate partial pressures of anaesthetic agents and oxygen.

In any situation where anaesthesia is not normally administered, flammable or explosive agents should be avoided. Even additional oxygen or nitrous oxide should be used with care, as increased concentrations of either of these gases may increase the flammability of materials normally considered to be safe. Naked flames such as coal fires or even domestic electric heaters may become extremely dangerous in the presence of increased concentrations of either of these gases.

The use of parenterally administered agents, such as ketamine must be considered to be much safer under these conditions.

## The Major Accident

In this situation there may be many casualties and the incident always occurs unexpectedly. The territory is often unfamiliar to those working, and this can often pose problems to all concerned. Exposure to high temperatures and dehydration in the tropics can be matched in its importance by extremes of cold climate, which may be found even in so-called temperate zones such as the UK. Low temperatures may not only incapacitate those working and harm the injured, but may also preclude the use of some anaesthetic agents, such as Entonox. Altitude may also pose problems with the administration of nitrous oxide and the volatile agents.

The lines of communication between the rescue workers and their patients, and the removal of the patients to safety, may be rendered very difficult by local conditions, as, for example, in an underground railway disaster or a mining accident. Darkness, dust and cramped conditions may preclude the carrying or employment of sophisticated equipment. If emergency amputation or disentanglement of patients from wreckage is required, this may well be achieved under intravenous or intramuscular anaesthesia with ketamine, but even so oxygen

(bearing in mind flammability) and Entonox, may be required. The greatest need may be for resuscitation, including endotracheal intubation, and this should be borne in mind when selecting equipment.

# Triservice Anaesthetic Apparatus

This compendium of anaesthetic and resuscitation equipment (Fig. 27.1) has been designed by the three British armed forces in order to provide a versatile but standardized system which, with the

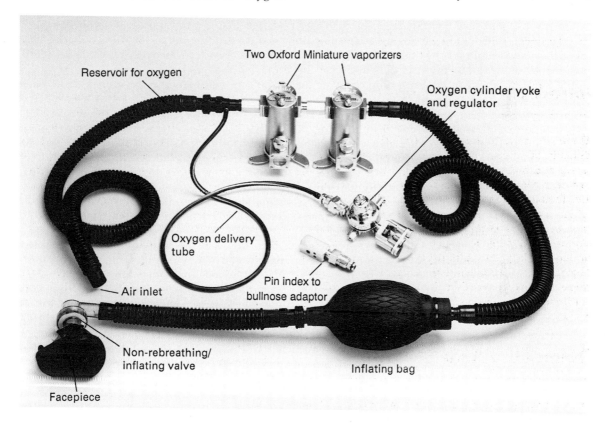

**Figure 27.1** The Triservice apparatus. The patient may breathe spontaneously, drawing air through the two Oxford Miniature vaporizers and the inflating bag. There is a valve mounted on the facepiece that prevents rebreathing. The air drawn in through the inlet may be enriched with oxygen from a cylinder which is attached to the cylinder yoke, with the pin index to bullnose adaptor if required. During expiration, the oxygen is stored in the reservoir tubing. The two Oxford Miniature vaporizers may be used for a variety of anaesthetic agents, there being interchangeable calibration labels for each. In the case of induction with ether, with spontaneous ventilation, both vaporizers will be required so as to produce an adequate vapour concentration. However, with spontaneous ventilation, if halothane is employed in the first vaporizer, it may be found convenient to use trichloroethylene in the second in order to make good the deficiency of analgesia caused by the exclusion of nitrous oxide. These vaporizers may be easily cleaned to remove traces of previous anaesthetic agents.

For controlled or assisted ventilation, the inflating bag may be squeezed manually or it may be replaced by a mechanical ventilator of the bag-squeezing type. The choice is dictated to some extent by the type of power source available. As an alternative to the inflating bag shown, the Laerdal folding silicone rubber bag may be used.

exception of the oxygen cylinder, is all housed in a box of rugged construction that can be dropped by parachute and weighs no more than 25 kg.

The basis of the compendium is a breathing system which includes a Laerdal folding manual resuscitator and two Oxford Miniature vaporizers (OMVs) (see Figs 12.1 and 6.28). During spontaneous ventilation the patient draws in air through the OMVs, and if it is desired to enrich it with oxygen the reservoir tubing is added to conserve the oxygen during the expiratory phase. During expiration the exhaled gases are voided to air through a valve mounted adjacent to the facepiece.

The OMVs are a modified version: they have three folding feet which enable them to be stood on a flat surface, and their capacity has been increased to 50 ml. The calibration scale for one agent may be detached and replaced by that for another — halothane or trichloroethylene (Trilene) may be used. Since the wicks in the vaporizing chamber are of metal, and therefore non-absorbent, one agent may be drained out, and after 'rinsing out' the vaporization chamber with a little of the new agent and then discarding it, it may be immediately filled with the new agent. When the control is turned to 'O' (off) the contents wil not spill if the vaporizer is accidentally inverted — although during transport it is preferable to empty out the agent. If the control is not turned to 'O', the vaporizer should be maintained stationary and upright, in the vertical position, for a few minutes before use, so that any liquid agent that has entered the bypass or the vapour control mechanism may drain back into the sump. Although the OMV is not temperature compensated, it does contain a heat sink, which helps to keep the output concentration relatively stable. Two OMVs are included in the system so that a quick change can be made from one agent to another, and also so that by using both, in series, for halothane or ether, a high enough concentration of those agents may be obtained for induction (as opposed to maintenance) of anaesthesia.

If the patient is apnoeic for any reason, whether arising from collapse or from the anaesthetic technique, IPPV may be instituted by manual compression of the resuscitator bag or by a ventilator, if available.

# Situations in Under-developed and Geographically Isolated Regions

In some underdeveloped countries problems may arise not only on account of apparatus but also due to the experience and training of the anaesthetist. It is not within the scope of this book to discuss the desirability of employing nurse-anaesthetists, but it seems certain that in many countries anaesthetics will have to be given by these 'medical assistants' for many years to come. Furthermore, it may well be argued that a medical assistant who has been well trained may be more efficient at anaesthetizing patients than a doctor who has received little or no training in anaesthesia.

Let us consider the personnel first. In many hospitals there may be one doctor who is helped by several medical assistants. In these cases he may well induce anaesthesia and intubate the patient himself and then hand over to the assistant while he performs the operation, returning to the role of anaesthetist at the end. It is quite obvious that the maintenance of a clear airway is one of the paramount duties of the assistant and this will be greatly facilitated if the patient has been intubated. Therefore, under these conditions, endotracheal intubation may be more common than elsewhere, and this should be borne in mind when considering the provision for endotracheal equipment. The anaesthetic apparatus used should be as simple as possible so that there are few controls to operate and the least possible chance of malfunction or maladjustment. A combination of the EMO vaporizer, the OMV (equipped and calibrated for both halothane and trichloroethylene (Trilene)), together with a means of inflation such as manual resuscitator or Oxford bellows, a Ruben or similar valve, and a facepiece or endotracheal connector may well be the most practical equipment available under these circumstances. The facility for the addition of a supply of oxygen would be desirable. The provision of equipment and supplies to these areas is prejudiced by long lines of communication and very often unreliable means of transport. Whilst much equipment can be delivered by air, this is expensive and may be precluded in certain weather conditions, and also it must be remembered that there are problems concerned with the delivery of agents such as ether by air.

## Restricted Articles Regulations

The International Air Transport Association publishes regulations concerning the precautions to be taken when transporting by air the following: flammable gas, oxidizers, corrosives, explosives, poisons, non-flammable compressed gas, flammable liquids and radioactive material. These regulations are accepted throughout most of the world, and are concerned with the labelling, the general packing requirements and the handling and loading of restricted articles. The labels are all diamond shaped, of different colours, and bear both a word and a symbol to denote the danger.

Agents such as trichloroethylene and chloroform may be carried in both passenger and cargo aircraft, but subject to a restriction in quantity; in both cases 40 litres. Halothane, unfortunately, is not as yet mentioned. Ether is not accepted at all in passenger aircraft and a maximum of 40 litres may be carried in cargo aircraft. One litre of ethyl alcohol may be carried in a suitable container in passenger aircraft and up to 40 litres in cargo aircraft. Up to 70 kg of both nitrous oxide and gaseous oxygen may be carried in passenger aircraft and up to 140 kg in cargo aircraft. Liquid oxygen is not acceptable as cargo in any aircraft, in either a non-pressurized or pressurized package. Up to 70 kg of gaseous or liquefied carbon dioxide may be carried in passenger aircraft and up to 140 kg in cargo aircraft; there is no restriction for solid carbon dioxide.

## Maintenance of Equipment

In some countries there are good standards of equipment and work, but maintenance may be a problem. One of the author's experiences in an island in the Indian Ocean with a population of less than one million was that the personnel in all categories were well trained. However, problems arose owing to the distance that had to be travelled by service engineers, and so even relatively small matters of maintenance became a problem. It would be difficult to justify the full-time employment of an engineer for just an occasional task, and yet the cost of transporting an engineer by air to perform his work is very expensive. For this reason it is better to avoid complicated and sophisticated equipment such as the larger ventilators, which may need frequent attention and adjustment. Supplies of oxygen and nitrous oxide may be available but very expensive, and consideration should be given to the use of closed, low-flow breathing systems and oxygen concentrators.

When ordering equipment for these areas, consideration should be given to the provision of adequate spares and it might well be deemed advisable to have one of the anaesthetists trained in some of the less-complicated mechanical manipulations required in servicing.

# Appendix I Further Reading

## PHYSICAL PRINCIPLES

Hill, D. W. (1980) *Physics Applied to Anaesthesia*. 4th edn. London: Butterworths.

Mushin, W. W. & Jones, P. L. (1987) *Physics for Anaesthetists*. 4th edn. Oxford: Blackwell Scientific Publications.

Padmore, G. R. A. & Nunn, J. F. (1974) SI units in relation to anaesthesia. *British Journal of Anaesthesia*, **46**, 236–243.

## ELECTRONICS

Horowitz, P. & Hall, W. (1989) *The Art of Electronics*. 2nd edn. Cambridge: Cambridge University Press.

Morris, N. M. (1983) *Control Engineering*. 3rd edn. Maidenhead: McGraw Hill Book Company.

## MEASUREMENT OF FLOW

Hayward, A. T. J. (1979) *Flowmeters*. London: Macmillan Publishers Ltd.

## VAPORIZERS

Carter, K. B., Grey, W. M., Rallton, R. & Richardson, W. (1988) Long-term performance of TEC vaporizers. *Anaesthesia*, **43**, 1042–1046.

Gray, W. M. (1988) Dependence of the output of a halothane vaporizer on thymol concentration. *Anaesthesia*, **43**, 1047–1049.

Leigh, J. M. (1985) Variations on a theme splitting ratio. *Anaesthesia*, **40**, 70–72.

Palayiwa, E., Hahn, C. E. W. & Sugg, B. R. (1985) Nitrous oxide solubility in halothane and its effect on the output of vaporizers. *Anaesthesia*, **40**, 415–419.

Schaefer, H. G. & Farman, J. V. (1984) Anaesthetic vapour concentrations in the EMO system. *Anaesthesia*, **39**, 171–180.

## ANAESTHETIC MACHINES

British Standards Institution: BS 4272 (1989) Anaesthetic and analgesic machines, part 3 specifications for continuous flow anaesthetic machines. Available from the Sales Department, Lynford Wood, Milton Keynes, Bucks, MK14 6LE.

*Check Out; a guide for preoperative inspection of the anaesthetic machine*, American Society of Anaesthesiologists, 515 Busse Highway, Park Ridge, Illinois 60068.

Editorial (1990) Carbon dioxide cylinders on anaesthetic apparatus. *British Journal of Anaesthesia*, **65**, 155–156.

McQuillan, P. J. & Jackson, J. B. (1987) Potential leaks from anaesthetic machines. *Anaesthesia*, **42**, 1308–1312.

Ritchie, J. R. (1974) A simple and reliable warning device for failing oxygen pressure. *British Journal of Anaesthesia*, **46**.

Schreiber, P. (1985) *Safety Guidelines: Anaesthesia Systems*. Telford, Penn. USA: North American Dräger.

## PIPELINE SYSTEMS

BOC Ltd (1990) *GAS SAFE – in the hospital, A guide to the safe use of Medical Gas cylinders*. Guildford, Surrey: BOC Ltd.

Brancroft, M. F., du Moulin, G. C. & Hedley-Whyte, J. (1980) The hazards of hospital bulk oxygen delivery systems. *Anaesthesiology*, **52**, 504–510.

British Standards Institution: BS 5682 (1984) Terminal units, hose assemblies and their connectors for use with medical gas pipeline systems. Available from the Sales Department, Lynford Wood, Milton Keynes, Bucks MK14 6LE.

Grant, W. J. (1978) *Medical Gases: Their Properties and Use*. Aylesbury: HM&M.

Howell, R. S. C. (1980) Piped medical gas and vacuum systems. *Anaesthesia*, **35**, 676–698.

HTM 22. Piped Medical Gases, Medical Compressed Air and Medical Vacuum Installations. London: HM Stationery Office.

HTM 22 (Suppl.) Permit to Work Systems. London: HM Stationery Office.

International Standards Organization (ISO) 5359. 1st edn (1989). Low pressure flexible connecting assemblies (hose assemblies) for use with medical gas systems.

International Standards Organization (ISO) 9170. 1st edn (1990). Terminal units for use in medical gas pipeline systems.

Jones, P. E. (1974) Some observations on nitrous oxide cylinders during emptying. *British Journal of Anaesthesia*, **46**, 534–538.

## BREATHING SYSTEMS

Anderson, P. K. (1981) Control of carbon dioxide in modified Mapleson A and D (Hafnia) anaesthetic systems. An experimental model. *Acta Anaesthesiologica Scandinavica*, **25**, 344–348.

Barnes, P. K., Browne, C. H. W. & Conway, C. M. (1977) The work of ventilating semi-closed rebreathing systems. *British Journal of Anaesthesia*, **49**, 1173.

Bracken, A. & Cox, L. A. (1968) Apparatus for carbon dioxide absorption. *British Journal of Anaesthesia*, **40**, 660–665.

Chan, A. H. S., Bruce, W. E. & Soni, N. (1989) A comparison of anaesthetic breathing systems during spontaneous ventilation. *Anaesthesia*, **44**, 194–199.

Christensen, K. N., Thomsen, A., Hansen, O. & Jorgensen, S. (1978) Flow requirements in the Hafnia modifications of the Mapleson circuits during spontaneous respiration. *Acta Anaesthesiologica Scandinavica*, **22**, 27–32.

Department of Health (1989) Anaesthetic and respiratory equipment: the use of 22 mm breathing system connections. *Safety Action Bulletin* no. 52.

Dorrington, K. L. & Lehane, J. R. (1989) Rebreathing during spontaneous and controlled ventilation with 'T' piece breathing systems: a general solution. *Anaesthesia*, **44**, 300–302.

Henville, J. D. & Adams, A. P. (1976) The Bain Anaesthetic System. *Anaesthesia*, **31**, 247–256.

Holmes, C. McK. & Spears, G. F. S. (1977) Very nearly closed circuit anaesthesia: a computer analysis. *Anaesthesia*, **32**, 846–851.

Humphrey, D. (1983) A new anaesthetic breathing system combining Mapleson A, D & E principles. *Anaesthesia*, **38**, 361–372.

Mapleson, W. W. (1954) The elimination of rebreathing in various semi-closed anaesthetic systems. *British Journal of Anaesthesia*, **26**, 323–332.

Mapleson, W. W. (1960) The concentration of anaesthetics in closed circuits, with special reference to halothane. *British Journal of Anaesthesia*, **32**, 298–309.

Miller, D. M. (1988) Breathing systems for use in anaesthesia. *British Journal of Anaesthesia*, **60**, 555–564.

Morris, L. E. (1974) The circulator concept. *International Anaesthetic Clinics*, **12(3)**, 181–198.

Murphy, P. M., Fitzgeorge, R. B. & Barrett, R. F. (1991) Viability and distribution of bacteria after passage through a circle anaesthetic system. *British Journal of Anaesthesia*, **66**, 300–304.

Neff, W. B., Burke, S. F. & Thompson, R. (1968) A Venturi circulator for anaesthetic systems. *Anaesthesiology*, **29(4)**, 838–841.

Revell, D. G. (1959) A circulator to eliminate mechanical dead space in circle absorption systems. *Canadian Anaesthetists' Society Journal*, **6(2)**, 98–103.

Thomsen, A. & Jorgensen, S. (1976) The Hafnia A Circuit. *Acta Anaesthesiologica Scandinavica*, **20**, 395–404.

## DENTAL ANAESTHESIA

Green, R. A. & Coplans, M. P. (1973) *Anaesthesia and Analgesia in Dentistry*. London: H. K. Lewis.

Naimby-Luxmore, R. C. (1967) Some hazards of dental gas machines. *Anaesthesia*, **22**, 595.

## ANAESTHETIC VENTILATORS

Adams, A. P. & Henville, J. D. (1977) A new generation of anaesthetic ventilators, the Pneupac and Penlon A–P. *Anaesthesia*, **32**, 34–40.

Editorial (1982) *Anaesthesia*, **37**, 987–989.

Editorial (1986) High frequency ventilation. *Lancet*, **March**, 477–479.

Fletcher, I. R., Carden, E., Healy, T. E. J. & Poole, T. R. (1983) The M & IE ventilator, a description and laboratory assessment. *Anaesthesia*, **38**, 1082–1089.

James, M. F. M. (1978) The use of a Cape Minor ventilator with the circle absorber system. *Anaesthesia*, **33**, 945–949.

Jones, P. L. & Hillard, E. K. (1977) The Flomasta, a new anaesthetic ventilator. *Anaesthesia*, **32**, 619–625.

Mushin, W. W., Rendell-Baker, L., Thompson, P. W. & Mapleson, W. W. (1980) *Automatic Ventilation of the Lungs*. 3rd edn. Oxford: Blackwell Scientific.

Sjostrand, U. & Eriksson, I. (1980) High rates and low volumes in mechanical ventilation—not just a matter of ventilatory frequency. *Anaesthesia and Analgesia*, **59**, 8.

Smith, B. E. (1985) The Penlon Bromsgrove high frequency ventilator for adult and paediatric use.

(A solution to the problems of humidification.) *Anaesthesia*, **40**, 790–796.

Smith, B. E. (1990) High frequency ventilation: past, present and future? *British Journal of Anaesthesia*, **65**, 130–138.

Sugg, B. R. & Prys-Roberts, C. (1976) The Penlon Oxford ventilator. *Anaesthesia*, **31**, 1234–1244.

## PAEDIATRIC ANAESTHESIA

Hatch, D. J. (1978) Tracheal tubes and connectors used in neonates—dimensions and resistance to breathing. *British Journal of Anaesthesia*, **50**, 959–964.

Hatch, D. J. (1985) Paediatric anaesthetic equipment. *British Journal of Anaesthesia*, **57**, 672–684.

Hatch, D. J., Yates, A. P. & Lindhahl, S. G. E. (1987) Flow requirements and rebreathing during mechanically controlled ventilation in a 'T' piece (Mapleson E) system. *British Journal of Anaesthesia*, **59**, 1533–1540.

## MONITORING

Gravenstein, J. S. (1990) *Gas Monitoring and Pulse-oximetry*. Oxford: Butterworth-Heinemann.

Gravenstein, J. S., Paulus, D. A. & Hayes, T. J. (1989) *Capnography in Clinical Practice*. Oxford: Butterworths.

Maynard Ramsey III (1991) Blood pressure monitoring: automated oscillometric devices. *Journal of Clinical Monitoring*, **7**, 56–67.

Merilainen, P. T. (1990) A differential paramagnetic sensor for breath by breath oximetry. *Journal of Clinical Monitoring*, **6**, 65–73.

Ralston, A. C., Webb, R. K. & Runciman, W. B. (1991) Potential errors in pulse-oximetry. *Anaesthesia*, **44**, 202–212, 291–295.

Sykes, M. K., Vickers, M. D. & Hull, C. J. (1991) *Principles of Clinical Measurement*. 3rd edn. Oxford: Blackwell Scientific.

Weinfurt, P. T. (1990) Electrocardiographic monitoring: an overview. *Journal of Clinical Monitoring*, **6**, 132–138.

## POLLUTION

Askrog, V. & Harvald, B. (1970) Teratogenic effects of inhalation anaesthesia. *Nordisk Medicin*, **3**, 490.

Austin, J. C., Shaw, R., Crichton, R., Cleaton-Jones, P. E. & Moyes, D. (1978) Comparison of sampling techniques for studies of nitrous oxide pollution. *British Journal of Anaesthesia*, **50**, 1109–1112.

British Standards Institution: BS 6834 (1987) Anaesthetic Gas Scavenging Disposal System. Available from the Sales Department, Lynford Wood, Milton Keynes, Bucks MK14 6LE.

Bruce, D. L. & Bach, M. J. (1976) Effects of trace anaesthetic gases on behavioural performance of volunteers. *British Journal of Anaesthesia*, **48**, 871.

Cohen, E. N. (1980) *Exposure in the Workplace*. Littleton, MA: PSG Publishing Company.

Deacon, R., Perry, J., Lumb, M., Chanarin, Minty, B., Halsey, M. J. & Nunn, J. F. (1978) Selective inactivation of vitamin B12 in rats by nitrous oxide. *Lancet*, **II**, 1023.

Hatch, D. J., Miles, R. & Wagstaff, M. (1980) An anaesthetic scavenging system for paediatric and adult use. *Anaesthesia*, **35**, 496–499.

Health and Safety Commission (1988) Control of Substances Hazardous to Health Regulations 1988. Approved code of practice.

Knill-Jones, R. P., Moir, D. D., Rodrigues, L. V. & Spence, A. A. (1972) Anaesthesia practice and pregnancy: controlled survey of women anaesthetists in the United Kingdom. *Lancet*, **II**, 1326.

NIOSH, National Institute for Occupational Safety and Health (1977) Criteria for a recommended standard: occupational exposure to waste gases and vapours. DHEW Publication No. (NIOSH) 77–140. Cincinnati, Ohio, USA.

Spence, A. A. & Knill-Jones, R. P. (1978) Is there health hazard in anaesthetic practice? *British Journal of Anaesthesia*, **50**, 713.

## CLEANING & STERILIZATION

Johnson & Johnson (1964) *The Concept of Sterility in Medical Products*. Slough: Johnson & Johnson.

## MEDICAL VACUUM

HTM 22, HTM 22 (Supplement) See under Pipeline systems.

Rosen, M. & Hillard, E. K. (1960) The use of suction in clinical medicine. *British Journal of Anaesthesia*, **32**, 186–503.

## ACCIDENTS (GENERAL, PSYCHOLOGY) SAFETY AND MORTALITY

Allnutt, M. F. (1987) Human factors in accidents. *British Journal of Anaesthesia*, **59**, 856–864.

Cooper, J. B., Newbower, R. S., Long, C. D. & McPeek, B. (1978) Preventable anaesthesia mishaps. *Anaesthesiology*, **49**, 399–406.

Dinnick, O. P. (1964) Deaths associated with anaesthesia. *Anaesthesia*, **19**, 536–556.

Dinnick, O. P. (1973) Hazards in the operating theatre. *Annals of the Royal College of Surgeons of England*, **52**, 349–354.

Edwards, G., Morton, H. J. V., Pask, E. A. & Wylie, W. D. (1955) Deaths associated with anaesthesia. *Anaesthesia*, **11**, 194–220.

Hurst, R. L. (ed.) (1982) *Pilot Error — the Human Factors*. St Albans: Granada.

Harrison, G. G. (1978) Death attributable to anaesthesia. *British Journal of Anaesthesia*, **50**, 1041–1046.

Hawkins, F. R. (1987) *Human Factors in Flight*. Aldershot UK: Gower Technical Press.

Holland, R. (1970) *Safety in Operating Theatres*. Royal Australian College of Surgeons Seminar.

Holland, R. (1970) Special committee investigating deaths under anaesthesia. Report on 745 classified cases 1960–8. *Medical Journal of Australia*, **1**, 573–594.

Hopkin, D. A. B. (1980) *Hazards and Errors in Anaesthesia*. Berlin: Springer-Verlag.

Schrieber, P. (1972) *Anaesthetic Equipment: Performance, Classification and Safety*. Berlin: Springer-Verlag.

Schreiber, P. (1985) *Anesthesia Systems — Safety Guidelines*. Telford, Penn., USA: North American Dräger.

Schreiber, P. & Schreiber, J. (1987) *Anaesthesia System Risk Analysis and Risk Reduction*. Telford, Penn, USA: North American Dräger.

Utting, J. E., Gray, T. C. & Shelley, F. C. (1979) Human misadventure in anaesthesia. *Canadian Anaesthetists' Society Journal*, **26(6)**, 472–478.

Vickers, M. D. (1970) Explosion hazards. *Anaesthesia*, **25**, 482.

Vickers, M. D. (1971) Explosion hazards. *Anaesthesia*, **26**, 155.

Ward, C. S. (1968) The prevention of accidents associated with anaesthetic apparatus. *British Journal of Anaesthesia*, **40**, 692–701.

Ward, C. S. (1981) *Electrical Safety in Hospitals*. London: Henry Kimpton.

Wyant, G. M. (1978) *Mechanical Misadventure in Anaesthesia*. Toronto: University of Toronto Press.

## DIFFICULT SITUATIONS AND SCENE OF THE ACCIDENT

Boulton, T. B. (1966) Anaesthesia in difficult situations, III. *Anaesthesia*, **21(4)**, 513–545.

Boulton, T. B. & Cole, P. (1966) Anaesthesia in difficult situations, I. *Anaesthesia*, **21(2)**, 268–276.

Boulton, T. B. & Cole, P. (1966) Anaesthesia in difficult situations, II. *Anaesthesia*, **21(3)**, 379–399.

Jowitt, M. D. (1984) Anaesthesia ashore in the Falklands. *Annals of the Royal College of Surgeons of England*, **66**, 197–200.

Leatherdale, R. A. L. (1966) The EMO ether inhaler. *Anaesthesia*, **21(4)**, 504–512.

Penlon (1975) *Instruction Booklet: EMO Outfits and EMO Ether Inhaler*. Abingdon, Oxford: Penlon.

# Appendix II  SI Units and Table of Conversions

Although SI units (Système International d'Unités) have been adopted for scientific purposes, they are not yet universally used in anaesthetic practice. As many pieces of anaesthetic and oxygen therapy apparatus will survive for many years, the older units in which they are calibrated have been retained throughout this book.

## SI Units

The SI units applicable to anaesthesia are as follows:

| Function | SI Unit |
|----------|---------|
| Mass | kilogram (kg) |
| Length | metre (m) |
| Force | newton (N) — accelerates a mass of 1 kg by 1 m/s$^2$ (1 N = 10$^5$ dynes) |
| Pressure | pascal (Pa) = 1 N/m$^2$ (NB 1 bar = 10$^5$ Pa) |
| Energy | joule (J) — force of 1 newton acting through 1 metre (1 J = 10$^7$ ergs) |
| Power | watt (W) = 1 J/s |
| Temperature | kelvin (K) = °C (0 K = −273°C) |
| Frequency | hertz (Hz) = 1 cycle/s |
| Capacity | litre (l) |

## Table of Conversions

| | |
|---|---|
| 1 metre | = 1.0936 yards = 3.2808 feet — 39.3696 inches |
| 1 kilogram | = 2.2046 pounds = 35.2736 ounces |
| 1 litre | = 0.22 (imperial) gallons = 1.76 pints<br>= 35.2 fluid ounces<br>= 0.27 US gallons |
| 1 kilo Pascal | = 0.146 p.s.i. |
| [1mmHg | = 1.36 cmH$_2$O = 133.3 N/m$^2$ = 0.0194 p.s.i.] |
| 1 joule | = 10$^7$ ergs = 0.239 calories |
| 0 kelvin (K) | = −273° Celsius ('absolute zero') |
| 273.15K | = 0°C = 32°F |
| 373.16K | = 100°C = 212°F |
| °C | = (°F−32) × 5/9 |
| °F | = (°C × 9/5) + 32 |

# Appendix III Standards

Standardization in design and manufacture of medical equipment is intended to promote safety for operator, safety of the patient, compatibility, interchangeability, ease of use, and protection of the environment.

All the industrialized nations have their own standards organizations, in the case of the United Kingdom this is the British Standards Institution (BSI). These organizations publish Standards that to the clinician often seem to have a language of their own. The complexity of the language used is necessary, however, as it is essential to ensure that designers and manufacturers can interpret the text in one way only.

British Standards contain:

1. A *Scope*, which describes what that particular Standard covers and what it *excludes*.
2. Definition of *terminology* and *classifications*.
3. *Specifications* for materials, function, dimensions, weight (if relevant), performance and safety.
4. *Tests* and *methods* of testing to ensure compliance with the rest of the Standard.
5. Instructions as to what must be written in the *instruction manual* and the *labelling* of the equipment.

The syntax of Standards includes *shall*, which implies that compliance is mandatory, and *should*, which is a 'strong suggestion'. The text of Standards has to be written carefully to avoid 'design restriction' and to avoid stifling of new developments.

Standards in the UK are written by Technical Committees that are set up by the BSI, which also supplies advice on wording and the secretariat. Technical Committees for medical equipment are usually chaired by a clinician and include representatives from the manufacturers' trade associations (e.g. the British Anaesthetic and Respiratory Manufacturers' Association (BAREMA) and the Scientific Instrument Manufacturers' Association), the Department of Health, and the users — that is clinicians.

In order to provide international standardization there are several international standards bodies. These international bodies try to produce Standards that may be used worldwide, both to improve international trade and to improve safety when equipment is imported and exported. Until recently there were two international standards bodies namely: the International Standards Organization (ISO), which deals with anything non-electrical and the International Electrotechnical Commission (IEC), which deals with equipment having *any* electrical components or connection. Unfortunately, the EC has found it necessary to increase the bureaucracy by introducing two more organizations, namely the Comité European de Normalisation (CEN) and its electrical equivalent to the IEC, CENELEC. When international agreement is gained, many national standards organizations agree to 'dual-number' their Standards, making them identical to the International documents and giving them a National number for example: BS 5724: Part 1 = IEC 601: Part 1.

Appended below is a list of relevant Standards published by the BSI with their equivalent International numbers. It should be realized that some standards come in several parts; part 1 contains general requirements that are necessary for the understanding of the relevant part 2, which contains the specific requirements for a particular piece of equipment.

## Anaesthetic and Breathing Equipment

**BS 1319**: 1976 (1986)              ≡ ISO/R 32, ISO 407
**Specification for medical gas cylinders, valves and yoke connections**
Cylinders, their valve outlets and connections of the pin index type. Appendices give recommendations for the care and handling of the equipment.

**BS 1319C**: 1976
**Colours for the identification of the contents of medical gas cylinders**

**BS 2050**: 1978    ≠ ISO 2878, ISO/DIS 2882, ISO/DIS 2883
**Specification for electrical resistance of conducting and antistatic products made from flexible polymeric material**
Limits and corresponding tests for products for hospitals and industrial use.

**BS 2718**: 1979 (1984)
**Specification for gas cylinder trolleys**
Specifies materials, dimensions and constructional and performance requirements for three sizes of gas cylinder trolleys to take steel cylinders of 1360, 3400 and 6800 litre capacities for use in hospitals.

**BS 3353**: 1987    ≡ ISO 5362
**Specification for anaesthetic reservoir bags**
Reservoir bags for use with anaesthetic or breathing apparatus. Includes requirements for the design of the neck, size designation, compliance and for electrical conductivity.

*BS 3487: TRACHEAL TUBES*

**BS 3487: Part 1**: 1989    ≡ ISO 5361–1
**Specification for all types of tubes**
General requirements for tracheal tubes, whether made of rubber or other elastomeric material.

**BS 3487: Part 2**: 1986    ≡ ISO 5361/2
**Specification for orotracheal and nasotracheal tubes of the Magill type (plain and cuffed)**
Tubes of the Magill type, whether made of rubber or of other elastomeric material. Specifies a range of designated sizes from 2.5 mm to 11.0 mm nominal inside diameters, and gives requirements for inflating tubes and cuffs, if provided.

**BS 3487: Part 3**: 1986    ≡ ISO 5361/3
**Specification for tubes of the Murphy type**
Tubes of the Murphy type, i.e. the type with an eye near the tip, with or without cuffs.

**BS 3487: Part 4**: 1988    ≡ ISO 5361–4
**Specification for tubes of the Cole type**
Tubes with a small patient end for use with infants. Covers designated sizes from 1.5 mm to 4.5 mm nominal inside diameter of the tracheal portion.

**BS 3487: Part 5**: 1986    ≡ ISO 5361/5
**Specification and methods of test for tube collapse and cuff herniation**
Requirements for a type test to be carried out on new unused tubes for evaluation of tube collapse and cuff herniation of cuffed tracheal tubes.

**BS 3622**: 1975 (1989)
**Specification for general-purpose stools and anaesthetists' chairs for hospital use**
Materials, dimensions and construction, electrical safety precautions and finish. Additional requirements for a top to form a chair. Two height ranges.

**BS 3806**: 1964
**Specification for breathing machines for medical use**
Classification, terms and definitions; lung ventilators; connectors for lung ventilators; hoses and hose connectors for cabinets; hoses for cuirasses.

*BS 3849: CONICAL CONNECTORS FOR ANAESTHETIC AND RESPIRATORY EQUIPMENT*

**BS 3849: Part 1**: 1988    ≡ ISO 5356–1
**Specification for cones and sockets**
Basic dimensional and gauging requirements for 15 mm, 19 mm, 22 mm, 23 mm and 30 mm size intended for use in breathing systems, anaesthetic gas scavenging systems and vaporizers.

**BS 3849: Part 2**: 1988    ≡ 5356–2
**Specification for screw-threaded weight-bearing connectors**
Requirements for conical connectors intended for use with inhalation anaesthetic apparatus and ventilators for mounting heavy accessories.

**BS 4068**: 1977 (1989)
**Specification for hospital trolleys for instruments, dressings and for anaesthetists' use, including angular trolleys**
Materials, dimensions, construction and electrical safety for instrument trolleys and dressing trolleys of four sizes, and for angular trolleys, with rectangular loose shelves.

*BS 4272: ANAESTHETIC AND ANALGESIC MACHINES*

**BS 4272: Part 1**: 1968
**Anaesthetic machines of the on-demand type supplied with nitrous oxide and oxygen from separate containers**
Basic requirements from the standpoint of performance and safety, for machines used in dentistry and midwifery. An appendix gives recommendations for periodic field testing of apparatus.

**BS 4272: Part 2**: 1968
**Analgesic machines of the on-demand type supplied with pre-mixed nitrous oxide–oxygen from a single container**
Basic requirements for machines supplied with a 50/50 mixture by volume. One field of application will be the self-administration of analgesic in domiciliary obstetric practice.

**BS 4272: Part 3**: 1989                                      ≠ ISO 5358
**Specification for continuous-flow anaesthetic machines**
Basic design and performance requirements.

*BS 5724: MEDICAL ELECTRICAL EQUIPMENT*

**BS 5724: Part 1**: 1989
**General requirements for safety**
Implements CENELEC HD 395.1.

**BS 5724: Part 2**
**Particular requirements for safety**
   **BS 5724: Section 2.23**: 1989              ≡ ISO 8359
   **Specification for oxygen concentrators**
   Devices which by separating out nitrogen from ambient air provide oxygen-enriched air for supply to a patient. To be read in conjunction with BS 5724: Part 1.

   **BS 5724: Section 2.24**: 1989              ≡ ISO 8185
   **Specification for humidifiers**
   Vaporizing and nebulizing humidifiers, including those suitable for inclusion in breathing systems, for use with both intubated and non-intubated patients. To be read in conjunction with BS 5724: Part 1.

   **BS 5724: Section 2.27**: 1989              ≡ ISO 7767
   **Specification for oxygen analysers for monitoring patient breathing mixtures**
   Both sampling and non-sampling oxygen analysers are covered. To be read in conjunction with BS 5724: Part 1.

**BS 6015**: 1980 (1987)                                      ≡ ISO 4135
**Glossary of terms used in anaesthesiology**
Establishes a vocabulary of terms used in connection with anaesthesiology and medical ventilation.

*BS 6149: TRACHEOSTOMY TUBES*

**BS 6149: Part 1**: 1987                                      ≡ ISO 5366/1
**Specification for connectors**
Connectors for tracheostomy tubes for use on patients undergoing surgical operation and/or those

for whom artificial ventilation or other respiratory support may be required.

**BS 6149: Part 2**: 1986                                      ≡ ISO 5366/2
**Specification for tubes (excluding connectors)**
Basic requirements for tracheostomy tubes made of plastics materials designed for patients who may require anaesthesia, artificial ventilation or other respiratory support, but not restricted to these uses. Includes requirements for size designation, size range and for such optional features as cuffs and inner tubes. Requirements for connectors are specified in BS 6149: Part 1.

**BS 6153**: 1987                                      ≡ ISO 5364
**Specification for oropharyngeal airways**
Size designation and basic requirements for materials and design.

**BS 6155**: 1981 (1988)
**Specification for tracheal tubes for large animals in veterinary anaesthesia**
Cuffed oral tracheal tubes; dimensions, size range, design of inflating tube, marking.

**BS 6546**: 1984                                      ≠ ISO 7228
**Specification for tracheal tube connectors**
Includes size designation, size range, materials and design.

*BS 6578: LARYNGOSCOPIC FITTINGS*

**BS 6578: Part 1**: 1985                                      ≡ ISO 7376/1
**Specification for hook-on type handle-blade fittings**
Specifies basic dimensions for the parts of the joint between any blade and any handle of a hook-on type laryngoscope, used mainly for tracheal intubation, in which an electric lamp in the blade is supplied with power through the handle.

**BS 6578: Part 2**: 1985                                      ≡ ISO 7376/2
**Specification for screw threads for miniature electric lamps and sockets**
Specifies requirements for screw threads for miniature electric lamps and lamp sockets used in laryngoscopes specified in Part 1 of this British Standard. Also specifies the contact form and general dimensions of the lamps.

**BS 6834**: 1987
**Specification for active anaesthetic gas scavenging systems**
Minimum performance and safety requirements for active anaesthetic gas scavenging systems and their component parts, intended to reduce the exposure

of hospital personnel to anaesthetic gases and vapours.

**BS 6850**: 1987                                    ≠ BS 6850
**Specification for ventilatory resuscitators**
Requirements for resuscitators intended for use with all age groups. Covers both operator-powered and gas-powered resuscitators that are portable and intended for use in emergency situations to provide lung ventilation to individuals whose breathing appears to be inadequate.

**BS 7143**: 1989
**Specification for catheter mounts (flexible adaptors) for use with medical breathing systems**
For connection of anaesthetic and ventilator breathing systems to tracheal tubes.

# Electromedical Equipment

*BS 4199: SPECIFICATION FOR SURGICAL SUCTION APPARATUS*

**BS 4199: Part 1**: 1967 (1988)
**Electrically operated surgical suction apparatus of high vacuum and high air displacement type**
Basic requirements for mobile apparatus intended for use on d.c. or on single-phase a.c. supplies of up to 250 V, for use in hospital operating theatres and wards.

**BS 4199: Part 2**: 1968 (1988)
**Electrically operated surgical suction apparatus for continuous drainage**
Basic requirement intended for equipment for use on d.c. or on single-phase a.c. supplies up to 250 V and capable of producing a reduced pressure (vacuum) of at least 150 mmHg below an atmospheric pressure of 760 mmHg (i.e. an absolute pressure of 610 mmHg (813 mbar)) for the continuous drainage of body cavities. Provision is made for both low and high air flow types of equipment.

**BS 4376**: 1982
**Specification for electrically operated blood storage refrigerators**
Particular requirements for refrigerators of the closed reach-in type constructed according to BS 2502, and for sectional cold rooms of the walk-in type, constructed according to BS 2502, which are intended for the preservation of whole blood and fluid blood plasma and its derivations at temperatures between 4°C and 6°C.

*BS 4803: RADIATION SAFETY OF RADIATION PRODUCTS AND SYSTEMS*

**BS 4803: Part 1**: 1983                           ≠ IEC 825
**General**
Gives definitions. Contains algorithms for calculation of radiation hazards. Biological considerations are discussed.

**BS 4803: Part 2**: 1983                           ≠ IEC 825
**Specification for manufacturing requirements for laser products**
Specifies manufacturing requirements for radiation safety of laser products. Defines laser product classes and gives requirements for classification procedure. Based on the latest information available including data from ANSI Z-136.

**BS 4803: Part 3**: 1983                           ≠ IEC 825
**Guidance for users**
Gives guidance on the safety precautions required for the use of laser products and systems. Contains information for calculation of radiation hazards. Based on the latest information including data from ANSI Z-136.

*BS 5724: MEDICAL ELECTRICAL EQUIPMENT*

**BS 5724: Part 1**: 1989                           ≡ IEC 601–1
**General requirements for safety**
Covers constructional requirements, accompanying documentation, transport, storage, installation and maintenance of medical electrical equipment used to diagnose and treat the patient.
Implements CENELEC HD 395.1.

*BS 5724: Part 2: PARTICULAR REQUIREMENTS FOR SAFETY*

**BS 5724: Section 2.2**: 1983                      ≡ IEC 601–2–2
**Specification for high-frequency surgical equipment**
Requirements for the safety of high-frequency surgical equipment used in medical practice. Some equipment having a rated output power not exceeding 50 W is exempt from several of the requirements of this standard and these exemptions are indicated.
Implements CENELEC HD 395.2.2.

**BS 5724: Section 2.4**: 1985                      ≡ IEC 601–2–4
**Specification for cardiac defibrillators and cardiac defibrillator-monitors**
Specifies safety requirements for equipment intended to defibrillate the heart by an electrical impulse via electrodes applied either to the patient's skin or to the exposed heart.

**BS 5724: Section 2.10**: 1988          ≡ IEC 601–2–10
**Specification for nerve and muscle stimulators**
Safety requirements for equipment intended for use in the diagnosis and/or therapy of certain neuro-muscular disorders. Does not apply to equipment implanted or permanently attached to the patient nor to equipment intended to stimulate the brain. To be read in conjunction with BS 5724: Part 1.

**BS 5724: Section 2.22**: 1987
**Specification for general operating tables**
Requirements for fixed-pedestal and mobile general operating tables whether or not having electrical parts.

**BS 5724: Section 2.23**: 1989          ≡ ISO 8359
**Specification for oxygen concentrators**
Devices which by separating out nitrogen from ambient air provide oxygen-enriched air for supply to a patient. To be read in conjunction with BS 5724: Part 1.

**BS 5724: Section 2.24**: 1989          ≡ ISO 8185
**Specification for humidifiers**
Vaporizing and nebulizing humidifiers, including those suitable for inclusion in breathing systems, for use with both intubated and non-intubated patients. To be read in conjunction with BS 5724: Part 1.

**BS 5724: Section 2.27**: 1989          ≡ ISO 7767: 1988
**Specification for oxygen analysers for monitoring patient breathing mixtures**
Both sampling and non-sampling oxygen analysers are covered. To be read in conjunction with IEC 601–1.

*BS 6902: CARDIAC PACEMAKERS*

**BS 6902: Part 2**: 1987          ≡ ISO 5841/2
**Method for reporting the clinical performance of populations of pulse generators**
Describes procedures whereby the performance of different types of pulse generators can be reported and assessed statistically.

**BS 7139**: 1989          ≡ IEC 878
**Guide to graphical symbols for use on medical electrical equipment**
A list of symbols, with their meanings, which has been derived from various sources including BS 6217. The 5 sections present general symbols and symbols for specific groups of equipment.

# Appendix IV Checklist for Anaesthetic Machines: A recommended procedure based on the use of an oxygen analyser*

## Section I—Introduction

Improvements in safety must be an important goal in anaesthetic practice. One very important aspect of safety is the checking of equipment before use. There is now a need for a more formalized procedure to govern the pre-use check of anaesthetic equipment and of anaesthetic machines in particular. It is regrettable that it often takes a serious accident with an anaesthetic machine to stimulate action.[1-3] One cause of these misadventures is the use of a machine which is not checked by an anaesthetist for proper function beforehand. The frequency of this has been reported as between 18 and 33% although sometimes another trained person may have completed a check.[4-7]

Various check procedures have been published;[8-11] that devised by Newton[12] is a practical revision of procedures issued after a disaster in 1975 involving 'crossed-over' pipelines;[1] these are the origins of the 'tug' and 'single hose' tests. Checklists have been published by various professional and commercial organizations in several countries over the last few years. The recommendation of a checklist by the Association of Anaesthetists of Great Britain and Ireland is in accord with current opinion where standards of audit and performance are required.

Anaesthetists are required to rely heavily on their memory for essential facts when carrying out routine and emergency procedures. In contrast, airline pilots do not rely solely on memory but use standard checklists. A series of pre-anaesthesia equipment checks has been developed for the Dräger NS650 machine by anaesthetists in The Netherlands working in conjunction with the Chief Pilot of KLM Royal Dutch Airlines;[13] items are called out by one anaesthetist and an assistant is responsible for checking that the relevant functions are correctly set. These authors emphasize the importance of training in checklist procedures as an integral part of training in anaesthesia.

A literature survey was undertaken and we have reviewed various published checklists. These include: the Faculty of Anaesthetists of the Royal Australasian College of Surgeons,[14] the Food and Drug Administration Checkout Procedure,[15] the Canadian Anaesthetists' Society,[16] The Colombian Academy of Anesthesia, North American Dräger,[17] The Merton & Sutton Health Authority;[2] also checklists prepared by commercial companies specific for particular anaesthetic machines. We have also considered several checklists prepared by various individuals and organizations which remain unpublished. Many manufacturers include very detailed check procedures (often known as 'Operation Verification Procedures') in their service manuals intended for use by service engineers which may take up to one hour to complete; these checks are not designed for daily use. We started by compiling a comprehensive user check based on various published lists, manufacturers' information, and on

* Reproduced by kind permission of The Association of Anaesthetists of Great Britain and Ireland, 9 Bedford Square, London WC1B 3RA, UK.

the anaesthetic machine standard of the American Society for Testing and Materials (ASTM) F116–88. However, this check took over 15 minutes to perform by one anaesthetist and an assistant; the checklist we have designed takes only a few minutes to perform and represents a reasonable investment in patient safety.

Our endeavour is to produce a checklist which, although it may not apply to every type of anaesthetic machine, will cover the vast majority of machines in current use, including those designed to prevent delivery of a hypoxic mixture. It is not the intention to supplant any pre-anaesthetic checking procedures issued by manufacturers. The aim is to strike the right level of checking so that it is not so superficial that the value is doubtful or so detailed that the procedure is impracticable. The Working Party has attempted to consider the problem from a completely new viewpoint using the oxygen analyser on the anaesthetic machine.[18] This approach will detect misfilling of oxygen cylinders[19] or contamination of liquid oxygen reservoirs.[20,21] Existing checks[12] designed to avoid 'crossover' would not detect these dangerous situations.

A record of the checks performed should be kept; this can be done by use of a specific logbook[2] for each anaesthetic machine or by making an entry in the patient's anaesthetic record. It is recognized that, rarely, situations may occur of an emergency nature when it is not possible to perform checks as laid down here. This document relates only to anaesthetic machines (with medical gas cylinders and/or pipelines, and vaporizers); it does not specifically detail the checking of other essential items. However, there is an outline check for breathing systems, lung ventilators and suction equipment. Common sense dictates that labels and instructions attached to the apparatus should be noted (e.g. 'first-user' notices attached by service engineers).[22]

The Association of Anaesthetists of Great Britain and Ireland cannot be held responsible for failure of an anaesthetic machine as a result of a defect not revealed by the following procedures.

It is recognized that the trend towards microprocessor-controlled anaesthetic machines and modern technology may lead to future revision of this document.

# Section II—Procedures

The following full check procedures should be performed at the beginning of each operating theatre session. The checks are the responsibility of the anaesthetist. They may be performed by the anaesthetist or the anaesthetist working with an assistant, prior to procedures under general anaesthesia or regional anaesthesia/analgesia. In the event of a change of anaesthetist, the checked status of the anaesthetic machine must be agreed.

## A. Oxygen analyser

The first step is for the analyser to be placed, checked and calibrated according to the manufacturer's instructions. The analyser should monitor the gases leaving the common gas outlet for the purpose of these checks.

## B. Medical gas supplies

1. The check procedure should start with the machine disconnected from all pipeline supplies and all vaporizers turned to 'off'. The electrical supply to the machine should be switched on.

2. Check that only cylinders which contain gases to be used are present on the machine, that they are securely seated and that they are turned off. A blanking plug should be fitted to any empty cylinder yoke.

   **Note**: Carbon dioxide and cyclopropane cylinders should not normally be present on the machine unless specifically requested by the anaesthetist.

3. Open all flowmeter control valves.

4. Turn on the reserve oxygen cylinder and check the contents gauge. Oxygen should flow through the oxygen flowmeter. If there is another 'in use' oxygen cylinder turn off the reserve oxygen cylinder and repeat the test.

   Check that the oxygen flow control valve can adjust the flow over the full range of the flowmeter, and set a flow of approximately 5 litres/minute.

   The oxygen analyser display should approach 100%.

5. Turn on the reserve nitrous oxide cylinder and check the contents gauge. Nitrous oxide should now flow through the nitrous oxide flowmeter. If there is an 'in use' nitrous oxide cylinder, turn off the reserve nitrous oxide cylinder and repeat the test.

   Check that the nitrous oxide flowmeter control valve can adjust the flow over the full range of the flowmeter, and set a flow of approximately 5 litres/minute.

6. Turn off the oxygen cylinder(s) and empty the oxygen from the system by operating the oxygen flush valve. The cylinder gauge(s) should return to zero.

The primary audible alarm should operate while the oxygen pressure is decreasing.

When the supply of oxygen fails, observe that the appropriate oxygen failure protection device (if fitted) functions correctly to prevent the delivery of a hypoxic gas mixture.

7. Connect the oxygen pipeline. This should restore the flow of oxygen and cancel the oxygen failure protection device. Perform a 'tug test' and check that the oxygen pipeline pressure gauge reads 400 kPa.

8. Turn off the nitrous oxide cylinder(s). Connect the nitrous oxide pipeline. This should restore the flow of gas through the nitrous oxide flowmeter.
   Perform a 'tug test' and check that the nitrous oxide pipeline pressure gauge also reads 400 kPa. Turn off the nitrous oxide flowmeter control valve.

9. If the anaesthetist has requested specifically that other cylinders be fitted, these should also be checked in a similar manner.

10. Turn off **all** the flowmeter control valves.

11. Operate the emergency oxygen flush valve and ensure there is no significant decrease in the pipeline supply pressure. Confirm that the oxygen analyser display approaches 100% during this test.

## C. Vaporizers

1. Check that the vaporizer(s) for the required volatile agent(s) are fitted correctly to the anaesthetic machine, that any backbar locking mechanism is fully engaged[23,24] and that the control knob(s) rotate through their full range(s). Turn off the vaporizer(s).

2. Check that the flow through any vaporizer is in the correct direction.

3. When charging each vaporizer ensure that the correct anaesthetic agent is used, and that the filling port is left tightly closed.

4. Where the anaesthetic machine is fitted with a pressure relief valve the following tests should be performed. (There may be a dangerous increase in pressure if these tests are performed in the absence of such a valve.)

   (i) Set a suitable test flow of oxygen (6–8 litres/min), and, with the vaporizer in the 'off' position, temporarily occlude the common gas outlet. There should be no leak from any of the vaporizer fitments, and the flowmeter bobbin will dip.

   (ii) Repeat this test with each vaporizer in the 'on' position. There should be no leak of liquid from the filling port.

Turn off the vaporizer(s), and the oxygen flowmeter control valve.

## D. Breathing systems

1. Inspect the configuration of the breathing and scavenging systems to be used, and check that they function correctly. Ensure there are no leaks or obstructions in the reservoir bag or breathing system.

2. The 'push and twist' technique[25] should be employed for connecting conical fittings.

3. Check that the adjustable pressure-limiting 'expiratory' valve can be fully opened or closed.

4. Each breathing system poses separate problems. Make a visual check, and perform an occlusion test on the inner tube of the Bain type co-axial system. Check the function of the unidirectional valves on the circle system.

## E. Ventilator

1. Check the normal operation of the ventilator and its controls.

2. Occlude the patient port and check that the pressure relief valve functions correctly.

3. Check that the disconnect alarm is present and operational.

4. Ensure that there is an alternative means to ventilate the patient's lungs in the event of ventilator malfunction.

## F. Suction equipment

Check all components relating to the anaesthetic suction equipment and test for the rapid development of an adequate 'negative' pressure.

## G. Leaks

The detection of small leaks is always a problem. Specific checks have been recommended.[26,27]

An oxygen analyser in the breathing system is a valuable safeguard against the delivery of a gas mixture which could result in hypoxia or awareness.[18]

# Section III—References

1. Leading article. The Westminster Inquiry. *The Lancet*, 1977; **ii**: 175–176.
2. District Instruction No. 60. Issued 1989. Merton & Sutton Health Authority, District Offices, 6 Homeland Drive, Sutton, Surrey SM2 5LY UK.
3. Brahams, D. Anaesthesia and the law. Awareness and pain during anaesthesia. *Anaesthesia*, 1989; **44**: 352.
4. Lunn, J. N. and Mushin, W. W. *Mortality associated with anaesthesia*. London: The Nuffield Provincial Hospitals Trust, 1982.
5. Cooper, J. B., Newbower, R. S. and Kitz, R. J. An analysis of major errors and equipment failures in anesthesia management: considerations for prevention and detection. *Anesthesiology*, 1984; **60**: 34–42.
6. Craig, J. and Wilson, M. E. A survey of anaesthetic misadventures. *Anaesthesia*, 1981; **36**: 933–936.
7. Report of the Survey of Anaesthetic Practice, 1988. Association of Anaesthetists of Great Britain and Ireland, 9 Bedford Square, London WC1B 3RA.
8. Ward, C. S. *Anaesthetic equipment. Physical principles and maintenance*, 2nd edn. London: Baillière Tindall, 1985, pp. 117–120.
9. Cundy, J. F. and Baldock, G. Safety check procedures in anaesthetic machines. *Anaesthesia*, 1982; **37**: 161–169.
10. Petty, C. *The anesthesia machine*. London: Churchill Livingstone, 1987, pp. 217–218.
11. Kumar, V., Barcellos, W. A., Mehta, M. P. and Carter, J. G. An analysis of critical incidents in a teaching department for quality assurance. A survey of mishaps during anaesthesia. *Anaesthesia*, 1988; **43**: 879–883.
12. Newton, N. I. In Adams, A. P. and Henville, J. In: *Recent Advances in Anaesthesia & Analgesia*, 13th edn. (eds. Hewer, C. L. and Atkinson, R. S.). London: Churchill Livingstone, 1979, pp. 50–51.
13. Spierdijk, J., Kooijman, J. and Bovill, J. G. Checklist procedures: aviation shows the way to safer anesthesia. *Scientific Exhibit, American Society of Anesthesiologists Annual Scientific Meeting 1987, Atlanta, Georgia*.
14. *Protocol for checking an anaesthetic machine before use*. Faculty of Anaesthetists of the Royal Australasian College of Surgeons, August 1980.
15. FDA Checkout procedure. Anesthesia Apparatus Checkout Recommendations. August 1986. In: *Anesthesia Patient Safety Foundation Newsletter*, 1986; **1**(3): 15. (September).
16. *Guidelines to the practice of anaesthesia as recommended by the Canadian Anaesthetists' Society 1987*. Toronto: The Canadian Anaesthetists' Society, 187 Gerrard Street E, Toronto, Ontario, M5A 2E5.
17. Anaesthesia apparatus checkout recommendations. Pre-use checkout and inspection procedure (based on North American Dräger Safety Guidelines). The North American Dräger Company: Pennsylvania, 1989.
18. *Recommendations for standards of monitoring during anaesthesia and recovery*. Issued 1988. London: Association of Anaesthetists of Great Britain and Ireland, 9 Bedford Square, London WC1B 3RA.
19. Safety Action Bulletin, No. 48. *Medical gas cylinders: safety and care in their storage, handling and use*. SAB(89)28. London: Department of Health, Russell Square House, 14 Russell Square, London WC1B 5EP. June 1989.
20. Sprague, D. H. and Archer, G. W. Intra-operative hypoxia from an erroneously filled liquid oxygen reservoir. *Anesthesiology*, 1975; **42**: 360–364.
21. Holland, R. 'Wrong gas' disaster in Hong Kong. *Anesthesia Patient Safety Newsletter*, 1989; **4**(3): 26. (September).
22. Health Equipment Information No. 98. Management of Equipment: 1982; para 66. London: Department of Health and Social Security, Russell Square House, 14 Russell Square, London, WC1B 5PE.
23. Health Notice, Hazard. *Health Service Management. Selectatec Vapouriser Systems*. HN(HAZARD)(84)13. London: Department of Health and Social Security, Russell Square House, 14 Russell Square, London, WC1B 5PE. 25 July 1984.
24. Safety Action Bulletin No. 43. *Anaesthetic Vaporizers: servicing*. SAB(88)72. London: Department of Health, Russell Square House, 14 Russell Square, London, WC1B 5PE. November 1989.
25. Health Equipment Information, No. 150. *Evaluation of breathing attachments for anaesthetic apparatus to BS 3849: 1965*. London: Department of Health & Social Security, Russell Square House, 14 Russell Square, London, WC1B 5PE.
26. Page, J., Testing for leaks. *Anaesthesia*, 1977; **32**: 673.
27. British Standards Institution. *A specification for continuous flow anaesthetic machines*. Part 3 BS 4272, 1989. British Standards Institution, 2 Park Street, London W1Y 3WA.

# Appendix V Directory of Manufacturers

Many of the products referred to in this publication bear registered trade marks or unregistered trade names of the various companies mentioned in this book and accordingly the publishers acknowledge this.

|  | Key |
| --- | --- |

AE *See* Ohmeda.     DW

**Ambu International UK Ltd**,    ERS
Charlton Road, Midsomer Norton, Bath BA3 4DR, UK. Tel: 0761 416868.
*or* **Ambu International A/S**, Sondre Ringvej 49, PO Box 215, DK 2600, Denmark. Tel: +45 43 63 01 11.

**Bedfont Technical Instruments Ltd**, PO   A
Box 42, Streatham, London SW16 1JH, UK. Tel: 081 769 7518.

**Bennett** *See* Puritan-Bennett   V
International Corp.

**Bird Products**, 8 Lansdown Place,   V
Lansdown Road, Cheltenham, Gloucestershire GL50 2HU, UK. Tel: 0242 250818.
*or* **Bird Products Corporation**, 3101 East Alejo Road, Palm Springs, CA 92262, USA. Tel: + 1 619 778 7200.

**Blease Medical Equipment**, Deansway,   GV
Chesham, Buckinghamshire HP5 2NX, UK. Tel: 0494 784422.

**BOC Ltd** , The Priestley Centre, 10,   CP
Priestley Road, The Surrey Research Park, Guildford, Surrey GU2 5XY, UK. Tel: 0483 579857.
*See* Ohmeda.

**British Fluidics and Controls Ltd**, Forest   F
Road, Hainault, Ilford, Essex, UK. Tel: 081 500 3300.

**Bruel and Kjaer (UK) Ltd**, 92 Uxbridge   AM
Road, Harrow Weald Lodge, Harrow, Middx, HA3 6BZ, UK. Tel: 081 954 2366.

**Cape** *See* Penlon Ltd.   V

**Carden** *See* M & IE.   V

**Childerhouse Developments Ltd**, 310A   G
Upper Richmond Road West, East Sheen, London SW14 7JN, UK. Tel: 081 876 6040.

**Cory Bros Co. Ltd**, 4 Dollis Park,   NT
London N3 1HG, UK. Tel: 081 349 1081.

**Criticon**, Broadlands, Sunninghill,   MZ
Ascot, Berkshire SL5 9JN, UK. Tel: 0344 27821.
*or* **Criticon Inc**, 4110 George Street, Tampa, Florida, USA. Tel: +1 813 887 2000.

**Cyprane** *See* Ohmeda.   DVX

**Dameca**, Isdlevdalvej 211, DK-2610   AGM
Rodovre, Denmark. Tel: +45 42 91 3480.

**Datascope Medical Co. Ltd**, 254   M
Cambridge Science Park, Milton Road, Cambridge CB4 4WE, UK. Tel: 0223 420333.
*or* **Datascope Corporation**, 580 Winters Avenue, PO Box 5, Paramus, New Jersey, 07653-005, USA. Tel: +1 201 265 8800.

**Dräger Ltd**, The Willows, Mark Road,   GKMPV
Hemel Hempstead, Hertfordshire HP2 7BW, UK. Tel: 0442 213542.
*or* **Drägerwerk**, Aktiengesellschaft, Postfach 1339, Moislinger Allee 53-55, D-2400 Lübeck 1, Germany. Tel: +49 451 8820.
*or* **North American Dräger**, 148B Quarry Road, Telford, PA 18969, USA. Tel: +1 215 723 9824.

East Health Care Ltd, Sandy Lane West,   GMV
Littlemore, Oxford OX4 5JT, UK. Tel:
0865 714242.

Engström, Gambro Ltd, Lundia House,   HMV
124 Station Road, Sidcup, Kent DA15
7AS, UK. Tel: 081 309 7800.
*or* Gambro Engström, AB, Box 20109,
S-161 20 Bromma, Sweden. Tel: +46 8
98 82 80.

Eschmann, Peter Road, Lancing, West   NS
Sussex BN15 8TJ, UK. Tel: 0903
761122

Ferraris Development & Engineering   M
Co. Ltd, 26 Lea Valley Trading Estate,
Angel Road, Edmonton, London N18
3JD, UK. Tel: 081 807 3636.

Flomasta *See* M & I E.   V

Franklin *See* Rusch.   T

Frazer Harlake (Now Matrx) *See*   D
Nesor.

Graseby Medical Ltd, Colonial Way,   Z
Watford WD2 4LG, UK. Tel: 0923 246
434.

Hamilton (GB) Ltd, Kimpton Link
Business Centre, Kimpton Road,
Sutton, Surrey, UK. Tel: 081 641 9008.
*or* Hamilton Medical AG, PO Box 26,
CH 7402, Bonadiez, Switzerland. Tel:
+41 81 37 2627.

Hewlett-Packard Ltd, Amen Corner,   M
Cain Road, Bracknell, Berkshire RG12
1HN, UK. Tel: 0344 363344.
*or* Hewlett-Packard Company, 3000
Hanover Street, Palo Alto, CA 94304,
USA. Tel: +1 415 857 1501.

Heine Optotechnik GmbH,   IY
Kientalstrasse, 7, D-8036 Herrsching,
Germany. Tel: +49 81 52 380.

Hoek Loos, Post Box No 663, 1000 A R,   G
Amsterdam, The Netherlands. Tel:
+31 20 581211.

Kay Pneumatics Ltd, Crescent Road,   GJV
Luton, Bedfordshire LU2 0AH, UK.
Tel: 0582 453303.

KeyMed, KeyMed House, Stock Road,   I
Southend-on-Sea, Essex SS2 5QH,
UK. Tel: 0702 616333. *See also*
Olympus.

Kingston Medical Gases Ltd, 121   CP
Clarendon Street, Hull, W. Yorks.
HU3 1AY, UK. Tel: 0482 24298.

IMED Kabi Pharmacia Ltd, Davy   Z
Avenue, Knowhill, Milton Keynes
MK5 8PH, UK. Tel: 0908 661101.
*or* IMED Corporation, 9775

Businesspark Avenue, San Diego, CA
92131-1192, USA. Tel: +1 619 566
9000.

Laerdal Medical Ltd, Laerdal House,   ERS
Goodmead Road, Orpington, Kent
BR6 0HX, UK. Tel: 0689 876634.
*or* Asmund S. Laerdal, PO Box 377,
N-4001 Stravanger, Norway. Tel: +47
4 511 700.

Leyland Medical International Ltd, *See*   T
Rusch.

Loosco *See* Hoek Loos.   G

3M Health Care Ltd, 3M House, Morley   N
Street, Loughborough, Leicestershire
LE11 1EP, UK. Tel: 0509 611611.
*or* 3M Inc, 3M Center, St Paul, MN 55144-
1000, USA. Tel: +1 612 733 1110.

McKesson Equipment Co. Ltd, Tradent   D
House, 110 Park Road, Chesterfield,
Derbyshire S40 2JX, UK. Tel: 0246
276111.

Mallinckrodt Medical (UK) Ltd, 11   MNT
North Portway Close, Round
Spinney, Northampton NN3 4RQ,
UK. Tel: 0604 646132.
*or* Mallinckrodt Medical
Incorporated, 675 McDonnell
Boulevard, PO Box 5840, St Louis,
MO 63134, USA. Tel: +1 314 895 2000.

Matrx Medical Incorporated, For UK *See*   DG
Nesor.
*or* 145 Mid County Drive, Orchard
Park, New York, NY 14127, USA. Tel:
+1 716 662 6650.

Medec International, Postbus 168, 15 20   U
AD, Wormerveer, The Netherlands.
Tel: +31 75 288899.

M G I, Orbit House, Albert Street,   PU
Eccles, Manchester M30 0LJ, UK. Tel:
061 787 8687.

M & I E (Medical and Industrial   GV
Equipment Ltd), Falcon Road,
Sowton Industrial Estate, Exeter,
Devon EX2 7NA, UK. Tel: 0392
431331.

Nesor Equipment Co, Gilmore House,   DG
166 Gilmore Road, London SE13 5AE,
UK. Tel: 081 852 8545.

Ohio *See* Ohmeda.   G

Olympus Optical Company Ltd, 1–22–2   I
San-ei, Building, Nishi Shinjuka,
Shinjuka, Tokyo, Japan. Tel: +81 340
2111.

Ohmeda, Ohmeda House, 71, Great   CGPV
North Road, Hatfield, Herts A19 5EN,

UK. Tel: 0707 263570. (Sales and Service).
Station Road, Steeton, West Yorkshire BD20 6RB, UK. Tel: 0535 656016 (Anaesthetic Equipment).
Telford Crescent, Staveley, Derbyshire S43 3PF, UK. Tel: 0246 474241 (Pipelines).
*or* **Ohmeda**, Ohmeda Drive, Madison, WI 53707, USA. Tel: +1 608 221 1551.

**Ollair Ltd**, Ollerton Research Laboratories, Nr Chorley, Lancs, UK. Tel: 0254 830565.   U

**Oxylitre Ltd**, Morton House, Skerton Road, Old Trafford, Manchester M16 0WL, UK. Tel: 061 872 6322.   PQS

**Pall Biomedical Ltd**, Europa House, Havant Street, Portsmouth PO1 3PD, UK. Tel: 0705 753545.   B

**Penlon Ltd**, Radley Road, Abingdon, Oxfordshire OX14 3PN, UK. Tel: 0235 554222.   GUV

**Physio Control**, Intec 2, Units 10–20, Wade Road, Basingstoke, Hampshire RG24 0NE, UK. Tel: 0256 474455.   M
*or* **Physio Control Corporate Headquarters**, 11811 Willow Road North East, PO Box 97006, Washington 98073–9706, USA. Tel: +1 206 867 4000.

**Pneupac Ltd** *See* Kay Pneumatics.   FGJV

**Portex Ltd**, 1–3 High Street, Hythe, Kent CT21 6JL, UK. Tel: 0303 260551.   NST
*or* **Concord/Portex**, 15 Kit Street, Keene, New Hampshire 03431, USA. Tel: +1 603 352 3812.

**Puritan-Bennett**, Unit 1, 152–176 Great South West Road, Hounslow, Middlesex TW4 6JS, UK. Tel: 081 577 1870.   PV
*or* **Puritan-Bennett International Corporation**, 9401 Indian-Creek Parkway, PO Box 25905 Overland Park, Kansas 66225, USA. Tel: +1 913 661 0444.

**Riken** *See* Weatherall.   A
*or* **Riken Keiki Fine Instrument Co. Ltd**, 2–7–6 Azusawa, Itabashi-ku, Tokyo, Japan. Tel: +81 3 966 1111.

**Rimer-Alco Ltd**, Dumballs Road, Cardiff CF1 6JE, UK. Tel: 0222 378421.   J
*or* **Rimer-Alco North America Ltd**, 15 Jefferson Street, Box 749 Morden, Manitoba, Canada, R0G 1J0. Tel: +1 204 822 6595.

**Rotameter Ltd**, KDG-Mobray Ltd, Crompton Way, Crawley, West Sussex RH10 2YZ, UK. Tel: 0293 525151.   MNQ

**Rusch UK Ltd**, Halifax Road, Cressex Industrial Estate, High Wycombe, Bucks HP12 3NB, UK. Tel: 0494 532761.   NT
*or* **Willy Rusch AG**, Strasse 4–10, Postfach 1633, D-7050 Waiblingen, Germany. Tel: +49 71514060.
*or* **Rusch Inc.**, 2450 Meadowbrook Parkway, Duluth, GA 30136, USA. Tel: +1 404 623 0816.

**Scott's Electrical**, Scott-Western Ltd, Dalling Road, Branksome, Poole, Dorset BH12 1DJ, UK. Tel: 0202 766066.   K

**Servomex (UK) Ltd**, Crowborough, Sussex TN6 3DU, UK. Tel: 0892 652181.   O

**Siemens plc**, Siemens House, Windmill Road, Sunbury-on-Thames, Middlesex TW16 7HS, UK. Tel: 0932 752421.   MV
*or* **Siemens Aktiengesellschaft**, Bereich Medizinische Technik, Henkestrasse 127, Postfach 3260, D-8520 Erlangen, Germany. Tel: +49 91 31 840.

**S & W Vickers Ltd**, Ruxley Corner, Sidcup, Kent DA14 5BL, UK. Tel: 081 309 0433.   M

**Tricomed Ltd**, Unit 2, Chiltonian Industrial Estate, Manor Lane, London SE12 0TX, UK. Tel: 081 463 0933.   GM

**Weatherall Equipment and Instruments Ltd**, PO Box 69, Tring, Herts HP23 6PL, UK. Tel: 024 029 8110   A
*or* **Riken Keiki Fine Instrument Co. Ltd**, 2–7–6 Azusawa, Itabashi-ku, Tokyo, Japan. Tel: +03 966 1111.

**Vitalograph Ltd**, Maids Moreton House, Buckinghamshire MK18 1SW, UK. Tel: 0280 822811.   M

**Xomed** *See* Zimmer.

**Warne Surgical Products Ltd** *See* Rusch   NT

**Zimmer Surgical Specialities**, Dunbath Road, Elgin Industrial Estate, Swindon SN2 6EA, UK. Tel: 0793 481441.

**Key to the principal products of the companies listed**

A  Analysers (gas and vapour)
B  Bacterial filters, etc.
C  Cylinders, etc. of medical gases
D  Dental anaesthetic equipment
E  Educational products
F  Fluidic and pneumatic equipment
G  General range of anaesthetic equipment
H  Humidifiers
I  Fibreoptic instruments
J  Oxygen concentrators
K  Sterilizing equipment
L  Leak detectors

M  Monitors
N  Disposables
O  Oxygen analysers
P  Medical gas and vacuum pipelines
Q  Flowmeters
R  Resuscitation equipment
S  Suction equipment
T  Endotracheal tubes, etc.
U  Scavenging equipment
V  Ventilators
W  Vaporizers
X  Pressure transducers
Y  Sundry instruments and aids
Z  Intravenous equipment
+  International code from country of origin

# Index